Quality of Life

It is not so important how many years you live
but how much life you put into living.

charm

**HELEN
WHITCOMB**

**ROSALIND
LANG**

GREGG DIVISION McGRAW-HILL BOOK COMPANY

New York St. Louis Dallas San Francisco Düsseldorf Johannesburg Kuala Lumpur
London Mexico Montreal New Delhi Panama Rio de Janeiro Singapore Sydney Toronto

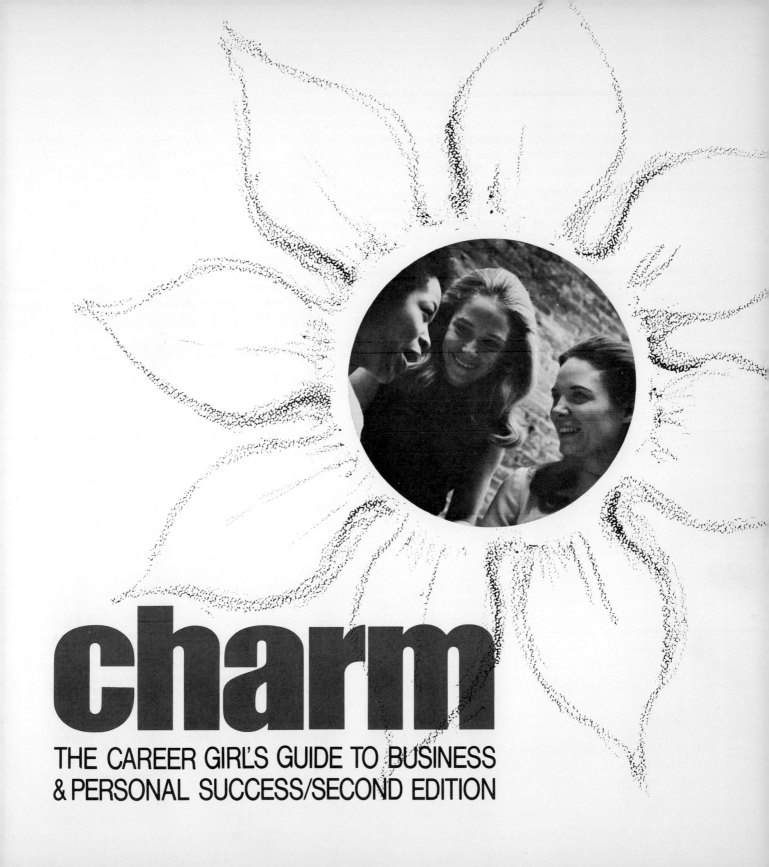

charm

THE CAREER GIRL'S GUIDE TO BUSINESS
& PERSONAL SUCCESS/SECOND EDITION

Helen Whitcomb, the former managing editor of *Today's Secretary,* is coauthor of several books, including *Charm for Miss Teen* and the *Charm for the Modern Woman Text-Kit.*

Rosalind Lang is a lecturer at colleges, business schools, and high schools. She has also been active in corporate training programs, notably for the New York Telephone Company.

DESIGNER: Barbara DuPree Knowles
SPONSORING EDITOR: Peggy Rollason Glick
EDITING MANAGER: Frank C. Wilkinson

ISBN 07-069655-1

Acknowledgments

The authors wish to thank the following companies and organizations for their help and cooperation: Abraham & Straus; Elizabeth Arden; The Bali Company, Inc.; Hazel Bishop, Inc.; Chesebrough-Pond's, Inc.; City Investing Co.; Helene Curtis Industries, Inc.; Clairol; Max Factor; General Motors; Dorothy Gray, Ltd.; Richard Hudnut; Le Pont Neuf; The Institute of Life Insurance; Lanolin Plus, Inc.; Manufacturer's Hanover Trust Co.; Helen Neushaefer Cosmetics; Revlon Inc.; Helena Rubinstein, Inc.; Shulton, Inc.; Tussy Cosmetics; Lugene, Inc.; Scarves by Vera, Inc.

The drawings are by Linda Lenkowsky Ericson with the following exceptions. The drawings on pages 11, 18-27, 40-49, 103-105, 114, 115, and 200 are by Nancy Reynolds Gamar. The drawing on page 75 is by Ray Porter. The art used for the cover, the part openers, and various ornaments has been adapted from the "Ladybug" design by J. Rahel, courtesy of Hallmark Cards, Inc.

PICTURE CREDITS: Page 2, B. D. Unsworth; p. 8, B. D. Unsworth; p. 28, B. D. Unsworth; p. 33 (upper left), courtesy of Tampax Inc.; (upper middle), courtesy of Bonne Bell Inc.; (right), courtesy of The Homestead; (lower left), courtesy of Bonne Bell Inc.; (lower middle), courtesy of The Homestead; p. 52, B. D. Unsworth; pp. 62 and 63, B. D. Unsworth; p. 66, B. D. Unsworth; p. 73, B. D. Unsworth; p. 86, B. D. Unsworth; p. 95 (upper left), courtesy of American Cyanamid Company; (upper middle), courtesy of Bonnie Bee Wigs; (upper right), courtesy of MADEMOISELLE. Copyright © 1970 The Condé Nast Publications Inc.; (lower left), courtesy of Helene Curtis Industries, Inc.; (lower middle), courtesy of Helene Curtis Industries, Inc.; (lower right), courtesy of Helene Curtis Industries, Inc.; pp. 100 and 101, courtesy of The Gillette Company; p. 108, courtesy of Helene Curtis Industries, Inc.; p. 110, courtesy of *Women's Day*—Photograph by Rudy Muller; p. 113, B. D. Unsworth; p. 118, B . D. Unsworth; p. 128, B. D. Unsworth; p. 142, courtesy of *Harper's Bazaar;* p. 160, courtesy of Fibers Div. Allied Chemical Corp.; p. 168, (upper right), courtesy of Lord & Taylor; (all others), courtesy of Helene Curtis Industries, Inc.; p. 170, courtesy of Villager; p. 194, courtesy of Lord & Taylor; p. 196, courtesy of Texize Chemicals Inc.; p. 210, courtesy of AT&T; p. 220, courtesy of AT&T; p. 226, courtesy of Benton & Bowles, Inc.; p. 230, courtesy of Selchow & Righter Co.; p. 233, B. D. Unsworth; p. 246, Richard McBride; p. 252, courtesy of Tampax Inc.; p. 258, B. D. Unsworth; p. 263, B. D. Unsworth; p. 268, *Ebony* Magazine; p. 280, courtesy of New York University; p. 288; B. D. Unsworth; p. 302, B. D. Unsworth; p. 316, courtesy of GLAMOUR ©1970 The Condé Nast Publications Inc.; p. 319 (upper left), courtesy of Saks Fifth Avenue; (upper middle), courtesy of American Cyanamid Company; (upper right), courtesy of Sugar Information, Inc.; (lower left), courtesy of *The College Store Journal;* (center), courtesy of Wrangler Jeans; (lower right), courtesy of GLAMOUR © 1970 The Condé Nast Publications Inc.; p. 321 (top), courtesy of *The College Store Journal;* (second), B. D. Unsworth; (third), B. D. Unsworth; (bottom), courtesy of Lincoln Center for the Performing Arts, New York—Photograph by Victoria Beller; p. 324, B. D. Unsworth; p. 340, courtesy of Lincoln Center for the Performing Arts, New York—Photograph by Bob Serating; p. 358, B. D. Unsworth; p.382, courtesy of Chanel Inc.; p.392, B. D. Unsworth; p. 400, courtesy of Peck & Peck.

Preface

Every young woman has exciting potential within her that can be discovered and nurtured to help her become an interesting, appealing, and more attractive person. *Charm,* Second Edition, has been planned and written to help the young woman make the most of her potential so that she can achieve success and happiness, both in her career and in her personal life. This second edition of *Charm* incorporates the best elements of the well-received first edition, and it has been updated for the career girl of the seventies.

The advice of experts in many fields has been brought together in this book and tailored to the needs of the career girl—to her problems, time limitations, financial status, and interests. The book is divided into six parts.

PART ONE considers posture and figure improvement, because these basic charm factors require time to develop. Much of any person's physical beauty depends on good posture and graceful movements, so detailed explanations, photographs, and drawings have been furnished. Tables are supplied to help the reader analyze her own figure problems, and advice is given on how to correct specific figure problems through exercise and proper diet.

PART TWO deals with beauty and cosmetics. It fully explores complexion analysis and tells how to care for the skin, how to use makeup to enhance facial assets and minimize imperfections, how to care for and style hair so that it is most flattering to the individual's basic face shape and height, and how to groom lovely hands. The full range of skin tones, features, and hair types are analyzed so that each student may identify her own special beauty assets and problems. New trends in grooming, such as the popularity of false eyelashes, wigs, and hairpieces, are also covered. In addition, because inner beauty is so necessary for a lovely countenance, personality improvement is also treated in this section.

PART THREE concentrates on the development of a personal flair for fashion. At a time when controversy is raging over skirt lengths and fashions are changing drastically from season to season, *Charm* concentrates on basics such as which lines, which fabrics and patterns, which colors, and which accessories will reveal the flattering fashion sense that marks a woman of taste.

PART FOUR explains how to develop a lovely voice and colorful, correct speech. Because so much of a young woman's charm is revealed by what she says and how she says it, both on-the-job telephone techniques and the art of social conversation are covered.

PART FIVE discusses the career girl's place in the business world. She learns how to make the best impression through an application letter and a résumé and during an interview. She also finds out how to get off to a good start on the job and how to become a success.

PART SIX deals with the out-of-the-office aspects of a career girl's life. Her home life—whether alone, with family, or roommates—is considered, and the problems of city living are evaluated. She is advised how to choose a suitable place to live, how to select compatible roommates, and how to manage her time, energy, and money. Dating is discussed, and special attention is given to the delicate handling required in the case of an office romance. An extensive chapter on etiquette equips the young woman with the poise that will enable her to handle possibly awkward situations—introductions, dining out, table etiquette, tipping, and others. Since increased charm often leads to matrimony, suggestions have been included for blending marriage and a career.

In short, *Charm* is a book that will show the modern career girl how to bring out the best in herself and how to be admired and liked by the people she meets—a prescription for happiness and success.

Helen Whitcomb

Rosalind Lang

Contents

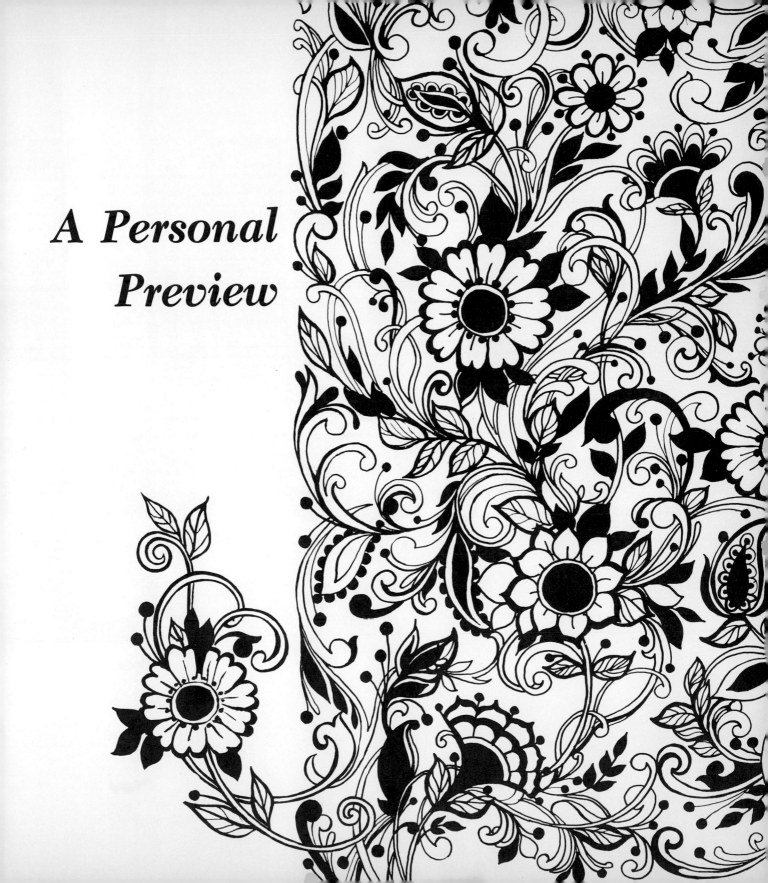

A Personal Preview

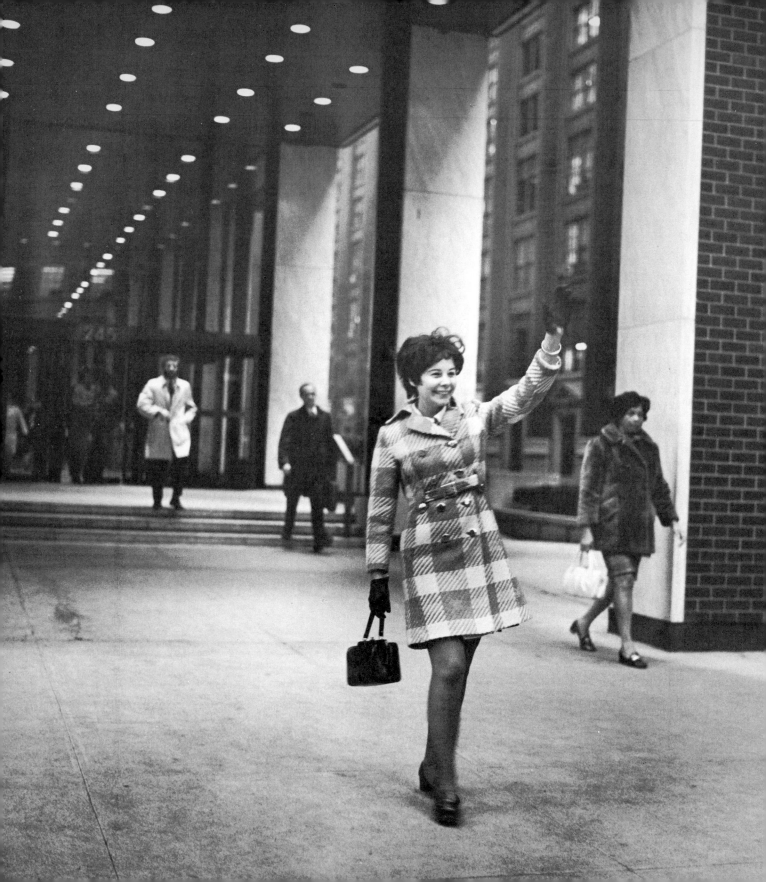

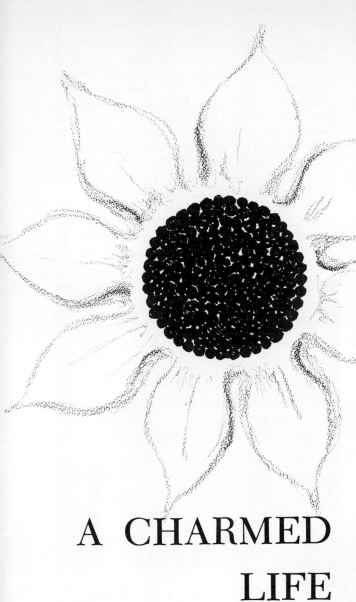

A CHARMED LIFE

If you're a career girl—or are about to become one—you're in for an exciting time. After years of being an onlooker, you're about to become an active participant in a dynamic world. This is a time when you can help with interesting and perhaps important work. It's a time when what you are and how you perform mean more than A's on a report card. Promotions, money, and opportunity are big stakes. This time you play the game for keeps—to find a job you'll enjoy, to move ahead to satisfying work, to make interesting friends, and probably to fall in love for good.

In these ventures, as with almost everything you do in life, one of your greatest assets is charm. In business you need skills, yes, but often the difference between the drone at the back desk and the executive in the front office is a matter of a charming personality. You must have ability, but to be promoted you must also look and act the part.

Charm is a difficult-to-pinpoint quality because it has so many different facets and is revealed in so many ways—a trim and tasteful appearance, a lovely way of moving, a pleasing voice, a good sense of humor, a sparkling smile, a warm and pleasant manner, tact, and thoughtfulness. Charm is a combination of all the qualities that make you a delight to be around and a pleasure to work with.

Although some girls are naturally blessed with physical beauty and an intuitively charming nature, these qualities can be nurtured and developed. All that is required is awareness. Once you have identified what is right and wrong for you, you can learn to play up your best features and to camouflage imperfections. Some of the world's most interesting beauties are the self-made variety, and some of our most charming personalities owe their ability to their own astute awareness and self-discipline. In these efforts nothing succeeds like success. The assurance that you look as pretty as possible and know how to act and what to say produces a subtle magic that boosts self-confidence and poise, making you all the more lovely.

Charm has no standard set of rules. One person's charm may be quite different from another's. You're a rather special individual, you know, unique in many ways. You must develop your own personal flair, based on your own attributes and abilities. And that's what this book is all about. Every chapter will help you discover your own beauty and charm and will tell you how you can best develop them. Whether you are tall or short, slender or plump, *femme fatale* or all-star athlete, or somewhere in between, you'll find helpful advice for your particular concerns.

In the chapters on posture, your figure, on care of the complexion, your hair, your hands, on grooming, makeup, and fashion, you'll find

When you work in an office, you will have the opportunity to make some wonderful friends.

B. D. Unsworth

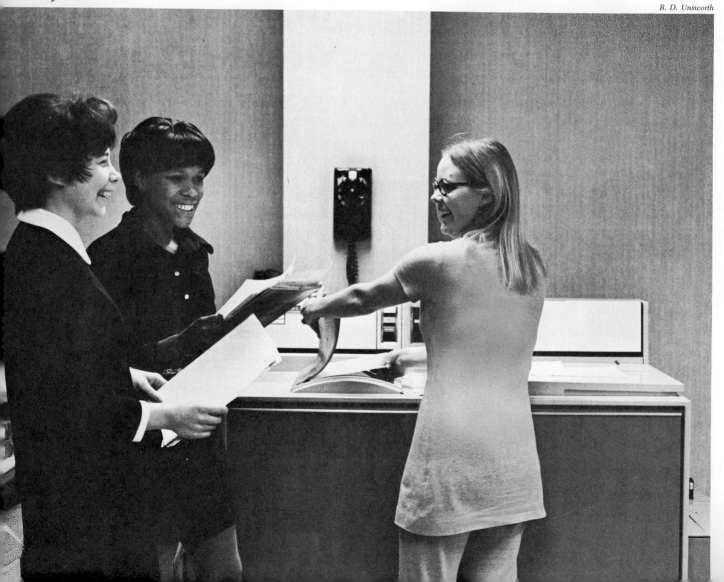

help for your problems and details for creating the loveliest YOU possible. You'll learn care and styling techniques, how to choose your most flattering fashions, what colors are yours, and how to develop a wardrobe that does the most for you. Then you'll go on to perfecting your voice and your speech and to learning how to delight others with your lively conversation and gracious manner.

Because a career is important, you'll learn how to hunt and obtain the right job, how to get off to a good start, and how to be well liked by everyone from distinguished executives to messenger boys. How a business girl lives often has such an important bearing on her success both as a person and as an employee that you'll also consider ways to make your life easier and more fun, ways to make the most of your time and money, and ways to enliven your social life.

You've an exciting course ahead, where good effort is clearly registered in your beauty and personality. Work well, for the subject is YOU. The reward: a charmed life.

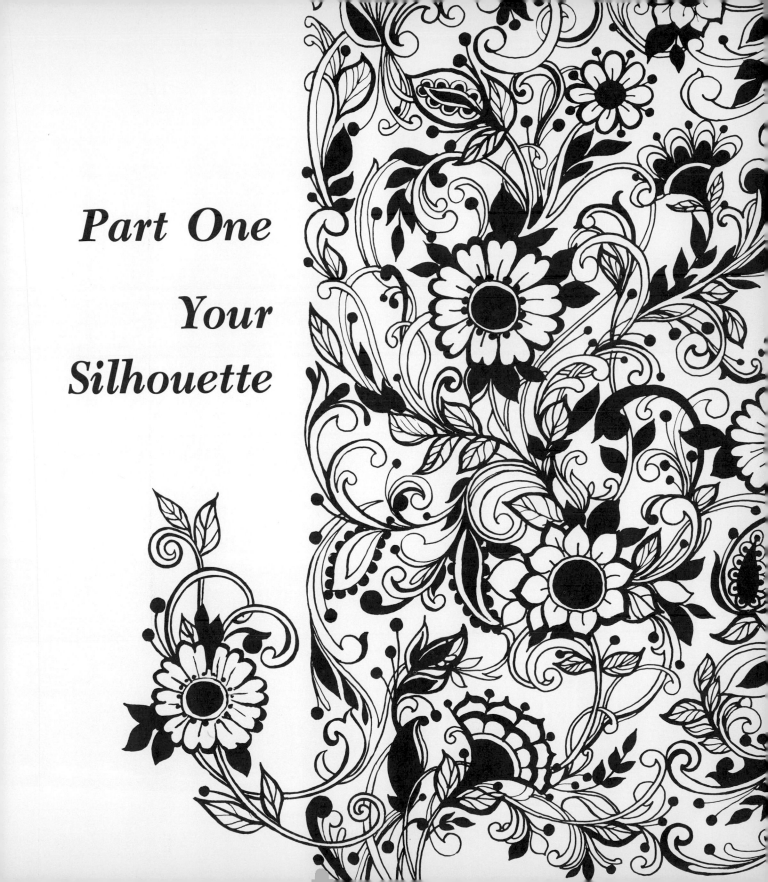

Part One

Your

Silhouette

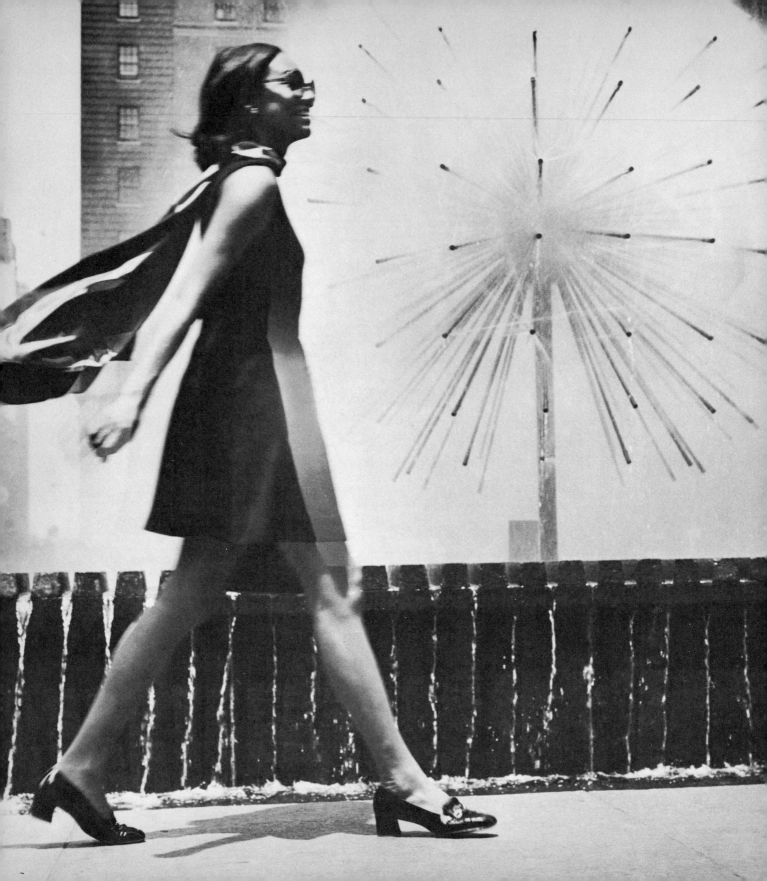

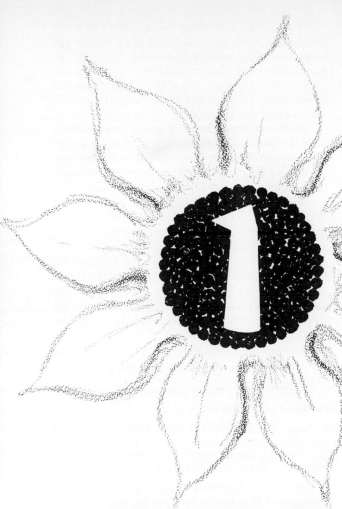

BEAUTY IN MOTION

The way you walk, the way you stand, sit, move, or manage your hands—these are major clues that help tell your public how you evaluate yourself as a person. Although you may not realize it, your posture can proclaim you as a bright, poised, assured young lady who knows the score—or it can label you as a droopy nonentity who's apt to be as awkward and slipshod in her manner as she is in her movements. A lithe, graceful body is one of your greatest assets.

The secret of a lovely, graceful body is posture. When you stand tall and carry yourself properly, your figure looks trimmer, your clothes fit better, and you seem more alert and vivacious. Posture is the foundation on which all good looks depend. A girl who possesses perfect posture and beauty of motion often is more appealing than a girl who has a pretty face but hasn't learned to move well.

Best of all, good posture helps you feel better. You have more energy, more pep. Your body was designed to operate most efficiently in a correct posture lineup. Digestive troubles, backaches, poor circulation, and just plain weariness can often be traced to posture difficulties. As if these disadvantages weren't enough to straighten us all up, there is also the grim prospect of the nasty things poor posture can do to a figure. When certain muscles are stretched unduly while others grow weak from disuse, such ugly silhouette saboteurs as protruding abdomen, broadened hips, midriff bulges, and rounded shoulders result. The way you stand today affects not only your present appearance but also determines the shape your figure will be in a few years from now.

Make a determined effort to remedy any posture imperfections. You'll be delighted with how much prettier you look.

❦ *Your Beauty Lineup*

To get the feel of perfect posture alignment, stand with your back to a wall, with your heels about two inches from the baseboard. Now press your head and back, shoulder blades, waist, and hips flat against the wall. Check these points:

• Your head should be level so that your chin is parallel to the floor. Keep your neck erect so that your ear lobes are centered over your shoulders.

• Each shoulder blade should be pressed flat for its entire breadth. If you hug the wall with your upper arms, your shoulders will be brought into position. Do not lift the shoulders. They should be back but should remain down and relaxed.

• The back of your waist should touch the wall. If you have difficulty, bend your knees and slide down the wall until the small of your back grips firmly. Then slowly move up the wall, digging as hard as possible with your waist to keep your torso hugging the wall.

As you move away from the wall, try to keep this perfect alignment by shifting your weight so that it centers over the main arch and ball of your foot. This is where your weight belongs in correct standing position (not back on your heels). Your knees should be slightly flexed, never back in a stiff, locked position.

Now you know how good posture feels. Try to become truly conscious of exactly how your body is positioned when it is correctly aligned so that you can practice this good posture until it becomes a habit. It may help to envision your body as a column of blocks, each of which must nest perfectly atop the other. When one block is out of line, the others must compensate by also tipping out of line so that sufficient balance is maintained. That is why good posture involves every inch and every muscle—and why one bad habit can spoil your total appearance.

If you walk with your head jutting forward like a duck after minnows, you have one of the most common posture problems. If you remember to keep your ears in line over the center of your shoulders and your chin in (but parallel to the floor), you'll avoid this unbecoming tendency—and the dowager's hump it can cause.

Rounded shoulders are most unattractive. Your shoulders should be held so that, in a side view, the shoulder blades are not visible but are concealed by your arm. If you stand with your arms folded, you will have to be especially careful, because this position pulls the shoulders around and forward. From time to time throughout the day, check the position of your shoulders. Perhaps you can't always stop to align your back against a wall, so instead try this: Rotate your shoulders forward, then up and back as far as possible; then let them drop suddenly. They will fall into a natural, attractive position. This is an inconspicuous movement, easy to do anywhere.

Another beauty destroyer is a jutting rear and its corollary, a protruding abdomen (the forerunner of weight accumulation in the waist and abdomen). These difficulties can be corrected if you remember to:

• Raise the top part of your body as high as possible (lift the waist up from the hips, the ribs up from the waist, the neck up from the shoulders, and hold your head up high).

• Keep your buttocks tucked in and under. Remember that column of blocks, each nesting perfectly atop the other, and see that your rib cage fits directly above the pelvic area (hips and abdomen).

• Keep your knees loose and properly centered. Often, poor alignment of the pelvic area is due to the habit of standing with the knees back in a stiff, locked position. Unless the knees are slightly flexed, the pelvis will tip out of line. When wearing heels, you will probably find it necessary to flex the knees just a bit more than you would in flats.

• Center your weight over the main arch and ball of your foot. (This applies no matter what heel height you are wearing.) If your weight is properly centered, you should be able to slide your heels slightly from side to side and, at the same time, wiggle your toes. This is possible because your heels and toes are free of weight.

Correct posture may feel a bit strained at first, but you should keep working at it. Don't try to keep your body rigid. Hold the proper alignment, but let your body relax.

If poor posture isn't corrected overnight, please don't become discouraged. You have misused your muscles all these years, and it will take some reeducation to make them behave properly. Soon good posture will be a habit and will be a completely natural part of the graceful new you.

❦ Take a Stand for Beauty

How do you place your feet while standing? Take a tip from actresses and models. They stand with one foot slightly behind the other, the back foot turned toe-out at a slight angle. This is a pose designed to show your legs at their prettiest—equally flattering to plump or slim legs. It also turns the body at a slight angle, which creates a curvaceous, long-stemmed look. *a long stemmed rose*

If you allow one foot to carry the body weight—always maintaining correct posture alignment—you have a lighter look than if your weight were plunked evenly on both feet. For development of a graceful stance, practice this movement: Assume that you are standing within a 16-inch square (average shoulder width), one foot a little behind the other. Imagine that your posture must remain correctly aligned and that your body must stay in the exact center of this 16-inch square. Now practice letting first one foot and then the other bear the body weight without allowing your body to shift from its center in the square or from its posture-perfect alignment. When you do this, your position can't help but be becoming. If you watch yourself in a mirror, you can see how the body automatically has more "lift" when the weight is on one foot. Your whole appearance will seem lighter and more graceful.

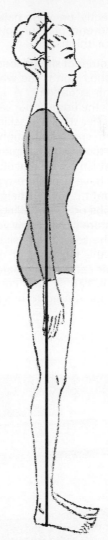

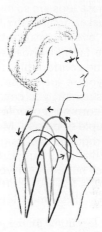

When you are standing straight, an imaginary line should pass through the tip of the ear, the center of the shoulder-arm joint, slightly behind the center of the hip, slightly in back of the center of the knee, and in front of the ankle joint. A good way to get your shoulder into the correct position is described on the preceding page.

❦ Sitting Pretty

Because most white-collar girls spend a good part of their nine-to-five hours seated, correct sitting posture is more important to them. It adds to their comfort and good looks. Attractive and healthy sitting posture depends on:

• Sitting tall—lift the whole upper part of your body out of your pelvic area.

• Sitting well back—your lower hip area should be touching the back of your chair.

• Sitting straight—sit directly on your pelvic bones, not slumped on the end of your spine or perched forward on your thighs.

When you are seated, your feet should touch the floor comfortably. If they don't, see what you can do to remedy the situation. A girl whose legs are so short that the edge of her seat presses against the back of her thighs is asking for circulation troubles and spreading thighs. The tall girl whose chair is too low must sprawl to be comfortable, and that isn't very graceful. If you're lucky enough to have a posture-type desk chair, you can custom-fit it to your height by turning a couple of knobs or push-pulling a couple of plugs. Most posture chairs allow you to regulate the height of the seat, the position of the back support, and the flexibility of the back support. If your chair can't be regulated and is too low, perhaps you can sit on a cushion. If it's too high, find something to use as

This model has her legs in the proper position, but how could she improve the way she is holding her head and back?

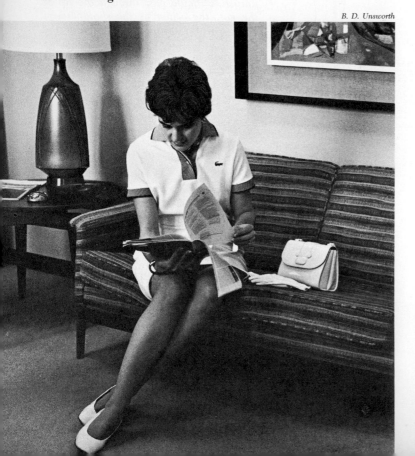

a footrest—maybe an unused mail tray or an old catalog.

A pretty pose for your nonworking moments is the diagonal sitting position models use. Place your legs diagonally across the seat of the chair. For example, arrange your feet at the right, with the left foot behind the right one and your knees at the left. This shows off your legs at their curvaceous best. It is also especially good for solving the problem of low-slung chairs or low car seats, where your knees would be too high for comfort. Positions to avoid:

• Sitting with knees apart.
• Sitting with legs strung out, grandpa-style, in front of you.
• Sitting with feet hooked around chair.
• Sitting in the morning-glory tangle, in which one leg crosses and entwines itself around the other.
• Sitting so that your skirt pulls up.

If you want to sit with your legs crossed, cross them either well above the knee or at the ankle. Crossing them directly at the knee flattens the calves, making them look fat and unattractive, as well as presenting a hazard to anyone forced to walk in front of your protruding foot.

❦ Take a Seat

The art of sitting down gracefully is easy to acquire. When you walk up to a chair, turn and place the back of your leg against the seat (this helps your balance and serves to guide you). With one foot slightly ahead of the other, lower yourself into the chair in one *smooth* movement. Keep your hips tucked under and your body erect. Put your calf and thigh muscles to work so that you go down evenly and gracefully. Your torso merely follows; it does none of the work. Nothing is worse (for beauty or the chair) than bouncing into a seat as if you'd been heaved for a forty-yard pass.

When you rise from your chair, make the same movements in reverse. Put one foot against the chair (or slightly under, if possible)

12

and keep your head and torso erect as you lift your body, using your calf and thigh muscles. Never pull yourself up by the arms of the chair. That makes you look like an old lady.

☙ *Take a Walk*

A good walk depends—once again—on good posture. It consists merely of moving about with as little unnecessary motion as possible.

Some do's. To learn how to walk gracefully, follow the step-by-step directions explained below. Practice each step until it feels relaxed and natural.

• Line yourself up properly—chin in and level, shoulders back and down, tummy pulled up and in, hips tucked under. Maintain this good alignment, keeping your body erect and *your torso as free from movement as possible.* Neither your shoulders nor your hips should sway. Your arms should be relaxed.
• Step forward, swinging your leg from your thigh-hip socket (not from your knee). If the action is correct, you will feel as if you are leading with the upper thigh. Your knees should be loose but not noticeably bent.
• As you move, center your body between the forward and back foot. (This is especially important and is how many walkers go wrong.)

Check the correct length for your stride by keeping your body in position over your left foot as you swing your right foot forward to the point where you can place it flat without moving your body forward. This is the best length stride for you. The distance between your feet should be about equal to the length of your foot.
• Aim your weight at the middle of your foot rather than at your heel. Your heel will then touch lightly and you will ride off it instantly. Your weight should pass along the *outer* border of the main arch to the ball of your foot and receive a final push-off from the big toe.
• Keep your feet parallel and close together (ankles about an inch apart), as if your footprints were to follow alongside a center line.

• Point your toes *straight* ahead.
• Walk without any up-and-down movement. Keep your feet close to the ground as you move, but avoid any tendency to shuffle. Flexing your knees will help to absorb shocks.
• Make your arm-swing a natural rhythmic accompaniment to your stride. It should not be too long, however. This keeps your profile neat.
• Keep the entire movement natural and easy. If the body is tense or the movement too vigorous, the effect of lightness and grace cannot be attained.

Some don't's. Here are some bad habits that are very common. You'll want to avoid them.

• Don't let your head bob from side to side as you walk. This fault can be corrected by learning to keep the weight of your body centered between your feet as you move instead of shifting your weight from one foot to the other. Centering your body sideways is as important as centering it front to back. To help you acquire this knack, focus your eyes on a spot on the wall as you practice walking toward it.
• Don't swing your shoulders. How ungainly is the person who seems to use her shoulders as an up-and-down or back-and-forth propeller to push herself along!
• Don't lead with your head. It won't get there any sooner than the rest of you. Hold it up proudly, like a princess.
• Don't lean back as you walk. This makes your legs seem to be running away from the rest of you.
• Don't bounce up and down on your toes. You want smooth, continuous, fluid movement. In modeling, the smoother and more natural a girl's walk, the more accomplished she is considered and the higher her rating. Top models seem almost to be gliding on wheels, as if pulled by invisible strings.
• Don't come down heavily on your heels. How horrible is the loud clap, clap, clap sound of heels coming down the corridor!
• Don't take too short a stride. A tiny, mincing gait makes you look prim and priggish and tends to give you the appearance of a mechanical doll.

13

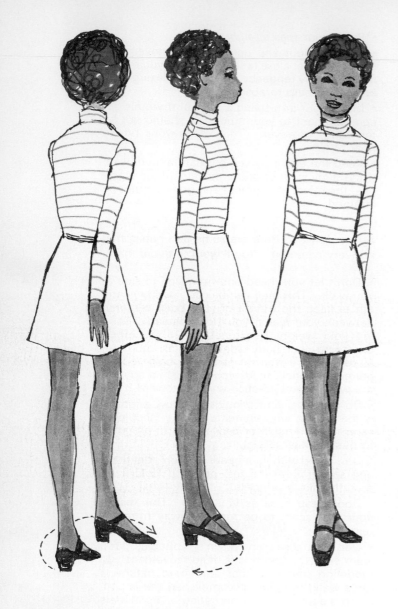

The Turn. Step forward, placing the right foot at a 45-degree angle, with the weight on the ball of the foot. Place the left foot beside it, turned slightly in, so that the toes of both feet point toward an imaginary spot. As the left foot touches the floor, pivot on the ball of the right foot, bringing the right heel against the left instep.

• Don't take too long a stride. It looks mannish.

• Don't stare at the floor. Keep your head erect. The person who studies the floor as she walks sees only the dirt and the dust. Look up and you'll be surprised at how many smiles you'll see.

• Don't pump with your arms. Keep them relaxed, palms turned in, and let them swing loosely in rhythm with your step. You won't look as if you're chugging along by means of their power if you maintain a short, natural swing.

• Don't let your arms flare away from your sides as you walk. Keep them close to your body.

❀ Feet First

A graceful walk begins with your feet. No one who is plagued by painful feet has an attractive walk. Weak feet can throw your entire posture out of line. And, conversely, poor posture can ruin your feet. Many common foot disorders arise from overtaxed muscles—the result of poor posture or poor walking habits. If you have any serious complaints about your feet, be sure to see your doctor.

Shoes that fit poorly also destroy good posture. When you purchase shoes, let comfort be your prime consideration. If high spike heels are painful, save them for your sitting-down occasions. Foot specialists urge the wearing of the lowest heel acceptable on the job. Many attractive low or midheel styles are available for both business and dress occasions.

Any girl who wears high heels all day should switch to flats when she gets home. A change of heel heights helps prevent leg cramps and keeps muscles more flexible.

The girl who isn't used to wearing high heels is wise to put in a little practice before she makes her public debut in them. You will notice that in order to keep good posture alignment when wearing heels, you must bend your knees slightly.

You can do much to strengthen your feet if you use odd moments for inconspicuous foot exercises. Just stretching and wiggling your toes is helpful, and this is an exercise you can do with your shoes on, even while making a phone call or riding in a bus. Another exercise for odd moments is rotating your foot at the ankle, pointing your toes up as high as possible and down as far as possible as you make the circle. On pages 25–26 you will find some excellent foot exercises that will help develop strong foot muscles for a lithe, attractive walk.

🌷 Strategy for Stairs

In climbing stairs, your objective is to look as if you were gliding upward smoothly and effortlessly. Your torso should move in a smooth line parallel to the banister—not in the bumpy zigzag of the steps. How is it done? By keeping all the action ''downstairs,'' in your legs. ''Upstairs,'' you'll keep your chest high, back straight, and hips tucked under. When climbing stairs, move that erect posture ahead, over the foot on the next step, before pushing up with your calf and thigh muscles. Your knee is bent, and as you push up from below, it will straighten out smoothly in one continuous motion. When almost all the weight is transferred, bring the lower leg up, place it on the second step above, and repeat the process.

Place your entire foot, not just your toes, on each step. Perching only the toes on each step is hazardous. Lift your foot lightly into position each time. Don't slide it onto the step.

When coming down stairs, keep your posture erect and step softly with your feet pointed straight ahead. If your foot is long and the step is narrow, you may find it helpful to turn your body slightly so that each foot touches the step at a right angle rather than pointing directly forward. You needn't look down at each step. Your brain will respond properly, judging the length and depth of the steps. Drop each leg to the next lower step, making a smooth transition from one foot to the next, using your knees and keeping your torso erect.

15

Practice going up and down stairs (good for the figure, you know) until you can achieve an attractive floating motion.

🌷 Beauty in Balance

Balance plays an important part in graceful movements. Some girls appear awkward merely because they have difficulty keeping their balance. With improved muscle tone, balance should improve.

B. D. Unsworth

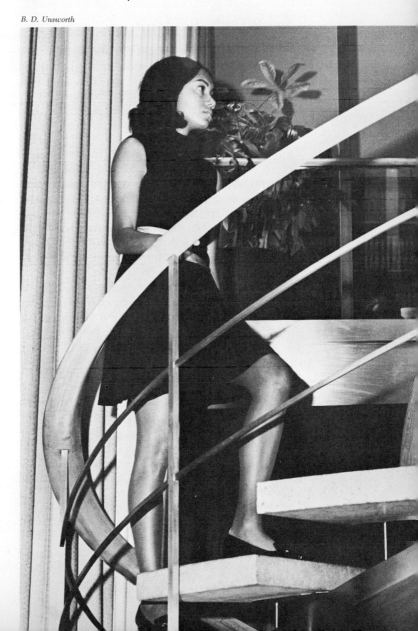

Here is an excellent exercise that dance studios suggest to help their pupils develop the good balance so important for smooth dancing. Stand on your right foot with your left foot hooked behind your right ankle. Place your hands on your hips and slowly move up and then down on the toes of your right foot. Do this ten times. Repeat, using your left foot. You'll find it easier to keep your balance as you move up and down if you concentrate on a spot on the wall at about eye level.

❦ Carriage for Cars

Getting into and out of cars is one of the most difficult maneuvers to do gracefully. Take your cue from the automobile commercials on television—watch how the models manage.

When climbing in, use the sideways method. Stand beside the open door, facing the front of the car. Rest your outer hand on the door handle or window if you wish, and bend your knee as you slide your nearest foot in sideways. Then slide the rest of your body onto the seat. Pull in your other foot as you move back on the seat. Avoid the forward lunge with its unattractive rear view. If you are carrying bundles, put them in first. It's difficult to make a graceful entrance when you're encumbered with packages.

Getting into the back seat of a two-door car can be performed gracefully. If you use the same sideways approach, put your nearest foot in, heel first, and then back your body onto the seat, it will be easy. Support yourself on the back of the front seat, if necessary, as you step in.

When you are coming out, a sideways movement is more graceful. Slide over to the end of the seat. Put your nearest foot out and a bit behind and touch the ground with your toe pointing toward the front of the car. Pushing against the foot on the ground, let your body and other leg follow smoothly as you clear the door and stand erect.

Buses are a different problem. When entering a bus with a high step, rise as high on your toe as possible while you lift your other foot. This is especially important if you are wearing a straight skirt. Disembarking is safer if you hold on to the rail at the side of the door and turn your body sideways toward this railing as you step down.

❦ Beauty at Hand

Are there times when your hands seem to be unnecessary appendages that you wish you could take off like a pair of gloves and park in a handbag for a while? Actually, they needn't be a source of trouble. The secret of graceful hands is to keep them *still* and to keep them *relaxed.* The fidgeter who twists a ring, toys with her gloves, or pats at her hair appears nervous, whether she is or not. The poised person learns to place—and keep—her hands in her lap (palms up, one hand on the other, is most attractive) or she rests them quietly on the arms of her chair.

When standing, you will find it comfortable and attractive to bring your arms across the front of your abdomen, resting your forearms on your pelvic bones as you clasp your hands loosely. Hold your elbows in close to your body. Another graceful position is keeping the hands down at your sides, with the insides of the wrists brushing your hips. Or, perhaps, you may prefer to keep one hand down at your side and to hold the other in front at the waistline. Your hands should always be relaxed, never stiff as if you were standing in a military lineup.

Many people stand with their arms entwined across their waists. This is comfortable and easy—but it looks unattractive and can lead to rounded shoulders. If you *must* cross your arms, turn one hand up along the inside of the opposite arm and let the other hand clasp the opposite elbow loosely. This gives you a more pleasing line and relieves much of the pull on your shoulders.

Your hand movements will have grace and beauty if you concentrate on making the major motions with your wrists. Don't grab! For instance, if you wish to pick something up, lead

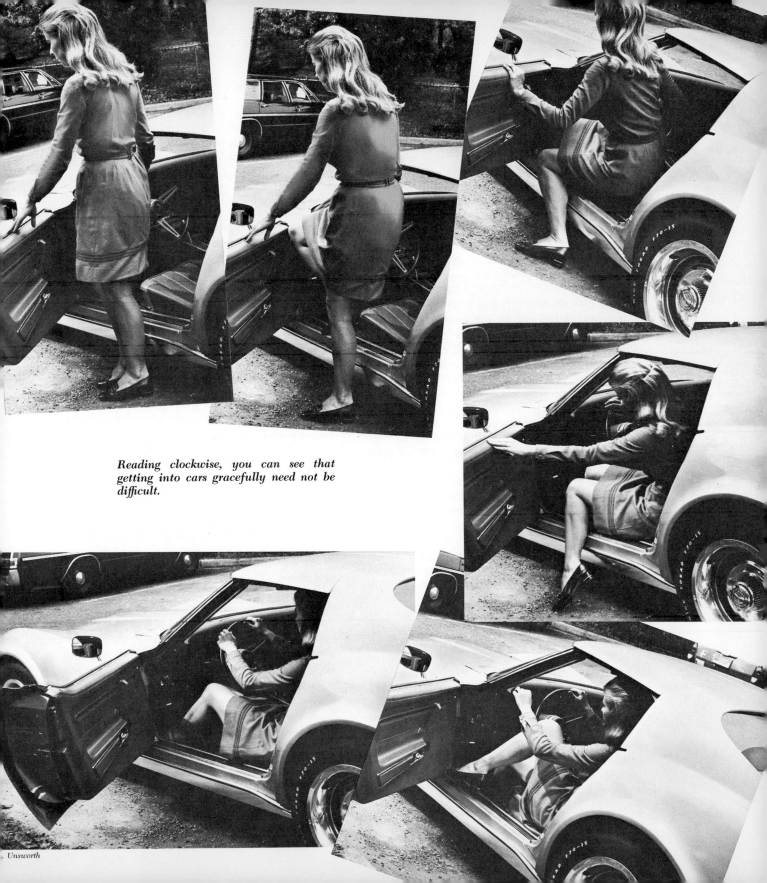

Reading clockwise, you can see that getting into cars gracefully need not be difficult.

Unsworth

with your wrist, keeping your fingers relaxed until they are just about to touch the object. This is much prettier to watch.

🌸 Bending with Beauty

Some business girls find their jobs require quite a bit of bending and squatting—there are the files in the bottom drawer, the needed book is on the lowest shelf of the boss's bookcase, and so on. *Down* may seem to be your major motion some days. Take cheer: all this squatting can do very nice things for your hip and leg muscles if you do it correctly. When you want to pick up something, keep your back straight and erect and bend your knees to go down. Then make your leg muscles push you up again. Not only is this more attractive than a bottoms-up stoop, but it prevents the back strain that can easily occur when heavy items are lifted incorrectly.

When carrying something heavy, be kind to your back. Carry packages in front of you just below the waist—not at chest level—so that the strong muscles in the lower part of your torso can share the work.

If you must frequently tote books, groceries, or any similar parcels in your arms, carry them well up on your arms and to the side, so that you can keep your shoulders and back straight. Carrying parcels on your hips drags your posture out of line. You'll be wise not to carry things on the same side each time. The person who does this may end up with one shoulder slightly higher than the other.

🌸 Exercises for Grace and Posture

Shoulder straighteners. Two groups of muscles must be retrained to improve rounded shoulders. Rounded shoulders are caused by a stretching of the back muscles between the shoulder blades and also by a shortening of the chest muscles at the front of the shoulders. The following exercises will help to remedy this imbalance.

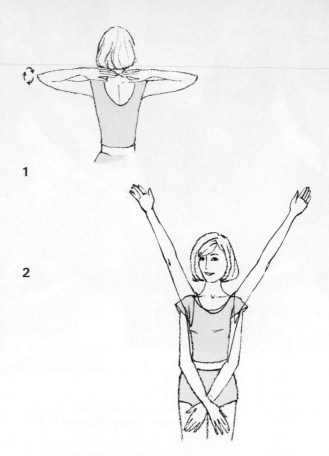

1

2

1 ELBOW TWIRL. Place your fingertips at the back of your neck just below the hairline. Keep the middle fingers touching.

Slowly circle the elbows forward, up, back, and down. Do five circles forward, five circles backward. Work up to a total of fifty circles—they only take about a minute.

You should feel pressure at the back in the neck muscles, a squeezing together of the shoulder blades, and a stretching of the front shoulder muscles.

2 HAND FLING. Stand with good relaxed posture, your arms crossed at the wrists in front.

Swing your arms up, out, and back as far as possible. Use brisk movements and keep the arms straight. Return to the starting position. Repeat ten times. Increase to twenty times.

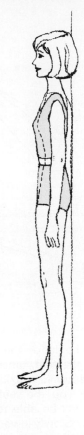

3

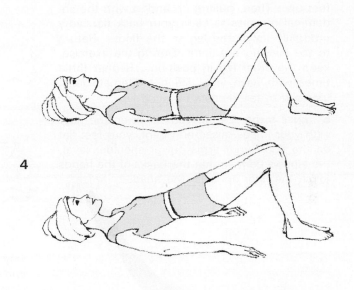

4

3 SHOULDER BLADE PRESS. Stand against a wall, body erect, knees loose.

Press your back against the wall, pushing the shoulder blades together. Concentrate on getting the entire shoulder area flat on the wall, but this time exaggerate the pull up and back on the chest and hold the chin-in position of a military cadet. Repeat this exercise at least three times and whenever possible throughout the day.

No sag, no sway. A protruding abdomen and a swayback go together. When there is an in-curve at the small of the back (swayback), there will be a compensating bulge of the abdomen. It is impossible to be sure whether the weakened back muscles or the weakened abdominal mus-les cause the trouble. (Incidentally, fat on the abdomen may not always be the cause of the

bulge—the bulge may be flabby muscles.) To correct this condition, both the back mus-cles and the abdominal muscles must be strengthened. These exercises will help to bring the body back into good posture.

4 ELEVATOR HIP LIFT. Lie on your back on the floor with your knees raised and bent, your feet flat on the floor, your arms down at your sides.

With the abdominal muscles, pull up and in, flattening the small of your back to the floor. Hold. Slowly raise the hips off the floor, con-centrating on making the end of the spine lift itself, one vertebra at a time. (Do *not* arch your stomach up, keep it as flat as it was.) Hold. Very slowly lower your back to the floor, one vertebra at a time. Dig in with the small of your back so that the tail bone touches last. Repeat twice at first. Work up to eight times.

19

5 LEG LOWERING. Lie on your back with your knees raised and bent, your feet flat on the floor, your arms down at your side. Relax your back muscles and your abdominal muscles.

Bring the right knee back towards the chest. Straighten out the knee as you raise the foot up. Then, pulling up and in with the abdominal muscles to keep your back flat, very gradually lower the leg to the floor. Return to the starting position. During the exercise, keep the other leg in position. Repeat three times with each leg. Do not alternate legs. Increase to ten repeats for each leg.

6 KNEE SLIDE. Lie on your back on the floor with your knees raised and bent, your feet flat on the floor, your arms out at shoulder level, the elbows bent so that the backs of the hands touch the floor opposite the head.

6

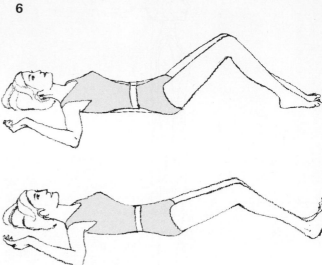

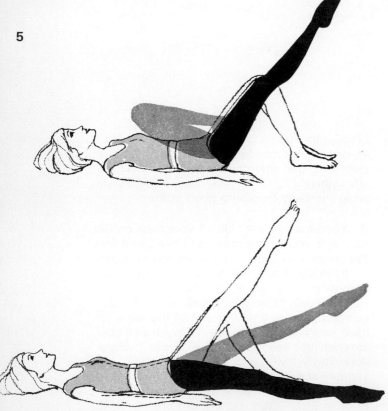

5

Force the spine to lie flat on the floor all the way from the neck to the seat, tensing the seat and abdominal muscles while relaxing the upper torso. This will give you the feel of perfect posture, so that you will be able to assume it when you are upright. Slowly lower both knees to the floor (by sliding the heels forward) until the point where you feel the arch returning to the back. Stop and bring the legs back to the starting position, still pressing down with the lower back. Repeat three times, later increasing to ten.

7 PELVIC TILT. This exercise to correct sway-back and the resulting abdominal droop can be performed in any of these four body positions.

a Make like a swayback nag on your hands and knees, keeping your head up and face forward.

Tighten the abdomen and arch the back high, dropping your face as low as possible. Hold for a count of five and then relax until the muscles release tension and resume the sway-back position. Repeat eight times.

b Lie flat on your back on the floor, with upper arms near the body and hands across the

7

a

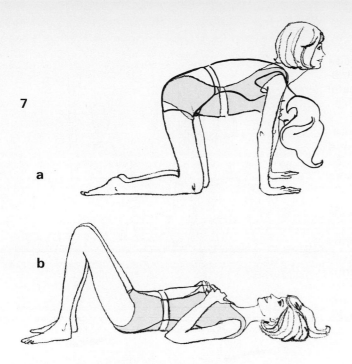

b

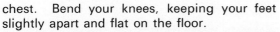

c

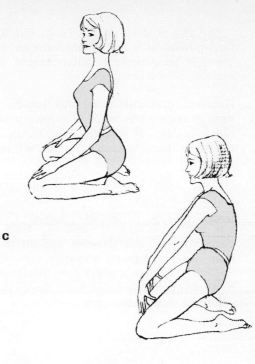

d

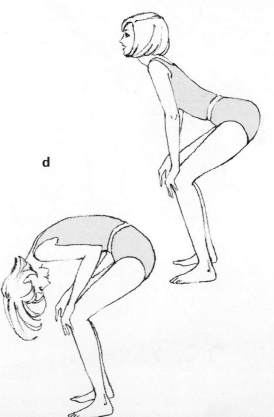

chest. Bend your knees, keeping your feet slightly apart and flat on the floor.

Arch the back, keeping shoulders and seat on the floor. Hold for a count of five. Then press the spine down flat on the floor, holding again for a count of five. Repeat eight times.

c Kneel with the legs apart and sit back on your heels, pointing your toes and resting hands on the thighs.

Lift your chest with head held high, and assume an exaggerated swayback position. Hold for a count of five. Let the shoulders and head round forward as you arch the back out. Restrain any upward motion of the head. Hold for a count of five and then relax to the original position. Repeat eight times.

d Stand with feet apart and knees bent. Lean forward to allow your hands to rest on your knees. Make an exaggerated sway with your back, keeping your head up and seat protruding.

Keeping knees bent, tuck your seat under your torso and tighten the seat and abdominal muscles while dropping your head and rounding your back. Hold for a count of five. Repeat eight times.

In any of the four positions, this exercise strengthens back and pelvic muscles, contributing to good posture, balance, and graceful motion.

Relaxed, graceful arms and hands. Tenseness is usually the cause of awkward arm and hand motion. If the arms and hands can be taught to relax, their movements will be more attractive.

8 ARM DROP. Stand erect and raise your arms above your head.

Keeping the hands relaxed, tense your arms and push up hard at the ceiling. Hold. Suddenly release your muscles and let the arms drop down and swing freely.

This exercise is helpful in loosening any tenseness in the shoulder joint. Doing this even once will relax the muscles.

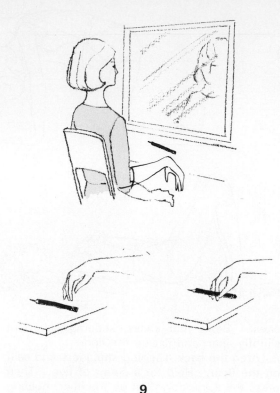

9

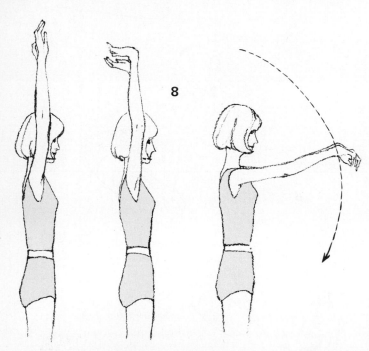

8

9 PENCIL PICKUP. Sit in front of a table with a mirror facing you. Place a pencil on the table.

Reach for the pencil with your right hand, concentrating on moving your wrist rather than your fingers. Keep your fingers relaxed and still until you are ready to pick the pencil up. Pick it up and hold it loosely. Reach out with your left hand and take the pencil. Return the right hand to your lap. Continue transferring the pencil ten times, checking your movements in the mirror.

Graceful leg control. To enable us to have graceful control of our bodies while walking, dancing, raising or lowering the body for sitting, or for climbing or descending stairs, the muscles of the legs, thighs, and feet must be strong. These exercises will strengthen and rehabilitate any muscles weakened through lack of use.

22

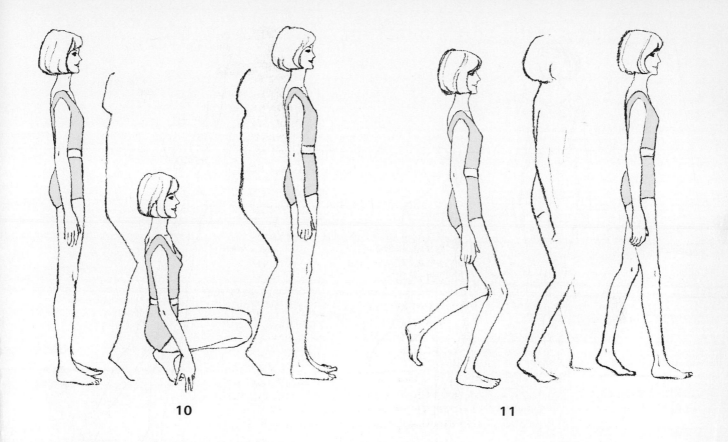

10

11

10 DEEP KNEE BEND. Stand with the torso erect and balanced. Be sure that your weight is properly centered over your arches. (Try swinging your heels and wiggling your toes without a shift in position.)

Slowly drop to the floor, bending the knees (and raising the heels) gradually until your seat rests at ankle level. Rise slowly to the starting position. Repeat five times, increasing to ten. Keep the torso relaxed and balanced throughout the exercise. The leg muscles should do the work. You should feel the tensing of the muscles in your calves and thighs.

The movements in this exercise are the same as those used to a lesser degree in all the various leg motions that involve lifting or lowering the body. The deep knee bend is one of the most valuable exercises in improving balance, grace,

and coordination—and also in producing shapely legs.

11 KNEE BEND GLIDE. Walk around the room in a half-way-down deep knee bend, torso upright.

As you walk, gradually unbend your knees until you are in a normal walking posture. Reverse the process, gradually walking down into the starting position. Repeat three times, increasing to six.

This exercise will help you adapt to the feeling of walking smoothly and gracefully and will help teach you to employ the knees as shock absorbers in order to keep the body gliding evenly.

Note: A good exercise for helping to correct bowlegs or knock knees is number 31 on page 46 of Chapter 2.

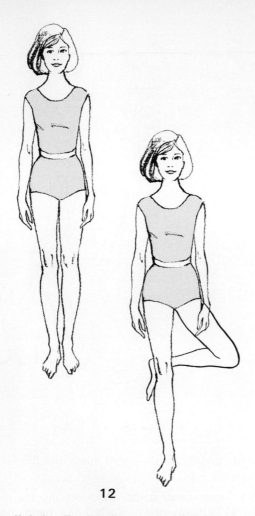

12

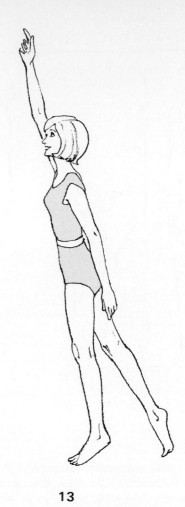

13

Step lightly. To develop a graceful carriage, you must improve your ability to balance yourself. You must also develop a feeling of lightness—of your body weight lifting off your feet—which is as essential in a graceful walk as it is in good dancing.

12 STORK STANCE. Stand in correct posture with your body weight centered directly over the main arch of each foot and evenly divided between both feet.

Without shifting your weight from its centered position, lift the left foot until the inside of its ankle touches the inside of the right knee. Hold this position as long as possible. Fixing your eyes on a spot on the wall will aid your balance.

Repeat the exercise with your right foot, again holding as long as possible. As your balance improves, you should be able to do this in high heels with your eyes closed for a count of 18.

13 BIRD-IN-FLIGHT WALK. As you walk around a room, imagine that you can take off and soar like a bird. As you step forward with your left foot, reach as high as possible over your head with the right arm. When the right foot leads, the left arm reaches high. Repeat as often as possible.

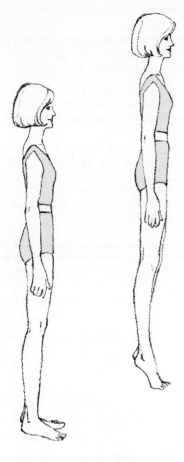

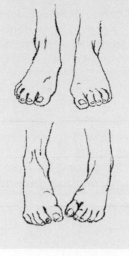

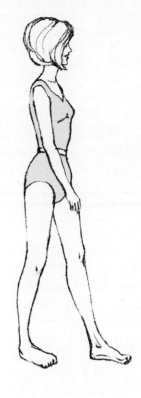

14

15

This exercise is helpful in acquiring the feeling of body lift, so that the feet are free to move as effortlessly as in dancing.

Strong footing. Tired, aching feet can make your whole outlook sour. These exercises will relax tense muscles and improve their tone, so that you will have stronger feet. They do lovely things for legs, too.

14 TIPTOES. Stand barefoot with your feet parallel, the weight slightly to the outside of the feet.

Slowly raise your body high on your toes. Then return as *slowly* as possible to the starting position. Do this slowly so that the arch muscles control the movement. This will give you the full benefit of the exercise. Repeat twenty times.

15 FOOT ROLL. Stand barefoot with your feet about an inch apart.

Raise the inner sides of the feet, rolling as far as possible over onto the outer sides. Curve the toes inward at the same time. Hold. Return to the starting position. Repeat twenty times. Then walk across the room and back on the outer sides of your feet. This exercise strengthens the main arch and is especially helpful for arches that roll in.

16 DOUBLE FOOT ROLL. Stand barefoot with your feet slightly apart. Keeping your upper body still, roll both feet to the left. Then roll both feet to the right. Repeat ten times. Move only your feet and legs. This exercise strengthens foot and calf muscles for greater flexibility and for ease in adjusting to different heel heights.

17 TOE LIFT. Stand barefoot with your feet flat on the floor about an inch apart.

Slowly raise the toes upward and backward as far as possible. Hold. Lower toes back to the floor as slowly as possible. Repeat ten times.

When this exercise is done properly you should be able to count to ten as you lift the toes and again as you lower them.

18 MARBLE PICKUP. Sit on a chair and practice picking up a marble or a pencil with your toes. Alternate feet. Repeat five times for each foot.

Note: A good exercise for correcting a walk that either toes in or out is number 31 on page 46 of Chapter 2.

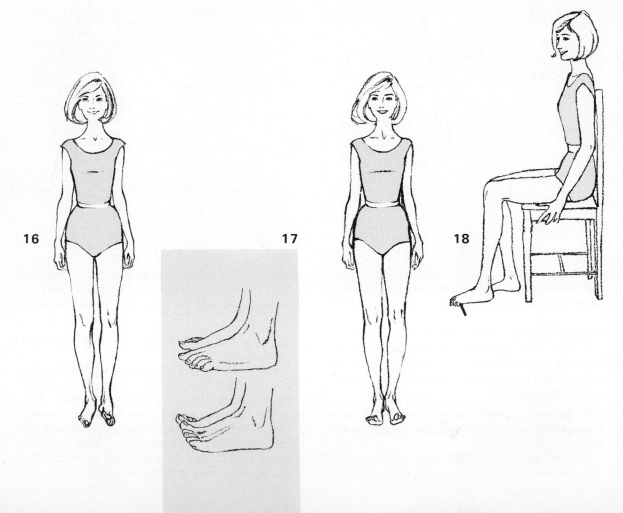

16 17 18

Select a few of the exercises from this group that will help you develop more grace or better alignment and do them regularly. If you're busy, you needn't spend a long time exercising. A five- or six-minute session each morning and bedtime should be enough to produce results. The important thing is to do your exercises regularly.

Throughout your day keep in mind your goal of beautiful, controlled action. In all your activities—as you work, walk, play—concentrate on maintaining good carriage and moving with a lithe smoothness. Thus all your actions serve as posture exercises also. Conversely, whenever you revert to bad posture habits, you are counteracting your efforts by reinforcing bad habits and making them all the more difficult to overcome.

Make good posture a total effort and you'll soon be delighted with the results.

1 *Line up three or four chairs with varying seat heights, some with legs, some with solid bases. Practice sitting and rising from these until you can manage them all gracefully.*

2 *Sit in front of a full-length mirror and devise five different comfortable and becoming ways you can place your hands and feet. Practice these until they become second nature. Then you will never feel ill at ease or awkward.*

3 *Before a full-length mirror, practice five graceful hand positions to use while standing. Practice these until they become a natural part of your posture.*

4 *If you have a car available, practice sliding in and out until you can do so in a smooth, attractive manner. Or use a low chair without arms, and simulate all the obstructions a car creates.*

5 *If you are a business girl who is lucky enough to have a posture desk chair, see if you can regulate yours for greater comfort. Even if it seems satisfactory now, experiment with different positions. Perhaps you can make it even more comfortable. You will also learn what to do in case you are ever switched to a chair adjusted to someone else's size.*

6 *To help remind yourself of good posture, resolve to check your posture each time you do some specific action such as combing your hair, waiting at a crossing, or walking through a certain doorway. Make good posture a habit for the future.*

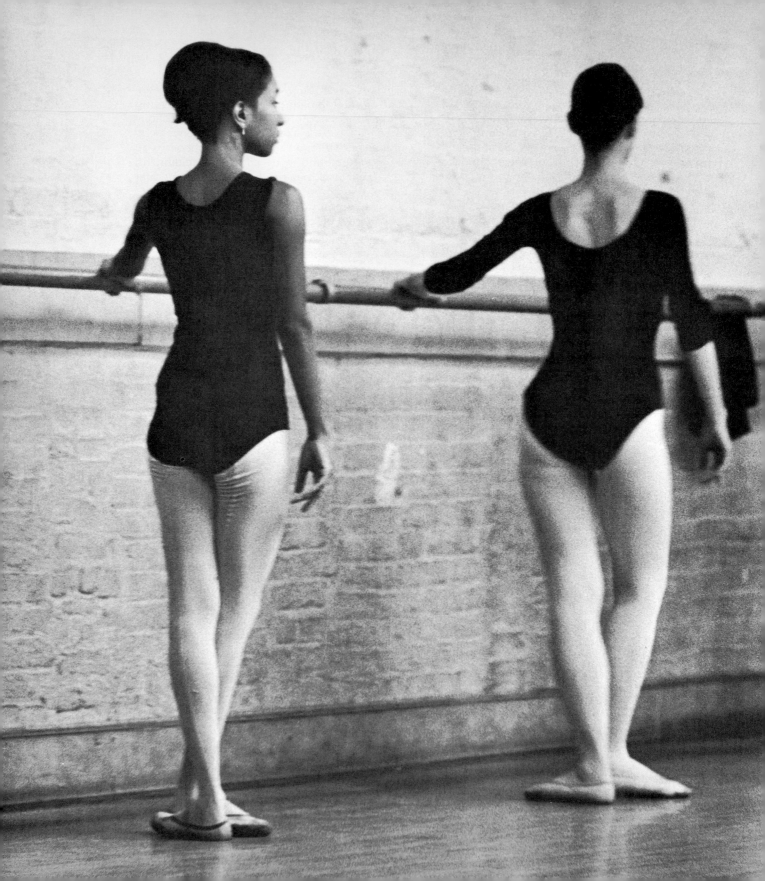

SHAPING UP

American standards of beauty call for a supple, well-proportioned figure that is slender but properly rounded. How well do you fit this image? Should you pare off a few inches here and there? Perhaps you would like to add a few curves? Or maybe a slight shift of padding would help?

Heredity has dealt each of us a certain body structure—tall or short, large- or small-boned, wide- or narrow-hipped. If your basic framework isn't quite a fashion designer's ideal, don't despair. True, your basic framework can't be changed, but usually the padding that surrounds it can be adjusted to produce a more svelte figure. Exercise can coax curves as well as reduce them. It can even cause less-than-perfect proportions to fade into obscurity by changing so-so legs into spectacular ones.

Any girl, whether ideally proportioned or not, looks best when her figure is smooth and trim. Excess pounds and slack muscles have a nasty way of emphasizing figure faults. Wise eating habits and a healthy, well-toned body help any girl to look prettier—and to feel great.

To see how your figure compares with the averages, let's do some measuring. In order to determine your ideal weight, you must first decide what type of bone structure you possess. Someone with delicate bone structure should necessarily weigh less than someone with a heavier body frame. To check on yourself, measure your wrist at the joint, just forward of the bone. Hold the tape snug and note the figure to the very last fraction of an inch. Then determine your structure from the chart on page 30. Mark this (and all other measurements that follow) on a personal record chart. Next, measure your height in stocking feet, being careful to credit yourself with every fraction of an inch. With these figures in hand, compute your ideal weight, using the weight chart appearing on page 31. Then weigh yourself to see how you compare.

Now bring out the tape measure again, and compare your statistics with the ideal measurement chart. All measurements are to be taken over the fullest part of the area. Check your side view to be sure the hip measurement is taken where your circumference is largest. Measure over a bra, but without a girdle, remembering to keep the tape measure straight and taut but not tight. The ankle is measured just above the ankle bone. Ideally, your bust and hips should measure the same, and your waist should be ten inches smaller.

If, after making allowance for your particular bone structure, you find that your weight is approximately correct and your pounds are properly distributed—lucky you! Guard your good figure jealously. If your weight is a few pounds below the suggested amount and you feel fit and healthy, don't feel that you must try to gain. Modern medical research indicates

that it is beneficial to be slightly underweight. Gaining weight is all too easy for most of us. Without realizing it, we develop careless habits—the scale reading starts to creep up before we know it.

❦ Good Habits, Good Figure

Ann Sawyer was a tiny girl who wore a size 9 dress and had a most enviable waistline. Her mother always prepared well-balanced meals, not too heavy in sweets and starches. When Ann went to work, she no longer ate lunches at home under Mother's watchful eye. A hamburger with French fries, a malted, and devil's food layer cake became a typical lunch, followed by a midafternoon snack of Coke and pie and possibly a candy bar. Of course, Ann's skin wasn't quite as clear as it should have been, but she didn't worry. She still didn't worry when she discovered a couple of her skirts were a bit too snug or that her new dress had to be size 11. But the woeful day arrived when even a size 15 was tight. Ann realized that something had to be done—she was rapidly slipping into the fat-girl category.

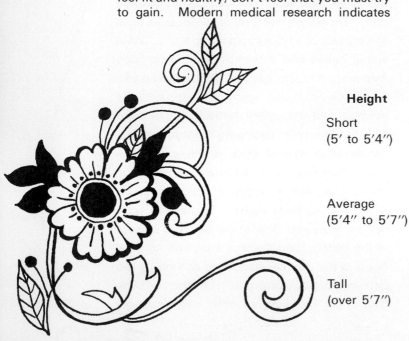

BONE STRUCTURE

Height	Wrist measurement	Bone structure
Short (5' to 5'4")	(a) 5¼" or less (b) 5¼" to 5¾" (c) 5¾" or more	(a) small (b) medium (c) large
Average (5'4" to 5'7")	(a) 5½" or less (b) 5½" to 6" (c) 6" or more	(a) small (b) medium (c) large
Tall (over 5'7")	(a) 5¾" or less (b) 5¾" to 6¼" (c) 6¼" or more	(a) small (b) medium (c) large

add 5" to ankle
6" to calf
for thigh

IDEAL WEIGHT

Height	Small frame	Medium frame	Large frame
4'10"	89–97	94–106	102–118
4'11"	92–100	97–109	105–121
5'0"	95–103	100–112	108–124
5'1"	98–106	103–115	111–127
5'2"	101–109	106–119	114–131
5'3"	104–112	109–123	118–135
5'4"	107–116	113–128	122–139
5'5"	111–120	117–132	126–143
5'6"	115–124	121–136	130–147
5'7"	119–128	125–140	134–151
5'8"	123–133	129–144	138–156
5'9"	127–137	133–148	142–161
5'10"	131–141	137–152	146–166
5'11"	135–145	141–156	150–171
6'0"	139–149	145–160	154–176

Note: This chart is based on figures from the Metropolitan Life Insurance Company. It shows ideal weight for girls of eighteen dressed in indoor clothing. If you are over eighteen, add one pound for each year up to the age of twenty-five, at which point ideal weight remains stationary.

IDEAL MEASUREMENTS

	Under 5'4"	5'4" to 5'7"	5'7" to 5'9"	Over 5'9"
Bust	32–33"	34–35"	35–37"	38–39"
Waist	22–23"	24–25"	25–27"	28–29"
Hips	32–33"	34–35"	35–37"	38–39"
Thigh	19"	19½"	20"	20½"
Calf	12½"	13"	13½"	13¾"
Ankle	7¾"	8"	8¼"	8½"
Upper Arm	9"	9½"	10"	10½"

Note: This chart is for the medium bone structure. To obtain ideal measurements for: Small frames, subtract 1" for bust, waist, and hips; ½" for thigh, calf, and upper arms; ¼" for ankle. Large frames, add 1" for bust, waist, and hips; ½" for thigh, calf, and upper arm; ¼" for ankle.

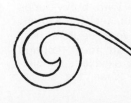

Fortunately, Ann had the wisdom to realize that her eating binge wasn't worth the toll in good looks. She also had the willpower to pass up the high-calorie foods until she had whittled her figure back to its former desirable proportions. When Ann's dieting days were over, she was quite pleased with herself for the strength of mind and determination she had shown. But she was well aware of how easy it was for her to gain weight and of how important it was to continue to eat wisely and moderately. She realized the shortsightedness of eating more than she really wanted, and she learned to substitute low-calorie treats for the routine of scale-sagging snacks she had formerly indulged in. When the gang stopped off for banana splits, Ann often voted in favor of raspberry sherbet. Instead of malteds, she ordered orangeade, limeade, or milk. She nibbled fruit instead of candy, celery instead of potato chips or peanuts. By eating properly, Ann not only regained her slim figure but also improved her skin. Her hair gleamed, and her fingernails lost their brittleness. She had more pep and energy, too, because her well-balanced meals gave her a good supply of all the food essentials—proteins, vitamins, and minerals.

Here are twelve good habits that can help you stay slim—and healthy.

1 Never skip a meal—breakfast, for instance. You'll only be tempted to fill up on doughnuts and similar nutritionless high-calorie snacks later on. Start the day right by refueling with a sound breakfast. It's been a long time since dinner and your body needs something to go on.

2 Eat slowly and chew your food well. The speedy eater may not realize how much she is consuming, and she always has time to be tempted by seconds before others are finished. Besides, we get the most flavor and satisfaction out of food that is eaten slowly and chewed thoroughly.

3 Begin lunch and dinner with bulky foods (such as a salad) to help you feel full sooner.

4 A crisp leafy salad is your figure's best friend. Salads with fresh fruit, meat, cottage cheese, or seafood are also excellent for dieters. Choose these rather than the soggy,

heavily dressed varieties, like coleslaw. Use lemon juice, which is an excellent calorie-free dressing, or use only a teaspoon of the richer dressings.

5 Avoid fried foods. The butter or fat used in cooking them adds an enormous number of calories.

6 Don't eat just because everybody else does. Perhaps you can become a bit of a secret gourmet snob about snacks—tell yourself that you don't really want to be bothered to eat unless you're offered something definitely out of the ordinary. This is rather helpful in passing up the mundane potato chips, pretzels, and so-so snacks that tempt us.

7 Don't eat while reading, studying, or watching TV—and skip the popcorn and ice cream at the movies. When your attention is diverted, you may consume more than you realize.

8 If you must tackle rich foods, eat only a little—a small taste of the chocolate cream pie, a sliver of seven-layer cake, and so on. When you are served rich foods while dining out, don't feel that you must finish your entire portion.

9 If you pal around with big eaters (boyfriends can be particularly detrimental), don't let yourself unconsciously match their consumption. Quit before you have that full feeling.

10 Get enough rest. When you are too tired, you often try to counteract your weariness by overeating.

11 Eat at regular hours. Delaying a meal may make you so famished that you will tend to eat more than you do normally.

12 Get enough regular exercise. Walk to work (or part of the way) if you can. Join a bowling team. Swim, play tennis, ski, go biking whenever possible.

❦ Eating for Beauty

A good diet consists of more than calories. Its primary function is nourishment. Beautiful skin, sparkling eyes, glossy hair, steady nerves, stamina, and often a good disposition and a cheerful outlook on life are strongly affected by what we eat. To maintain health and beauty, our bodies need a balanced diet with a full quota of protein, vitamins, and minerals. Each day

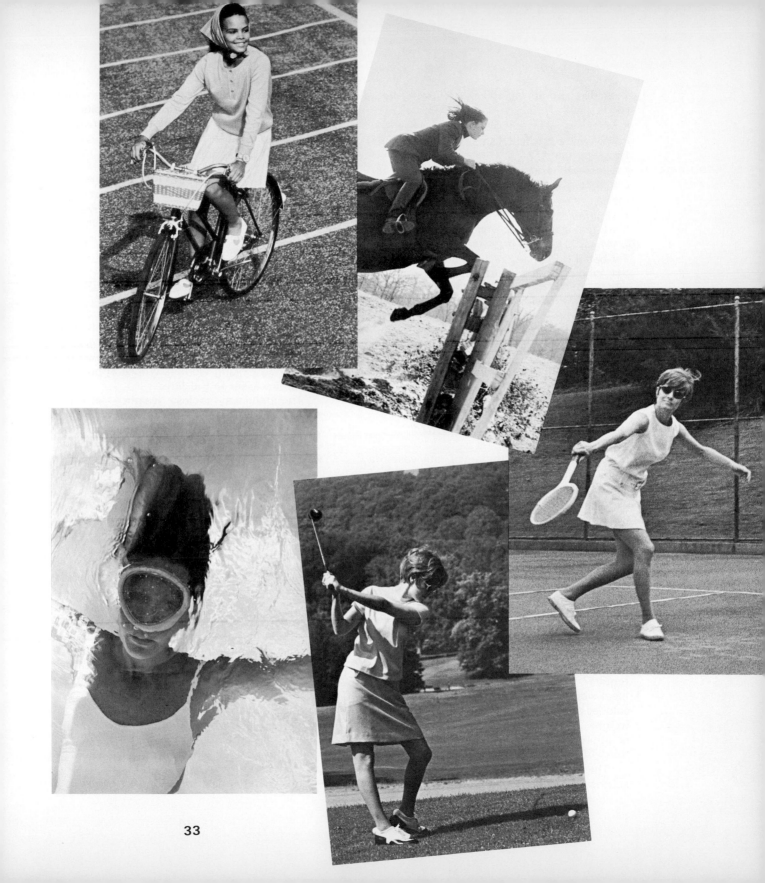

33

your diet should include the following beauty foods.

- *Milk*—at least two glasses.
- *Protein foods* (meat, fish, poultry, or cheese)—two servings.
- *Eggs*—at least three to five a week.
- *Fruit*—two servings (one a citrus fruit or tomato).
- *Vegetables*—two or more servings, especially leafy green and deep yellow vegetables.
- *Whole grain bread or cereal*—two servings. For better health and beauty, acquire a taste for the whole wheat, oatmeal, and other dark, whole grain breads that contain many vitamins and minerals lost in processing flour for white bread. Choose whole grain cereals—whole wheat, oat, or high-protein varieties—rather than corn flakes, puffed cereals, or rice crisps, which have a low nutritional value. When in doubt, check the cereal labels. They often list the vitamin content.

❦ How Much Do You Eat?

Make a list of everything you ate yesterday. Include not only what you ate at meals but also any between-meal snacks like cookies or soda. Every bite and every sip counts. Then check your calories. Most cookbooks contain sizable calorie charts, and dieting books with calorie charts are easy to find in libraries, dime stores, and supermarkets. Using such a chart, determine the caloric value of the various foods you eat and the total number of calories you consume in an average day. (You should also include the little extras, such as butter on your bread or potatoes, cream and sugar with your coffee, and dressing for your salad.)

How many calories does *your* body actually require? To obtain this amount, multiply your ideal weight by 20 (your body needs 15 to 20 calories per pound per day). If you want to lose weight, reduce your calorie requirements by one-third. If you want to gain, add on one-third. This gives your calorie quota for one day.

The results of your mathematics may be surprising. It isn't until you actually take the time to figure out your calorie intake that you get a clear picture of your eating habits. By counting calories and holding to a certain quota, most people can lose or gain as they choose.

❦ Trimming Excess Poundage

If your weight is ten pounds or more above what it should be, you ought to slim down while it's still relatively easy. Excess poundage not only sabotages your good looks, but it also creates an undesirable impression on others. Lack of willpower, laziness, self-indulgence, and slowness are attributed (although often wrongly) to stout people. The hefty girl may find it difficult to get a good job, and she is less likely to be considered for promotion to the more interesting meet-the-public jobs. Businessmen want attractive, smart-looking workers whose appearance will be an asset to the firm.

The only way to lose weight—let's face it—is to cut calories. You'd have to walk about thirty-six miles to lose one pound—exercise alone isn't enough. You must diet, in some way.

If the idea of dieting sounds like a torturous ordeal, take heart. There's no need to starve yourself. No fasting. It's merely a matter of substituting low-calorie foods for high-calorie ones. Many of the best-loved foods—steak, cantaloupe, some cheeses, asparagus—are ideal for dieters. Magazines and cookbooks contain many low-calorie versions of popular desserts. You need not deny yourself the pleasures of good eating just because you're on a diet.

Although it's true that reducers must usually eat less, it's amazing how appetite adjusts to habit. As you eat less, your appetite shrinks. Within about a week you will probably feel just as full, just as satisfied on your sensibly trimmed-down diet as on your usual fare. You may wonder how you ever managed to stow away so much before.

Before you undertake any diet, you'll be wise to check with your doctor and let him suggest what is best for you. For the sake of your health, steer clear of fast, fad diets. You need well-balanced meals every day. The wild dieter who goes on a crazy banana-and-hard-boiled-egg diet sheds pounds quickly. But her success may be short-lived. In order to prove her tremendous willpower, she may seriously jeopardize her health.

There are several food concentrates on the market that serve as low-calorie meal substitutes. While these products, with their 900-calories-a-day total, bring about a quick weight loss, many medical men consider them too drastic. They suggest using these concentrates for one meal a day, lunch perhaps, accompanied by a small salad. Then eat a normal, but low-calorie, breakfast and supper. As weight decreases, gradually work away from these products.

Resist the tempting appeal of appetite-chasing pills. Some types have been found to cause undesirable or even dangerous side effects. In many cases users were dismayed to find that once they discontinued using the pills, they ballooned back to their former dimensions. A better way to bolster willpower is to join a dieters' group such as Weight Watchers, which encourages its members to develop intelligent eating habits and to stick with them. Although depressants and low-calorie meal substitutes have value for some people, they do not help dieters develop the wise eating habits that will keep their figures slim. Users often return to their old ways after dieting and soon regain their old overweight figures. The aim of the intelligent dieter is to change her tastes so that she is satisfied with lower calorie dishes and no longer craves the fattening foods.

When you feel the urge to nibble, choose something that won't shatter your diet—celery, carrot sticks, fruit, unsweetened fruit juice. Even a drink of water can sometimes save you from disaster!

Try to keep mentally and physically active as you diet, for the lonely, bored individual is the one who beats a steady path to the refrigerator door. Keep your life so filled with absorbing activities that you haven't time to think

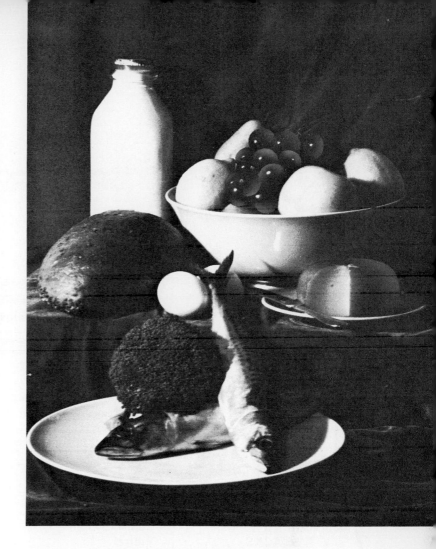

of food. Keep your mind on your goal of charm and beauty, and you'll easily shun the tempting figure-destroyers.

❦ How to Gain Weight

A slim figure may be the ideal today, but no woman is attractive if she is too thin. Gaining weight is often more difficult than losing it. It is well worth the effort, however, particularly if you have high hopes for your career. Girls who are extremely underweight may find themselves crossed off the list for desirable jobs because many employers feel that such girls are a health

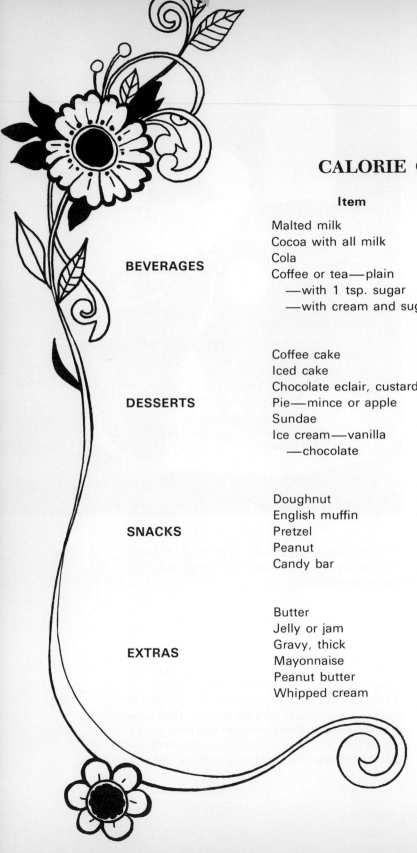

CALORIE CAUTIONS

	Item	Quantity	Calories
BEVERAGES	Malted milk	average glass	400
	Cocoa with all milk	8 oz.	235
	Cola	8 oz.	105
	Coffee or tea—plain	8 oz.	none
	—with 1 tsp. sugar	8 oz.	25
	—with cream and sugar	8 oz.	50
DESSERTS	Coffee cake	average slice	150
	Iced cake	average slice	300
	Chocolate eclair, custard	1	315
	Pie—mince or apple	average slice	400
	Sundae	average	400
	Ice cream—vanilla	1 scoop	150
	—chocolate	1 scoop	240
SNACKS	Doughnut	1	135
	English muffin	1	175
	Pretzel	1 medium	70
	Peanut	1 (!)	5
	Candy bar	average	255
EXTRAS	Butter	1 pat	50
	Jelly or jam	1 tbs.	50
	Gravy, thick	2 tbs.	100
	Mayonnaise	1 tbs.	100
	Peanut butter	1 tbs.	125
	Whipped cream	1 tbs.	50

SAMPLE REDUCING DIET

BREAKFAST

1 serving of fruit
1 egg (preferably boiled or poached)
   —OR 1 cup *whole grain* or high-protein cold cereal
   —OR ⅔ cup hot oatmeal or other whole grain hot cereal (use granulated or liquid sugar substitute)
1 glass of skimmed milk
   —OR 1 thin slice of toast (preferably whole wheat) with ½ tsp. butter
1 cup of coffee or tea, if desired (sugar substitute and skimmed milk, not cream, may be added)

LUNCH

1 small serving of lean meat, fish, poultry, cheese (for example, ⅔ cup cottage cheese)
   —OR two eggs
½ cup green vegetable
   —OR yellow vegetable (without butter or sauce)
1 serving of tossed green salad, with low-calorie dressing if desired
1 serving of fruit for dessert (preferably fresh fruit)
1 glass of skimmed milk or buttermilk
1 cup coffee or tea, if desired (sugar substitute and skimmed milk may be added)

DINNER

1 small serving of lean meat, fish, poultry
   —OR two eggs
½ cup green vegetable and ½ cup yellow vegetable (without butter or sauce)
1 serving of tossed green salad
   —OR tomato salad (low-calorie dressing)
1 serving of fruit
   —OR two small graham crackers
   —OR two gingersnaps
1 glass of skimmed milk
1 cup coffee or tea, if desired (sugar substitute and skimmed milk may be added)

risk and lack the physical stamina needed to meet the day-to-day demands of the work.

To put more meat on your bones, you need some calories to spare. This means eating more and burning up less energy. Easier said than done, perhaps. If your appetite is fickle, it may be due to a combination of things—faulty nutrition, irregularity of meals, or fatigue. If you frequently feel tired out, consult your doctor. You may have an iron or vitamin deficiency that prevents you from putting on weight. Here are some suggestions for adding pounds.

• Develop a healthy respect for good nutrition. Because your appetite is limited, make sure you eat a sufficient supply of the beauty-building essentials, such as milk, meat, green and yellow vegetables, fruits, and whole grain cereals. Indulge in the high-calorie desserts if you wish, but only after you've packed away a good nutritious meal.

• A between-meal pickup, such as a milk shake or ice cream, is excellent. Schedule snacks so that they won't interfere with meals, preferably two to three hours before your next meal. Too much nibbling of rich or starchy foods can spoil the appetite and fill you up to such a degree that you haven't room left for the vitamin-packed foods you need most.

• Don't skip a meal. Curiously enough, the only way to build up an appetite is to eat. If you eat three meals a day at approximately the same times, you become the victim of habit and your appetite responds. Another factor is that the B vitamins in food tend to spark your appetite and prepare you for the next meal. If you've been breakfasting on coffee only, try to educate your palate to better things. Perhaps at first you'll find that a milk shake with an egg in it (flavored with coffee if you wish) will give you early-morning nutrition you can enjoy or at least tolerate. Gradually, as you become accustomed to a morning meal, you can move up to a more substantial breakfast.

• Learn to relax. The girl who is tense and keyed up burns calories at a terrific clip. Avoid tension by trying to minimize crises—allow yourself enough time so that you are never rushed, don't let little things annoy you, steer a wide berth around unpleasant people whenever possible, and make an effort to remain calm and to keep your emotions under control.

If you don't squander your energy on trifles, you'll have more left for the fun of life.

• Get plenty of rest—eight or nine hours a night without fail—and don't allow yourself to become overtired.

• Allow plenty of time for your meal. Eat slowly and chew your food thoroughly.

• Don't smoke. If you must, smoke only moderately. Avoid smoking before meals because it will tend to kill your appetite.

• Develop an interest in food. Occasionally treat yourself to unusual exotic dishes at foreign restaurants. Try to learn more about cooking. Look for unusual recipes and learn to use herbs and spices to bring out flavors. Perhaps you'll become such a culinary artist that you won't be able to resist your own cooking.

❦ Adjusting the Curves

Although exercise doesn't make you lose much weight, it can help you to lose inches in some places and build up curves in others as you lose pounds by dieting. If your measurements are out of proportion when you *start* dieting and you don't exercise, you will end up smaller but *still* out of proportion. To put and keep the proper curves in the proper places, make exercise a habit. Many a slender girl still needs to flatten her tummy or improve her posture or tone up her thigh muscles. Even the girl who is attempting to gain weight may find that unless she exercises, her extra pounds all settle unbecomingly around her waist and tummy.

Before you begin a routine of exercises, have your doctor check your heart and blood pressure—not that you plan to undertake anything terrifically strenuous, but it is always important to know that your heart is in good condition before you undertake any unusual physical activity.

If you manage to get regular exercise of the bowling-swimming-tennis-biking variety, this may be sufficient to keep your muscles in tone. But just about every girl needs to do at least one waist and hip exercise, one shoulder and bust exercise, and one posture exercise each

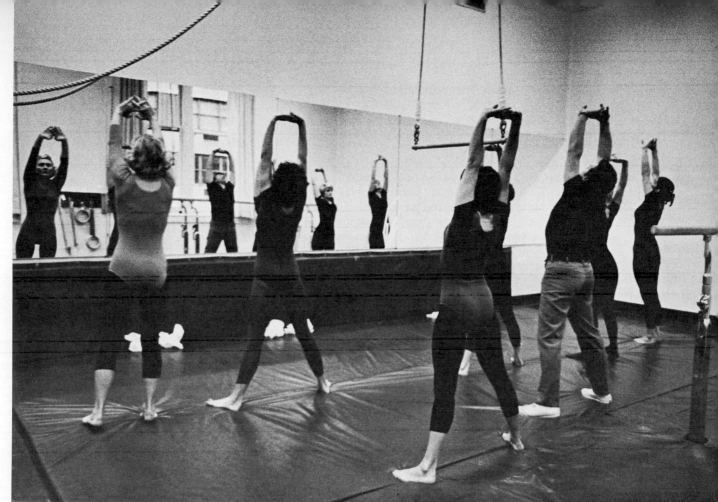

Courtesy of Tina Raver, Gala Fitness

day. Set aside five or ten minutes each morning or evening for a few exercise quickies. Once you get into the habit of exercising, you'll find it so relaxing and refreshing that no day will seem complete without your daily half dozen.

To get the most out of your exercises, go at them s-l-o-w-l-y and rhythmically, stretching gracefully as far as possible. The girl who madly flails about like a propeller does little more than wear herself out. Pretend that you are a ballet dancer. Kick and swing as smoothly and gracefully as a prima ballerina. If you can do your exercises to music—even humming a tune to yourself—so much the better. It's fun to kick around when you have peppy ballet music or show tunes playing in the background to heighten the illusion.

Exercise classes, like this one with Larry Lorence of Gala Fitness, provide a variety of equipment, but they should be supplemented with daily exercise at home.

In order to have exercises perform their toning and beautifying magic, you must keep at them regularly. A few minutes' worth each night is better than an hour's rugged workout every week or two. Keep up the good work and in a few short weeks your tape measure will indicate the pleasing results.

❦ Spot-Reducing Exercises

Waist whittlers. These will help to reduce your midway dimensions and are good for posture too.

19 BALLET BEND. Lift your arms overhead, holding them limply. Then stretch high. The stretch should be felt only through the midriff, not in the arms.

Hold the tension as you stretch high. Then relax and bend directly to the left, letting the right arm drop as far over the head as possible. Hold. Come back to your starting position. Stretch high, tense, relax, and bend to the right, with the left arm over your head. Your knees should be kept straight, and you should feel a good pull at the sides of your waist. Repeat five times on each side, increasing to ten.

20 FORWARD AND BACK BENDS. Stand erect with your feet a foot apart.

Drop forward, bending at the waist. Keep your knees straight and try to touch your hands to the floor. Hold. You should feel the stretch in your midriff and in the back of your thighs, not in your arms. Rise to the original position. Then bend backward as far as possible. Hold, then return to position. Repeat four times, increasing to eight.

You may not be able to touch the floor in the beginning, but make a good try.

21 TORSO TWIST. Stand erect in good posture, with your arms out at the sides and your feet about eighteen inches apart.

Keeping the feet firmly in place, twist the upper body as far to the left as possible. Try to follow your left hand with your eyes. Then reverse and swing to the right, following your right hand with your eyes. Repeat four times on each side, increasing to eight.

The effort should be felt in the waistline, which is only possible if you stand erect.

22 FORE AND AFT LEG SWING. Lie on your left side, your head on your outstretched left arm.

Keeping your left leg in position, swing your right leg forward as far as possible. Hold. Then swing it backward as far as possible. Hold, and return to starting position. Repeat four times with one leg. Roll over and repeat with the other leg. Increase to eight times.

Your torso must be straight throughout and the pull should be felt only in the waist, hip, and thigh areas (all of which benefit from this).

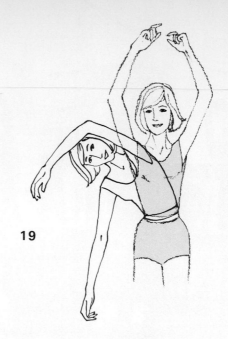

19

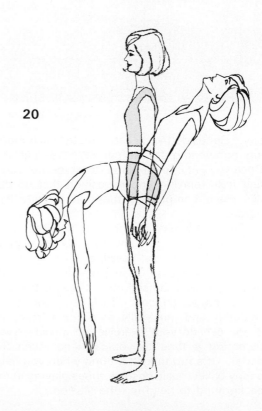

20

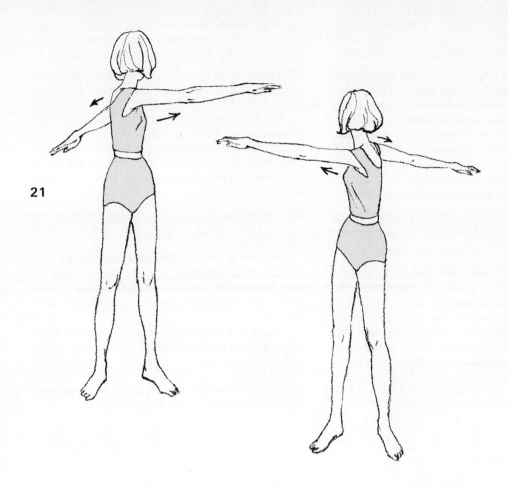

21

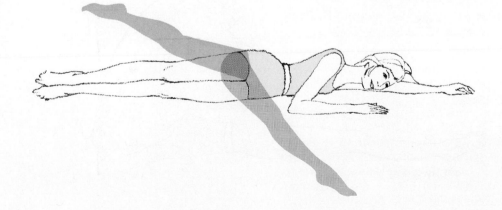

22

41

For a trim tummy. The exercises (4–7) suggested at the end of Chapter 1 for correcting a protruding abdomen or swayback will also trim excess fat while they improve posture.

23 SITUP. Lie on your back on the floor, legs straight, hands clasped at the back of the neck.

Sit up, letting your abdominal muscles do the work. When you are fully erect, straighten your back and hold your head high as you give your elbows a good backward push. Then, rounding your back, *slowly* roll down to the floor, trying to touch each vertebra in order as you go. Repeat twice, gradually increasing to ten times.

This is *the* best exercise for the abdomen and should be done regularly. If you have difficulty the first few times, tuck your feet under a low piece of furniture so that they stay on the floor.

24 ROCKER. Lie face down on the floor with your arms extended forward.

Raise the right arm and the left leg simultaneously. Then alternate, using the opposite arm and leg. Do ten times. If this is easy for you, try the more advanced version: raise both arms and both legs off the floor simultaneously—a few inches will do at first but lift higher as you become more supple.

Hips, hips away. One of the most common figure problems is heavy hips. A regular exercise routine can definitely trim inches from this area, so make a firm resolution and go to it.

25 ROLL OVER HANDS. Lie on your back with your hands at your sides, your knees drawn up to your chest.

Roll sideways over your arms and touch your knees to the floor. Use your hip, leg, and abdominal muscles (not your hands) to roll your body back to position. Then roll to the other side and back. Repeat eight times for each side.

26 BICYCLE RIDE. Lie on your back and roll up on your shoulders, supporting your hips with your hands.

Pedal big circles with your feet, *being sure that the inner borders of your knees touch as they pass each other.* Pedalling wildly or with your legs wide apart does no good. Pedal a minute.

There is a threefold purpose here: you work the legs into proper contact at the thigh joint, reduce the hips and thighs, and strengthen the muscles that keep your legs tracking properly for smooth carriage. (And good carriage automatically slims you as you walk!)

23

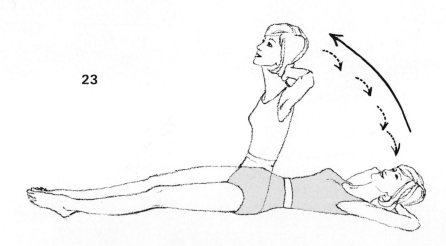

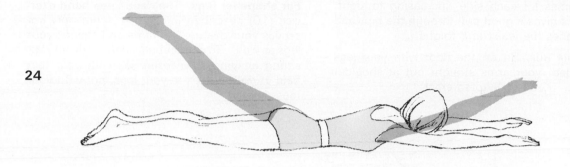

24

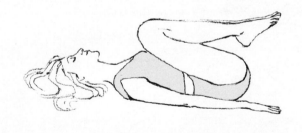

25

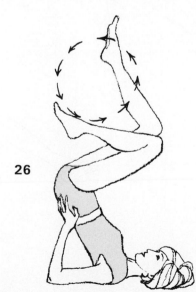

26

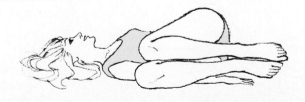

27 SPREAD EAGLE. Lie on the floor with your arms outstretched at shoulder level.

Swing the right leg across the body at hip level, stretching it as far to the left as possible. Hold. Keep the rest of the body in position. Then bend the right knee, and bring it up to touch your left elbow. Return to the starting position and repeat with the left leg. Repeat four times for each side, increasing to eight.

This gives a good pull through the hips and also tones the waist and thighs.

28 HIP HOP. Sit on the floor with your legs extended, your arms straight out at shoulder height. Keep your torso erect.

Using your buttocks as feet, "walk" forward pointing your toes. Then reverse and back up, curling toes up toward you. Take about 25 steps forward, then return.

You literally walk off fat pads with this exercise. Make sure you lift your legs from the hip joints.

For shapelier legs. The deep knee bend exercise (10) described in Chapter 1 not only improves your posture but firms and shapes your legs as well. To correct bulgy calves, do all your sitting or lying-down exercises with your feet held at right angles to your legs, *not* with your toes pointed.

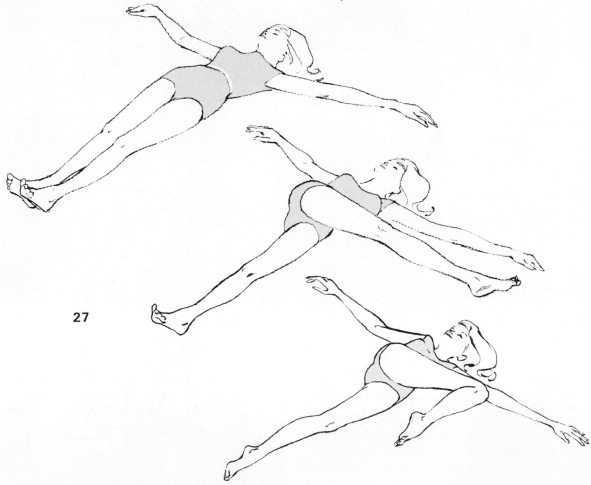

27

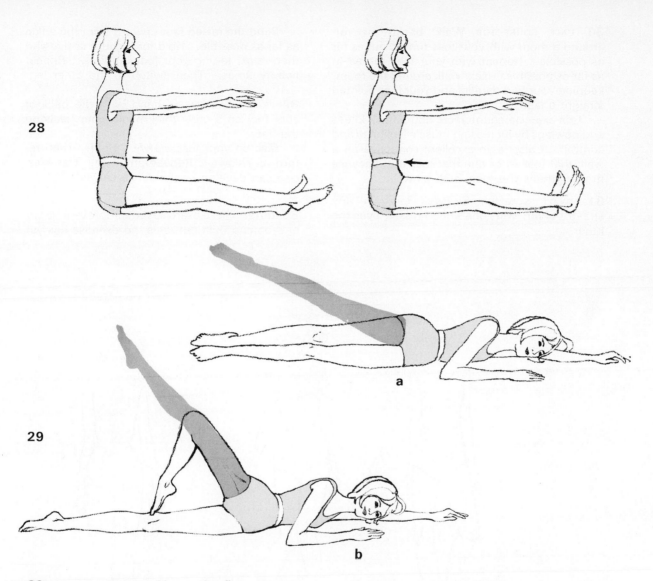

28

29

a

b

29 THIGH SLIMMER. Lie on the floor on your left side with your head on your outstretched left arm, your legs together.

a Slowly raise your right leg straight up from the hip joint until you feel the pull on the inside thigh muscles. Hold. *Slowly* return to position. Repeat five times before changing to other side.   Then do five times on right side. After a week or more, increase to ten times on each side.

b Using the same starting position, bend your right knee upward, pointing the right toe to the inside of the left knee.   Straighten your right leg, pointing the toe toward the ceiling. Hold.   Lower to a bent-knee position and then return to the starting position.   Repeat five times.   Change to the other side and repeat five times.   Gradually work up to ten times.

This exercise is especially good for front and inner thigh muscles, as well as for hips.

30 CALF CORRECTOR. Walk briskly or run around a room with your toes turned out as far as possible. Repeat with your toes turned in as far as possible. Next walk around the room, keeping your feet parallel and your toes pointed straight ahead.

This exercise counteracts both knock-knees and bowlegs by increasing muscle flexibility and control. It also is an excellent corrective for a walk that toes in or one that toes out, because it strengthens the main arch as well.

31 ANKLE SLIMMER. Sit well back in any straight chair, with one knee crossed over the other.

Bend the raised foot upward from the ankle as far as possible. Hold for a count of five and then relax, letting your foot fall limp. Repeat twenty times. Then switch to the other leg.

32 CALF BEAUTIFIER. Stand with the balls of your feet on a fairly thick book, your heels on the floor.

Rise on your toes *slowly.* Hold. Then return very slowly. Repeat ten times. This exercise can develop *or* slenderize calves.

Bustline. These exercises will improve a heavy or drooping bust but, alas, no exercise has yet

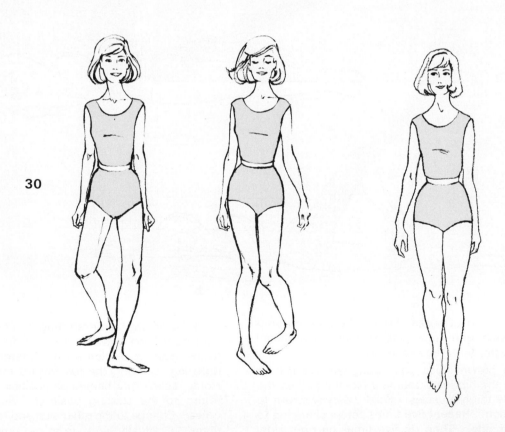

30

been found that actually increases the size of a small bust. These exercises will strengthen the chest muscles, however, and they will encourage better contours for either a small or large bosom.

33 PUSH-UP, LADIES' STYLE. Lie face down with the hands, palm down, at shoulder level.

Hold your torso rigid as you push away from the floor, straightening your arms so that your body is supported by your hands and knees. (Your knees should never leave the floor.) Next sit back on your heels. Hold. Then move your body forward and lower it to the floor. Start with two or three push-ups and work up to ten.

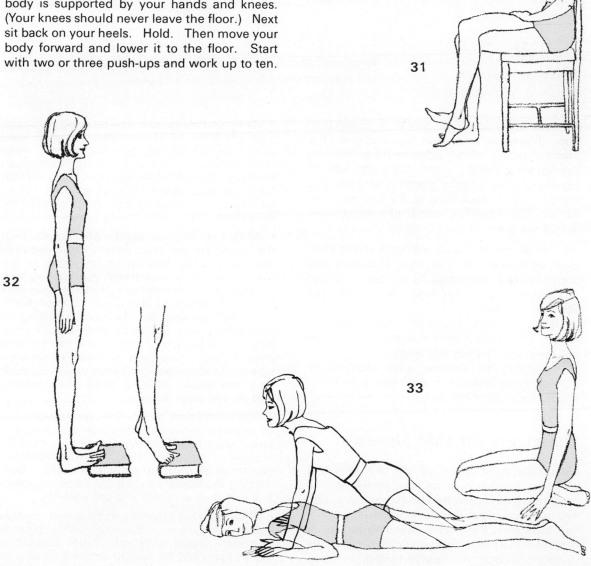

47

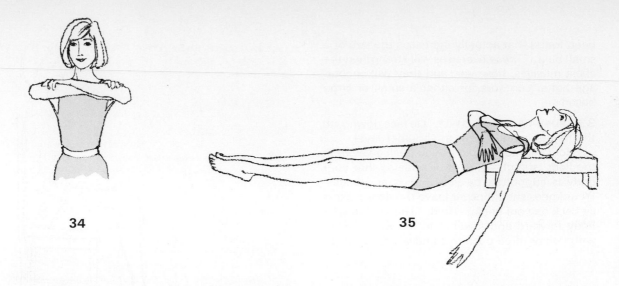

34

35

34 ELBOW CHUG-CHUG. Stand in good posture. Raise your arms chin-high and grasp the *inside* of each forearm just below the elbow with the opposite hand. Then push the elbows together as you resist by grasping hard with the fingers. Hold; then relax to the first position. Repeat fifty times—it won't take much more than a minute.

35 CRISS-CROSS. Lie on your back across a low stool or hassock so that your shoulders and upper back are supported by the seat and your feet are resting on the floor. Start with your arms on the floor.

Raise your arms up and cross them over your chest. Slowly drop arms straight back to original position. Repeat ten times.

To make this exercise more effective by offering more resistance, hold heavy books of equal size in your hands.

❦ Exercises for Odd Moments

Unlike the daily dozen variety, the following exercises involve only muscle stretching and contracting, and can often be sneaked in during ordinary activities. While you are riding in a car, talking on the phone, standing in line, or even seated at your desk, you can put your idle moments to work for muscle toning.

• When you wake up in the morning, recharge your muscles by giving them a good hard stretch before you struggle out of bed. Hold on to the headboard with one hand and push hard with the heel of the opposite foot. Stretch hard and push down as far as you can. Then switch to the opposite hand and push with the other foot.

• While toweling yourself dry after a bath, loop the towel behind your neck. Pull your chin back as you tug forward on both ends of the towel, resisting the towel with your neck as hard as you can to a count of ten. Relax. Then slide the towel down to the small of your back. Again pull forward on the towel, resisting by contracting your abdomen and buttock muscles. Push back hard against the towel as you count to ten. Now loop the towel under your toes and pull up with both ends while you push your toes down. Hold for ten counts, release, and do the other foot.

• Abdominal and hip muscle contractions are so inconspicuous that they can be done any time. Just tense the muscles tightly, hold for a count of ten, then relax. Do this whenever you think about it throughout the day. Contracting the buttock muscles is especially effective if it is done while you are walking.

• When you are standing in bare feet, try this variation to firm inner thighs as well as buttock muscles. Stand with your heels about two inches apart and the weight on the balls of your feet. Concentrate on slowly bringing the buttocks close to each other so that you feel their contraction. Also exert tension through the inner thigh by attempting to press your knees together. (Don't bend your knees, and be sure to keep your ankles straight and inner arches high.) Hold for a count of ten. Slowly release the tension. Do at least six times during the day.

• Twisting your hip while you stand creates a front-to-back hip stretch. Stand on your left foot and turn the right foot in as far as possible toward the inside of the left leg. At the same time try to look over your right shoulder at your right heel. Then turn that same foot outward and back as far as you can, still looking at the heel over your right shoulder. Repeat with the left foot and look over your left shoulder.

• To flatten the upper back and to overcome round shoulders, stand in perfect posture and put both arms behind your body, backs of hands toward each other, thumbs pointing to rear, elbows straight. Lift your arms up behind you as far as they will go, which will not be high. Hold while you count to ten. Release tension and relax.

• For correcting a double chin, a dowager's hump, or a problem of head posture, try this. Sit erect and slowly rotate your head in a circle—forward, around to the left, to the back, to the right, to the front. Then reverse the direction. Be sure to keep your neck and spine erect. You'll get the correct feeling if you imagine that you have a basin of water strapped on your head and that you are going to spill out a few drops in a complete circle around you.

• During a phone conversation, use your opposite hand to do an arm twist. Keeping your arm extended straight out to the side, rotate your hand back and forth. Do each arm separately, slowly at first and then doubling the tempo. This is good for the upper arm.

---

1 *After you've determined the calorie quota needed to maintain or change your figure, plan complete menus (plus snacks, if desired) for three days. Choose foods that you like, but be sure that your meals are well balanced and that your calorie tally is approximately correct. Each day's set of menus should include foods from each of the beauty-food categories.*

2 *If you need to reduce:*
   a Find recipes for at least two low-calorie dishes you would like to try.
   b Prepare a list of at least twenty high-calorie items that you eat frequently but that are taboo for reducers.

3 *If you wish to gain weight:*
   a Find at least two recipes for unusual dishes that tempt your appetite.
   b Make a list showing at least twenty high-calorie foods that you enjoy. Include not only desserts but also meats, fruits, vegetables, dairy products, and other foods.

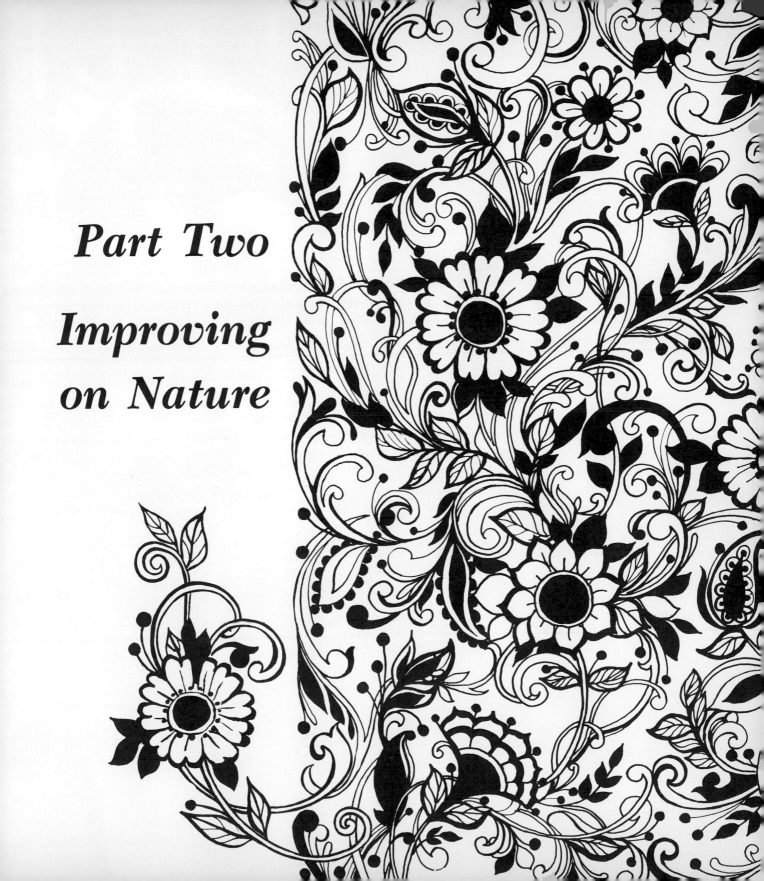

Part Two

Improving on Nature

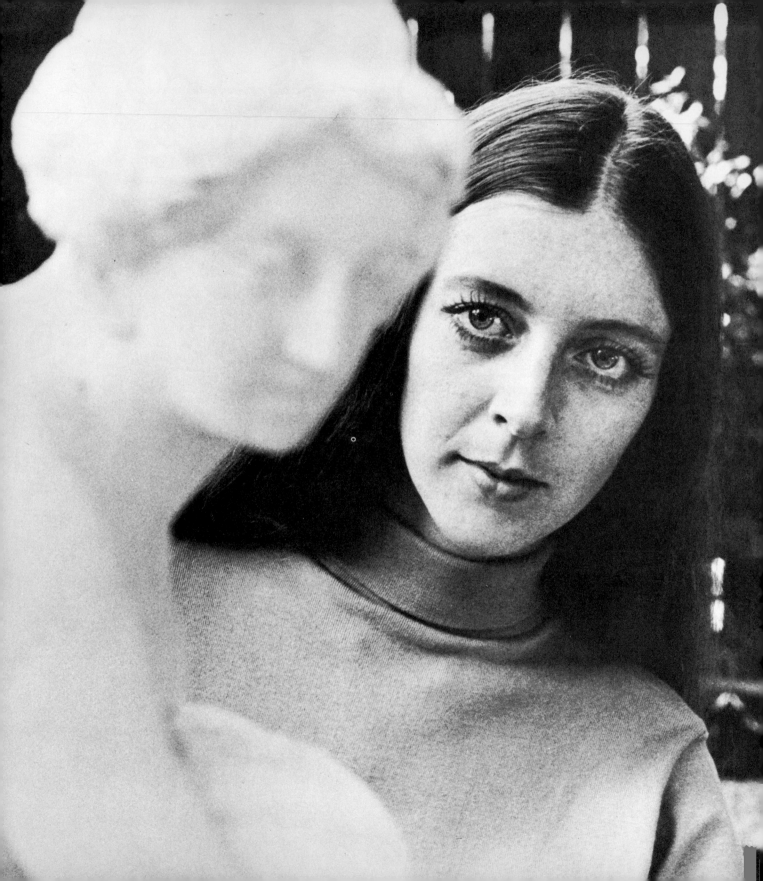

COMPLEXION CARE

There are many pretty girls whose features, if examined closely, are far from the most perfect, but because of a clear, glowing complexion, their faces seem beautiful. Lovely, smooth skin adds a radiance that magnifies beauty. A good complexion is so important that even a set of movie-queen features will never add up to beauty if their owner has poor skin. Very often complexion care is the vitally important detail that can turn a so-so face into an especially attractive one. But the only way to achieve a beautiful complexion is by taking good care of your skin. No makeup can create the loveliness of a natural glow nor truly compensate for the lack of it. Such a glow comes only from the healthy condition of the skin itself. Fortunately, skin is a living, growing thing that responds to proper care. Because the top layer is continually being washed or worn off and replaced by new cells, even neglected skin can be made to bloom within a reasonably short time. As we grow older, however, our skin responds less easily to our efforts to improve it. Now, while you are young, is the time to bring your complexion to its peak of beauty and to guard its health carefully so that it can better withstand the ravages of wear and age. As in everything else, there are fads and fashions in complexion care, but the basics still must be observed if you wish to develop an enviable complexion. Don't make the mistake of thinking that you will have a beautiful skin if you refrain from using cosmetics entirely. Sun, wind, and air pollution can ravage any girl's complexion if she does not guard against them by working out a program of care for her own skin type.

53

ꙮ Which Skin Type Is Yours?

To decide how your complexion should be treated, you need to know what type of skin you have. The care that is suitable for oily skin may be ruinous for dry skin, and vice versa. In addition, your skin may be oily in several spots but normal or dry in others—and your treatment, to be really effective, must then be special for each different area.

Normal skin. If you have a fresh reasonably clear complexion that is soft and smooth with no flaky patches, no dry, tight-feeling areas, no greasy shine, and no blemishes, thank your lucky stars. You have normal skin and should make every effort to keep it that way.

Oily skin. Oily skin is usually easy to identify. The most noticeable clue is its greasy shine, which may reappear within an hour or so after washing. This shine appears because the oil ducts are overactive and the pores cannot get rid of the excess oil. When oil remains on the surface of the skin, it acts like flypaper to hold dust and dirt—the perfect setting for the formation of nasty blackheads and pimples.

B. D. Unsworth

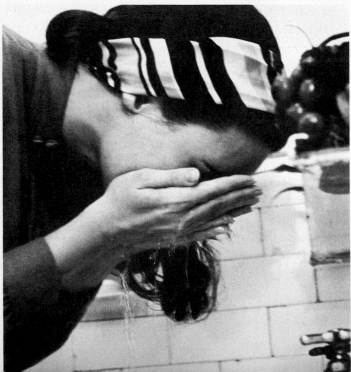

Blemished skin is almost always oily skin. Unless a vigorous battle for cleanliness is waged, blemishes are likely to be a problem.

Oily skin is usually most troublesome during the teen-age years. Gradually, as we grow older, the secretion of oil lessens. One pleasant prospect is that this type of skin usually resists wrinkles better than other types do.

Dry skin. Dry skin is characterized by a tight feeling and a tendency to develop little lines, particularly around the eyes and lips. Pores are small and fine. The skin may look drawn over the cheeks and may be rough and flaky in places.

Don't be misled by flaking skin on your nose. This is not a sign of dryness. We are constantly manufacturing new cells, and dead scales seem to cling to the nose longer.

Dry skin needs the gentlest of care. It must be pampered and protected or it will wrinkle at an early age.

Combination skin. If your skin type doesn't fit neatly into one of the preceding categories, you may be one of the multitude of girls who has combination skin. Many girls have skin that is normal or dry in some sections and oily in others. Usually the middle portion of the face is oily—the nose, chin, and center of the forehead—while the cheeks may be normal or even a bit dry. In such cases each section must be treated according to its type: gentler cleansing and protection for the drier areas, vigorous cleansing and no lubrication for the oily areas.

ꙮ Basic Care for All Skin Types

Proper care of your skin involves four important steps: cleansing, stimulating, lubricating, and protecting.

1 Keep skin clean, clean, clean. Cleanliness is the most important factor in obtaining and retaining lovely skin. Most of the lasting damage that is done to young skin is the result of insufficient cleansing. Blackheads, whiteheads,

54

blemishes, enlarged pores, and muddy complexions can usually be traced back to that arch villain—DIRT. For the sake of your beauty, promise yourself that you will never go to bed without first thoroughly cleansing your face. No matter how weary you are, take the extra few minutes to clean off all makeup and dirt. During the day remove old makeup before applying the new, whenever possible. Many business girls keep a cosmetic bag of cleansing and makeup essentials in their lockers or desk drawers for easy makeup changes. When you can't do a completely new makeup job, rub a moistened tissue (or your *clean* moistened hands) over your face to remove some of the previous makeup and accumulated grime before applying new cosmetics.

Do you know how to clean your face properly? Today's clinging cosmetics require thorough methods to remove them. Just soap and water were all right for the girl who never ventured near the cosmetic counter, but they can't do a good job of removing modern makeup. A cleansing cream or lotion must be used first and then followed by a second cleansing—either with soap and water (or other wash-off cleanser) or with a deep-cleansing lotion or a second creaming plus skin freshener. (The products you choose for your skin type will be discussed later.)

When applying cleansing cream or lotion, take a dab on the fingertips of both hands and use *upward and outward strokes* to massage the cream gently all over your throat and face (see diagram). Glide lightly over the skin; never push or stretch the skin in any way. Allow the cream to set for two or three minutes so it can do its work. Then tissue off very gently. Avoid dragging the skin downward and be particularly gentle in the area around the eyes. Age and the elements do enough to pull our faces out of shape and to cause wrinkles without our contributing to the damage.

If you wash your face with soap for your second cleansing, work up a good lather and rinse well with warm water. No soap should ever be left on your skin. Then follow with a stimulating cold splash.

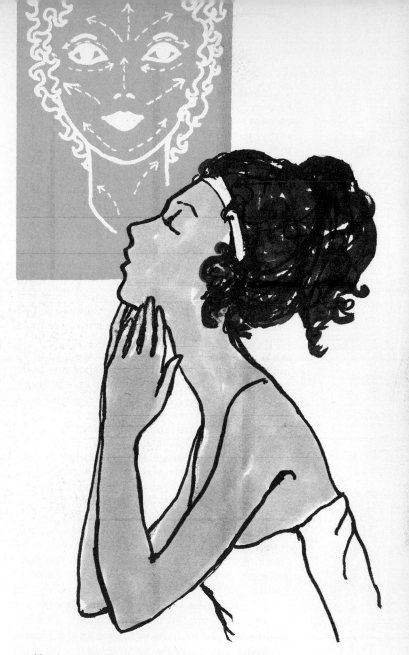

If you use two cream cleansings in place of soap, be sure to finish off with skin freshener (sometimes called skin lotion). This removes the last vestiges of dirty cleansing cream that would otherwise remain in the pores to cause trouble. In addition to its cleansing action, skin freshener gently tones your skin.

You probably know the old saw about the ounce of prevention. In regard to your face, it's certainly worth several pounds of cure. Protect your skin as much as possible from contact with dirt. If you tend to prop your chin with your hand or if you have any other habits that involve touching your face, better adopt a hands-off policy. You know how dirty your hands become during an ordinary day of reading, writing, and typing. When you transfer this dirt to your face, you're only inviting trouble.

Everything that comes in contact with your face should be immaculately clean. Always use a separate washcloth for your face, and change facecloths frequently. Your washbasin should be scrubbed and shining, your towel fresh and clean. Girls with blemished skin are wise to boil their facecloths and to dry linens in the sun to help prevent the spread of infection (which is what a pimple is). A soiled powder puff is another trouble causer. Using disposable puffs or tufts of cotton to apply makeup is a more sanitary method.

2 Stimulate your skin to beautify itself. Even the most expensive creams can do very little for complexions. Skin is nourished primarily from within. The bloodstream brings the important health nutrients supplied by the beauty foods in a well-balanced diet. Poor circulation means that the blood delivery system isn't working at full capacity—the skin is being deprived. You can improve your circulation by getting plenty of exercise, especially outdoor exercise, and also by giving direct stimulation to the skin.

Stimulate the skin directly by massaging it as you apply cream or soapy lather, stroking lightly in the directions indicated in the picture on page 55. Gently patting your skin with quick little slaps is especially good and will bring the blood rushing to the area. Exercise of facial muscles—pretend you are a man shaving, or blow your cheeks out—not only tones up these muscles but also provides stimulation for your complexion.

Cosmetic aids to stimulation include skin fresheners, astringent lotions (the latter for oily skins only), and facial masks, which, in addition to their cleansing benefits, are especially good for encouraging a pretty glow for big date nights.

Also good is plain cold water. After washing, try this stimulating finale to prod lazy circulation. Take two washcloths. Put one in warm water and then press it against your face for a few seconds. Meantime, place the other washcloth under the cold water tap and then exchange this for the warm cloth, pressing the cold cloth against your face. Continue alternating with warm and cold cloths three or four times. You'll love the tingle you feel in your skin and the healthy glow that results. Just don't let the water become too hot or too icy. Neither extreme is wise for delicate skin.

3 Lubricate your complexion. Protection is, of course, most important to those with dry skin. Use of lubricating creams and lotions that contain lanolin and other rich emollients can help compensate for the lack of natural oil production and keep dry skin soft and smooth. They can be used on dry skin nightly after cleansing and also under makeup for protection during the day, if necessary. In addition to the heavy lubricating products, there are also moisture creams and lotions, which soften skin and add moisture. If your skin is normal or oily, one of the greaseless moisturizers will be best for softening any chapped or rough areas; the rich lubricating products are intended only for dry skin. Moisture is needed on the surface of the skin to help spread the oil that is pumped up by the oil glands. Normally this moisture comes out through every pore, but cold air outdoors and hot, dry air indoors tend to retard this process, as well as to hold down oil production. Incidentally, after applying skin freshener in wintertime, those with dry or normal skin should wait fifteen minutes before beginning their makeup so that the new supply of oil and moisture can spread and create a fresh base for makeup.

Although lubrication is of greater concern to the girl with dry skin, there is one very important area that needs regular care even for girls with oily skin—the area around the eyes. Most girls over twenty-one—and some that are younger—begin to notice tiny lines forming beneath and at the corners of the eyes. This may occur even though the rest of the skin is oily. The eye area is generally the first to wrinkle. A tiny bit of eye cream or oil used nightly can help ward off the development of permanent crow's feet and lines. An eye cream is a heavy clinging cream especially designed to penetrate the pores in the eye area. These pores are almost totally closed and are not capable of absorbing regular creams. Only the tiniest touch of cream or oil is needed, and it should be patted on *very* gently so that the skin is not pulled or rubbed.

4 Protect your skin's loveliness. The onslaught of drying winds, hot sun, dry indoor heat, sooty outdoors, and pore-clogging cosmetics can all play havoc with your complexion. Any young woman who cares about her complexion knows how unwise it is to sunbathe without first using a protective suntan preparation. You should also help to shield your skin from the daily abuse of the elements by applying the proper type of makeup base under your makeup. Normal or slightly dry skin can use a film of moisture lotion; very dry skin benefits from a lubricating cream under makeup. Oily skins should use one of the corrective foundations designed to limit oil production and to impede growth of blemish-causing skin bacteria.

❧ How to Care for Your Skin

Normal skin. Your aim is to keep your skin just the way it is—healthy, lovely, and normal. You should use makeup sparingly and should choose light, nongreasy products that allow your natural beauty to show itself off. By all means, don't overtreat your skin. You needn't waste money on ''high-powered'' lubricating creams and lotions. You already have the skin that the ads extol, and rich creams are only likely to cause harm. The one exception might be an

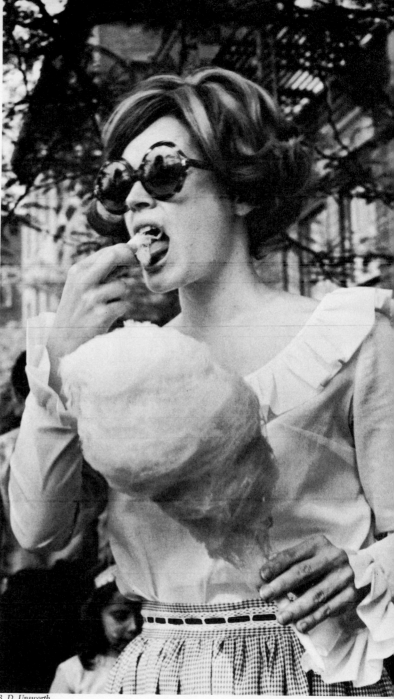

B. D. Unsworth

If you want to have beautiful skin, one of the things you have to watch is your diet. Sweets are enjoyable, but too many of them can ruin a good complexion, particularly if they replace more nutritious foods.

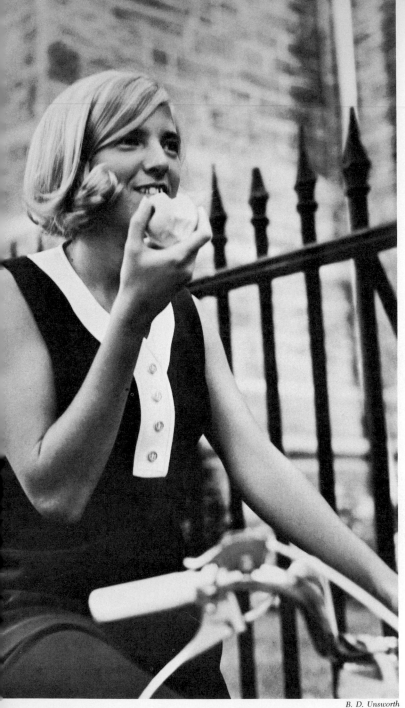

Fruit, leafy vegetables, whole wheat breads, milk, and meat are good for your complexion, especially if you are troubled with oily skin. Many complexion problems can be stopped before they start simply by eating a well-balanced diet.

B. D. Unsworth

eye cream. If your skin seems slightly dry in winter, you can use a light moisture cream or lotion under makeup. Other than this, the best rule for normal skin is to leave well enough alone.

Cleanliness, of course, is most important in maintaining your normal complexion. Cleanse your face twice, using a cleansing cream the first time and a deep-cleansing lotion or wash-off cleanser the second time. If soap doesn't cause your skin to feel tight, you may use a gentle facial soap after your cream cleansing. If you prefer to use only cream on your face, finish up with skin freshener to remove the last vestiges of cleansing cream. This is important, for the cream that remains in the pores has the same effect as excess secretions and will clog pores and attract dirt. Your morning cleansing routine can be a washup with either soap or a cleansing lotion.

Oily skin. When oil glands are overactive, skin usually loses its fresh, young look and becomes sallow and flabby. Oily skin is also the ideal site for the formation of blackheads and blemishes. Your aim is twofold: to help control this excess oil and to get rid of any oversupply before it can do damage. Good care can help alleviate an oily condition.

• Be a demon for cleanliness. By frequent cleansings you can remove excess oil.

• Eat a nutritious diet. Avoid greasy foods that stimulate overproduction of oil as well as blemish-causing rich or spicy foods. Some complexions register every gooey dessert or candy bar in the form of a pimple. Chocolate and nuts are particularly troublesome. The best prescription for oily skin is a well-balanced diet based on plenty of meat, milk, leafy vegetables, fruit, and whole wheat breads.

• Maintain regular elimination habits. The experts advise drinking six to eight glasses of liquid (noncarbonated) each day. It's also a good idea to include in your diet some raw fruits and vegetables (apples, whole oranges, and green salads) for roughage.

• Perk up your circulation. The overactivity of oil glands is often due to sluggish circulation.

Both exercise and cosmetic stimulants should be part of your beauty campaign.

• Bask in the sun. Sunshine is especially good for oily skins and a great boon in drying up blemishes.

• Use cosmetics sparingly. Naturally, you'll avoid all greasy creams and bases. Under makeup, use one of the medicated foundations designed to limit oil production and to limit the growth of blemish-causing skin bacteria. Any areas that become chapped or rough can be treated with a greaseless moisture lotion. Oily skin may flake off slightly at certain times of the year. This should not be considered a sign that lubrication is needed. Oil secretion has merely lessened sufficiently so that the *normal* scaling off of dead skin is occurring.

• Keep your hair scrupulously clean. Many infections on the face arise from dust, dirt, and oil transferred from the hair.

Cleansing routine for oily skin. To help counteract excess oil, you'll need to cleanse your face thoroughly at least three times a day, more if your condition requires it. All old makeup should always be removed before applying new. A light cleansing cream (one that liquefies easily) or a lotion is best for you. Follow this with either a medicated cleansing lotion or a soap-and-water scrub. If you use soap, try a soft-bristled complexion brush for extra stimulation and for help in removing any clinging dead scales. Finish off with an astringent lotion. An astringent provides the stimulation oily skin needs and also helps to tighten pores and to delay the return of a greasy shine. An economical homemade concoction is half witch hazel and half rubbing alcohol.

Your morning routine can omit the cream cleansing. You went to bed with a sparkling-clean, makeup-free face, didn't you? A soap-and-water sudsing followed by astringent lotion will remove excess oil and wastes secreted during the night.

For exceptionally oily or blemished skin, you may want to try washing with either a tar soap or tincture of green soap. Each has a helpful drying effect and can be used about twice a week. Calamine lotion applied to blemishes after your cleanup is helpful in drying up pimples.

If you are troubled by blackheads, you can use a cleansing grain preparation once or twice a week. Grainy cleansers have a gentle scouring action that tackles blackheads far more safely than your squeezing could. If you like to mix your own beauty aids, you can make quite acceptable cleansing grains by combining equal parts of uncooked corn meal (or almond meal) and mild granulated soap (soap beads). Take a teaspoonful in the palm of your hand and mix it with warm water so that it forms a soft paste. Spread this over your face and work it well into any blackhead areas. Avoid any pimples that might be scoured open, as this could spread the infection. Rinse thoroughly.

Dry skin. Dry skin, with its fine texture and delicate translucence, can be beautiful. It is seldom the victim of blackheads or blemishes. But it must be preserved carefully to keep it lovely. If nature is not given some assistance, your complexion may become rough, dull, and coarsened and will be subject to wrinkles.

• Avoid the things that dry your skin. Don't overexpose your skin to sun, wind, water, or hot indoor air. Dry, overheated rooms are a beauty menace. Try to keep the thermostat at 70 degrees or below.

• Eat a well-balanced diet. A poor diet not only means neglect for your skin but also means neglect for your nervous system. A nervous condition is often the cause of skin disorders— and there you have double trouble.

• Use cosmetics that contain plenty of lubricants. You need the heavier cleansing creams and rich lubricating and moisture creams. Use a moisturizer under makeup and choose a creamy foundation to help protect your skin during the day.

• Step up your circulation with exercise. Improved circulation helps a dry skin as well as an oily one, because it can do much to correct any imbalance in oil production.

Cleansing routine for dry skin. Cleanliness is important for dry skin. Pores must not become clogged, as that would interfere with the secretion of whatever oil is present. Your cleansing methods must be very gentle. Avoid soap and harsh cleansing agents.

Cleansing cream will be kindest to your skin. Use two applications, massaging lightly while you apply the cream, and then tissuing it off very gently. Cleansing *twice* is important. Finish off with a skin freshener designed for dry skin. Never use an astringent.

Your morning routine can be a single cream cleansing plus skin freshener. During the day try to remove makeup completely at least once.

Pamper and protect dry skin. Dry skin needs plenty of lubrication to protect its loveliness. If skin is very dry, a lubricating preparation can be used nightly after cleansing. A tiny dab of lubricating cream goes a long way. No need to slather it on—a light film will do. The cream should be gently massaged over your clean skin—using upward and outward movements. (See the illustration on page 55.)

Lubricating creams are best used during your daily bath time. The warmth and steam open the pores and help your skin absorb the cream. Occasionally you may want to give yourself a hot cream treatment. A heating pad is wonderful for this. Just place a sheet of waxed paper over your creamed face and hold the pad against it.

Don't butter your face with cream before going to bed at night. You get full benefit from a lubricating product in about fifteen or twenty minutes. Then you can blot off any residue and hop into bed without fear of smearing sheets and pillowcases. Your skin should be allowed time at night to breathe—free of cosmetics or treatments.

If your skin is very dry, a light film of moisture cream should be used after your morning cleansing to protect your skin under makeup during the day.

When choosing a lubricating preparation, pick one intended for your age category. Young girls, for instance, will steer clear of hormone or estrogen creams and other products designed for aging skin. Don't be tempted by alluring ingredients such as turtle oil, royal jelly,

placenta extract, or other exotic concoctions. These usually perform about the same as regular creams, the main difference being in what they do to your wallet.

Combination skin. Although combination skin should be treated as normal in most respects, your cleansing routine should include a vigorous soap-and-water scrub for the oily areas. At times the dry areas may need a little lubrication. You will be careful, of course, that none of the cream reaches the oily sections of your face, where it might cause skin eruptions.

❦ *Treat Yourself to a Facial*

When you want to look especially pretty, treat yourself to a facial! After your regular cleansing, apply a light film of cleansing cream to your face and give yourself a steam treatment to open pores. Steam treatments are an important part of a facial in the famous beauty salons. An at-home version can be created by leaning over a steaming pot of heated water (or run hot water in a basin). Cover your head completely with a towel to form a tent that will direct steam to your face, and lean over the steaming water. Continue this for five minutes and then wipe with tissues. Your pores will open, wastes will be excreted, and your skin will be receptive to further cleansing.

Next comes a deep-pore cleansing mask. A mask is an excellent pickup for a sallow complexion. Not only does it help draw out wastes, remove blackheads and whiteheads, but it also stimulates your skin and leaves it bright and glowing, with a soft, silky texture. A mask is not recommended, however, for those with severe acne or other skin infection, because the squeezing action that is so beneficial to other complexions may tend to increase the trouble by spreading the bacteria. If the skin is severely blemished, stop at this point and wash your face with soap and water or cleanse with an antiseptic cleansing lotion. Then apply astringent.

GOLDEN RULES FOR ALL COMPLEXIONS

• Cleanliness, we can't overemphasize, is the key to complexion beauty. Unless you have a special skin problem, keeping your skin clean will keep it bright, clear, and fresh.

• Get sufficient rest. Sleep, all too often neglected by busy young misses, is essential for skin to revitalize itself. A girl can manage to drag herself around and get by with too little sleep, but the dark circles under her eyes and her chalky countenance give her away all too easily.

• Eat a well-balanced diet, and drink a lot of water.

• Give your skin a vacation from makeup whenever possible. During your private hours, clean your face and let your skin breathe freely.

• Whenever you're tempted to squeeze a blackhead or pimple, *don't*. Treat blackheads with a facial instead, and apply a good medicated lotion to pimples. In a few days the blemish will probably cure itself, but squeezing is likely to spread the infection and may also injure the blood vessels, causing permanent, unsightly red marks.

• Choose treatment products for specific needs. A cleanser is not a substitute for a lubricating cream, nor should a hand cream be used for a face cream.

• Look at the brighter side of life and try to keep your emotions on an even keel. Complexion disorders often stem from emotional upsets.

• Adapt your beauty routine to the seasons. Temperature and humidity have such a strong effect on skin condition that it can vary with the weather. A girl whose complexion seems normal or even a bit dry in winter may find that she has an oily shine to contend with in summer. As you get older, your skin type can undergo several changes.

• If a well-planned routine of skin care doesn't leave you with a clear, fresh complexion, look for professional help. The advice of a good dermatologist may solve your problem quickly.

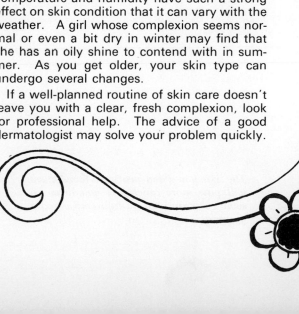

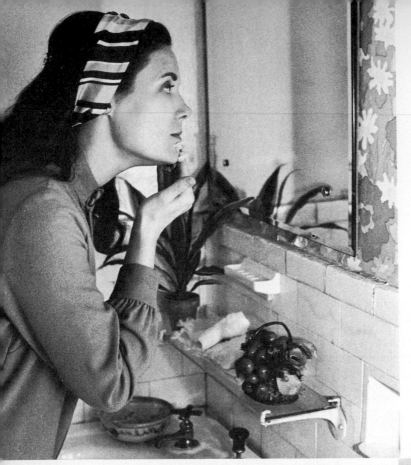

Homemade versions. You can buy excellent facial masks at cosmetic counters, but the following homemade versions are inexpensive and good.

OATMEAL MASK. Cook about half a cup of oatmeal. (The instant varieties are ready as soon as you add hot water.) Allow oatmeal to cool to a comfortable temperature. Hold your hair back with a kerchief or makeup band and apply a thin layer of the oatmeal to your thoroughly cleansed face, avoiding the eye area.

The mask will dry in about ten or fifteen minutes, but better results are gained by leaving it on for a total of twenty or twenty-five. Remove the mask with lukewarm water, followed by a cold splashing.

EGG-WHITE MASK. Use only the white of an egg. Beat it lightly with a fork and apply to the face, avoiding the eye area. Leave it on and rest with your feet propped up for about fifteen or twenty minutes, until the mask dries and begins to pull and draw your skin. Rinse with cool water, then with cold water.

The time you spend wearing a facial mask will pass more quickly if you listen to some good music or an informative radio program.

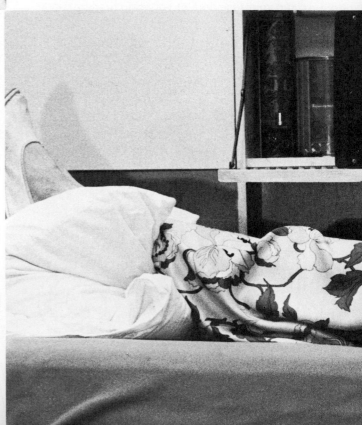

Use the waiting period for a beauty catnap. Moisten two cotton pads with cold water and place these over your eyes as you lie down to rest. The cool pads help soothe your eyes and make them clear and sparkling. If you place two pillows under your feet and one under your fanny—none under your head—this inclined position will stimulate circulation in your face for extra beautifying.

Skin Problems

Frustrated by freckles? Don't be! Freckles can be delightfully charming. They can create an interesting pixie-like quality or set you off as the all-American outdoor type. If you are concerned about your freckles reaching the too-many point, shield your face from the sun as much as possible and use a makeup foundation whenever you are outdoors. There are special sun protection products that coat your skin so that *none* of the sun's rays reach you. Use these at the beach.

If you feel disturbed by your freckles, you can lighten them by applying a bleaching face cream or by doing a little freckle painting with lemon juice. Apply the lemon juice with a paint brush or cotton swab to each freckle. Leave it on for half an hour; then rinse off with warm water. Lemon juice has a drying effect, as well as a bleaching one, and you will probably want to apply a lubricating cream afterwards.

Skin discolorations. Birthmarks, red marks, and eye shadows can often be masked by one of the heavy covering agents especially designed to hide discolorations. These are usually applied under a regular foundation. With these products, you choose the color nearest your own skin tone and apply according to directions. Some companies make a stick form of covering agent for use on small spots.

Too much suntanning sometimes produces a yellow or brownish shadow around the mouth and nose area or along the upper lip, a shadow that lingers long after summer tan has faded. Gradually this shadow should disappear, but

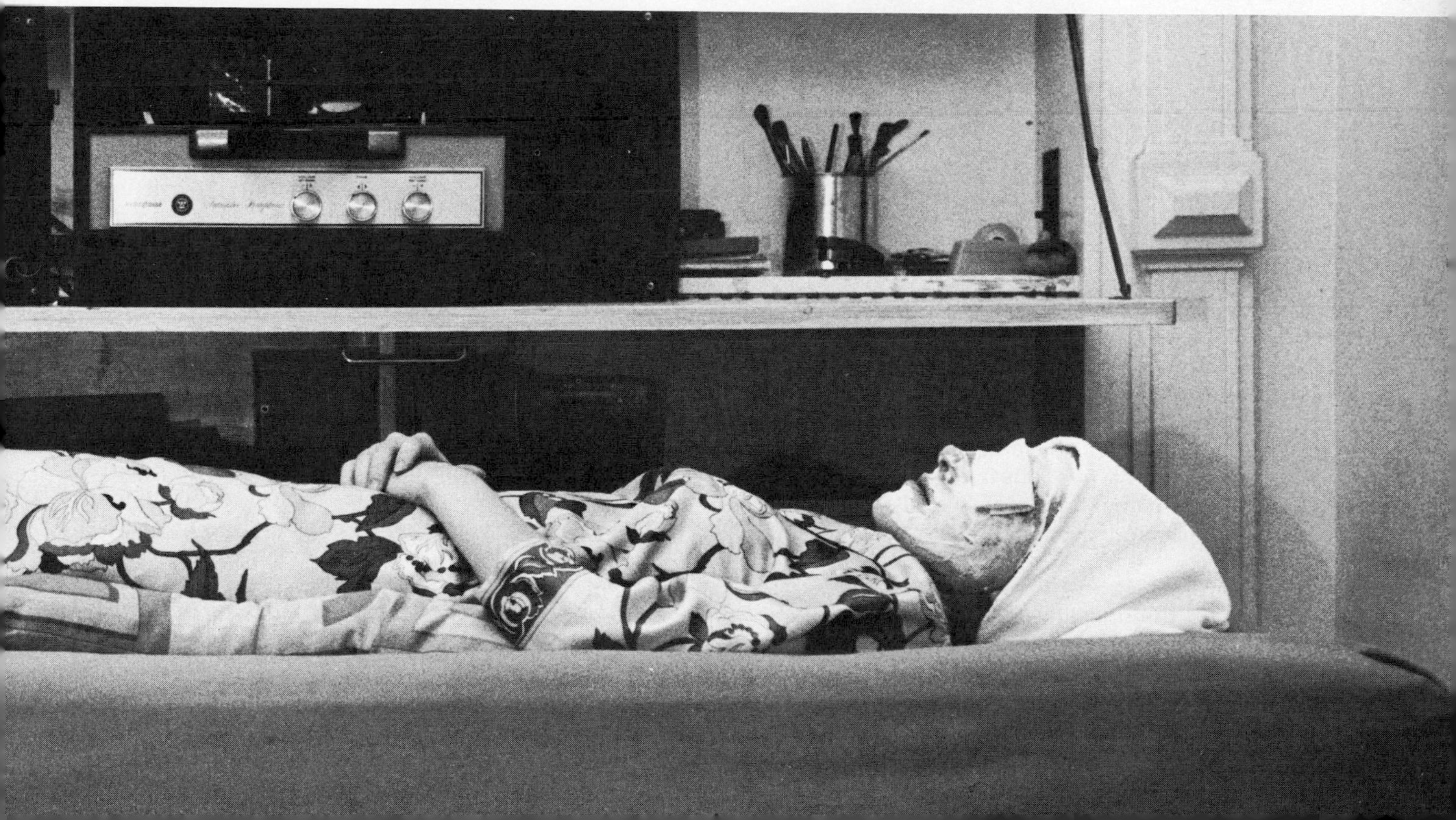

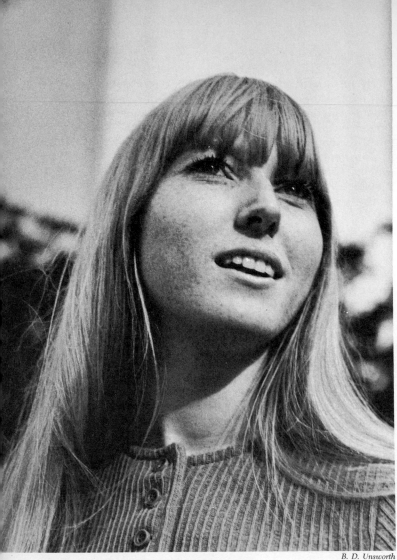
B. D. Unsworth

The girl with freckles may find that they are an asset, lending a pixie-like charm to her appearance. Over-freckling can be avoided, if you wish.

flaw without realizing that it could easily be removed or at least be made less visible. Severe scarring from acne and similar defects in skin texture can often be treated quite successfully by a dermatologist. Moles can be removed, while large scars or birthmarks can be concealed by plastic surgery. If you are considering such treatment, consult a highly qualified specialist who can judge how your particular problem can best be handled.

Facial hair. Every now and then a young woman is horrified to discover a long, bristly hair growing on her cheek or chin. This is nothing to worry about. Simply apply a bit of alcohol to the area and tweeze the hair out. There are a few exceptions, however. Keep hands off if the hair is growing from a mole or if it protrudes from the nose or ear. Serious trouble can be caused by such tweezing. Straggly nose and ear hairs can be trimmed shorter with scissors. Only a physician should remove mole hair.

When there is considerable dark fuzz on upper lips or cheeks, try bleaching to hide it. Here is a simple recipe for a gentle bleach. Mix together $\frac{3}{4}$ cup of gentle-action soap flakes, 4 tablespoons of 20-volume peroxide, and 3 drops of ammonia. (Be sure to ask your druggist for bleaching peroxide and for ammonia water diluted for facial use. *Never* use household ammonia or regular hydrogen peroxide.) Coat the hairs with this paste and allow it to remain for about fifteen minutes. Wash it off with lukewarm water and apply a lubricating cream to the area. If results aren't light enough, reapply the bleach in a day or two. (Never use bleach of any sort near your eyes or on your brows. It can cause blindness.)

If facial hair growth is too thick to camouflage with bleaching, it can be removed by waxing or electrolysis. Waxing lasts about six weeks. (The kind of lip wax that doesn't need heating is easier to use.) The only way to remove hair permanently and safely is by electrolysis. This should be done only by a qualified specialist.

Never use a razor on your face; the hair will grow back unbecomingly bristly and coarse.

use of a bleaching face cream or lemon juice, as described on page 63, will help. In the future, keep this area shielded by a hat or sun cream or an adhesive-tape patch. Using a lighter foundation on the discolored areas will help produce a more even coloring.

Moles, scars, birthmarks. All too many people go through life feeling self-conscious about a conspicuous mole or some sort of unsightly skin

Facial depilatories are sometimes a little risky for home use; if they are used, the instructions must be followed very carefully.

Allergies can be annoying. Certain hypersensitive skins will break out in blotches or become itchy or irritated when regular cosmetics are used. Fortunately, some excellent cosmetics are now being produced that are free from the ingredients that might prove irritating. If your skin seems to react adversely to regular cosmetics, or if your lips become cracked or swollen when you use lipstick, investigate the hypoallergenic brands. Of course, some skin disorders result from allergies of other types—allergies to various foods, to pets, to dust, and to other things we come in contact with. If the irritation persists, consult your doctor.

---

1 *Stand in good light while you examine your face closely. Based on what you have learned, decide what your skin type is.*

2 *Visit a cosmetic counter and study the various products available to decide which would be suitable for your particular skin. Find the items necessary for a complete cleansing, lubricating (if needed), stimulating, and protecting routine. As soon as your budget permits, purchase any of the essentials you lack so that you can enjoy the benefits a complete skin care program brings. Follow your beauty routine carefully. Treatment products must be used regularly to bring results. The cream that sits unused on a dressing table can't help anyone.*

3 *Pamper yourself with a complete beauty facial. Give yourself the "works" and see what a wonderful lift it adds to your appearance—and to your morale.*

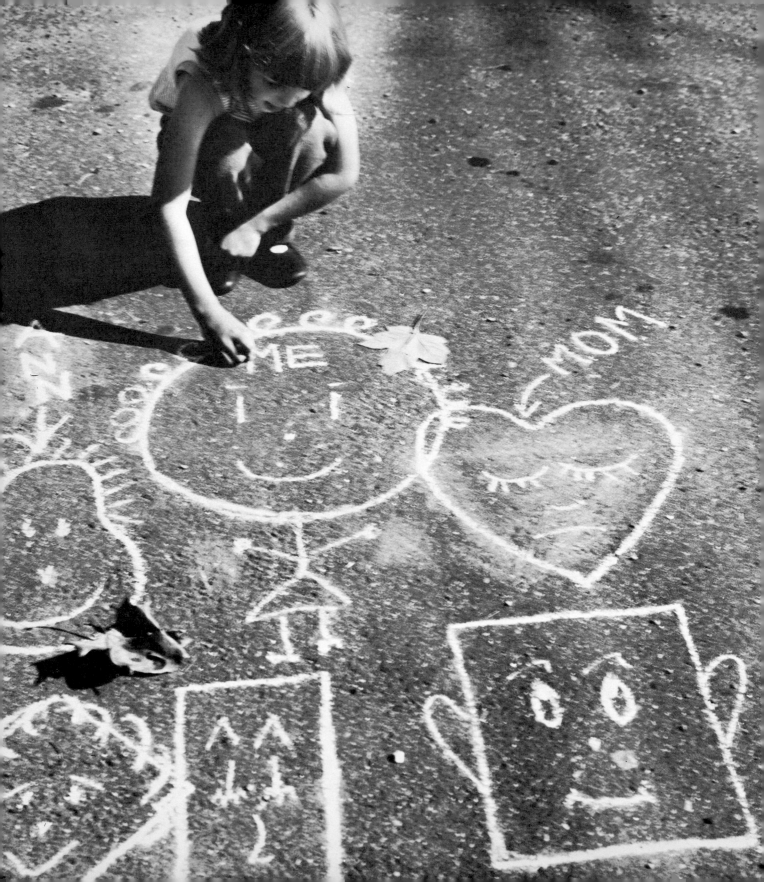

MAKE THE MOST OF YOUR MAKEUP

Some women are born beautiful, but a much larger percentage have made themselves beautiful, thanks to skillful use of cosmetics. When properly applied, makeup can smooth and brighten your complexion, conceal or camouflage your bad features. It can even seem to change the shape of a face or the length of a nose. But it must be used with wisdom and discretion, for that little touch of color here and pat of powder there can be read like a billboard, telling the world about your fashion know-how, your personal grooming habits, and your good taste. The girl who has learned to use a degree of artistry in putting on makeup has beauty power that can work magic for her all her life. The same skill can be yours.

Before you begin your study of makeup, you should examine your face and features to see what should be enhanced and what should be modified. Start with the shape of your face. Is it oval, round, square, oblong (long and narrow), heart-shaped (wider at the top), diamond-shaped (wider through the cheek bones), or pear-shaped (wider at the bottom)? If you're in doubt, have a private study session with your mirror.

Pull your hair straight back from your face so that your *entire* hairline is exposed, and pin or tie your hair flat. Then, closing one eye and looking straight at your reflection, trace the outline of your face on the mirror with a piece of soap. Now you have the general outline of your face. If you compare it with those illustrated in this chapter, you can identify the general shape. Possibly your face isn't a perfect example of one particular shape. Few faces are. A square face, for instance, may have a little pointed chin. A widow's peak may dip into a round face. What you need to know is what general category your face shape belongs in.

❦ The Ideal Face

An oval face is usually considered the ideal shape. It is two-thirds as wide as it is long and has perfect oval contours. However, one face type is as attractive as another if it is properly dramatized. Through makeup, hair styling, and choice of necklines, any face can be made to appear more oval.

If you are planning to lose or gain weight during this course, you will want to check your face shape again as your scale shows improvement. Weight loss can, for instance, change a square face into an oval one, while extra poundage might make a round face out of a triangular one.

Now give your features some close scrutiny to see how they compare with artistic standards. You may find it helpful in checking your facial dimensions to hold a book flat under your

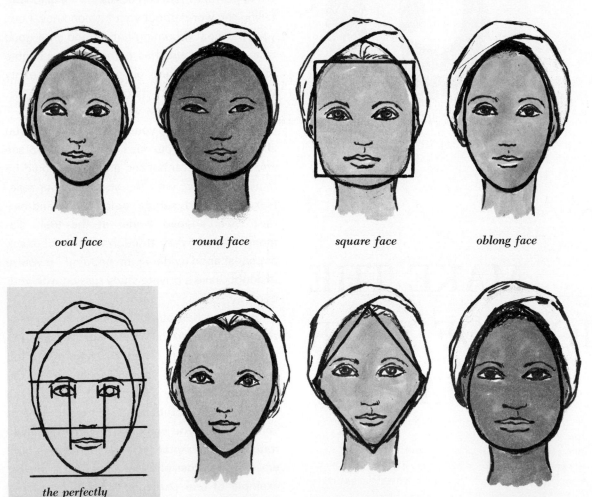

oval face   round face   square face   oblong face

the perfectly proportioned face   heart-shaped face   diamond-shaped face   pear-shaped face chin so that you have a flat surface on which to stand your ruler while reading your measurements in the mirror. Make sure that the ruler is straight, not tipped forward or backward.

• The perfectly proportioned face can be divided into three equal parts. This means that ideally the length of your nose from the base of your brows to nose tip is supposed to equal the distance from the eyebrows to the hairline and should also equal the distance from the tip of the nose to the tip of the chin.

• The space between the eyes should equal the width of one eye.

• When lips are closed, unsmiling, the corners of the mouth should be directly beneath the inner curve of the colored iris of the eye. When smiling, the lip corners should be directly beneath the pupils (centers of the eyes).

Don't forget your profile in this self-study. Check both left and right sides; they can be surprisingly different, you know. Examine your nose and forehead line. Does your chin recede or jut forward? Is it firm and straight? How about any facial hollows, puffiness, color irregularities, shadows, or lines? Because we don't see our profiles often, we may tend to disregard this view, but others are forced to judge us from this angle, too. In examining your profile, don't search for beauty as much as for character, strength, and individuality.

❀ The Art of Camouflage

Camouflage with cosmetics is the delicate art of "sculpturing" your features to more perfect form by the use of light and shadow. Deeper color minimizes, hides, and causes to recede; lighter color attracts, enlarges, and makes more prominent. For instance, full cheeks will appear more slender if a foundation that is just slightly darker than the shade used on the rest of the face is applied to the outer edges of the cheeks. A receding chin can be brought forward by applying a foundation that is slightly lighter than your regular shade to the front of the chin. Facial camouflage can be done, as

shown on page 70, with two shades of foundation—your regular color plus an extra shade that is one or two shades lighter or darker (depending on whether you wish to highlight or shadow). For shadowing, blushers are also good, though not so long-lasting as foundations. For highlighting, there are a variety of special, pale-tinted or light-reflecting cosmetics, as well as iridescent products and glosses that can play up a feature. Whenever camouflage shading is employed, care must be taken that the two colors blend inconspicuously. This is important for achieving subtle camouflage rather than an obvious, marble-cake effect.

❀ Order of Procedure

Before you can begin your makeup, your face must be immaculately clean. Then, depending on your skin type, apply a "primer coat"—a lubricant for dry skin, a moisturizer for normal skin, an oil controller for oily skin, or a medicated lotion for blemished skin. No need to use gobs; the lightest film will do. The application of makeup will be as follows:

1 Protective base
2 Tinted foundation
3 Cream blusher or cream or liquid rouge, if used
4 Powder
5 Cake blusher or rouge, if used
6 Lipstick
7 Eyebrow coloring
8 Eyeshadow, if used
9 Eyeliner, if used
10 Mascara, if used

❀ Foundation for Makeup Magic

Just as its name implies, a foundation (or base, as it is sometimes called) is the foundation of good makeup. It is the first cosmetic you apply, and probably the single cosmetic that does the most to simulate a perfect complexion. It gives

69

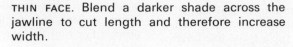

CAMOUFLAGE WITH FOUNDATION

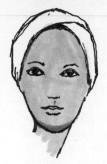

thin face

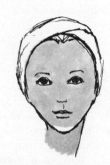

receding chin

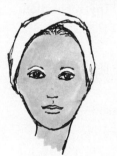

deep-set eyes

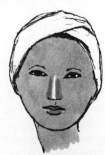

broad nose

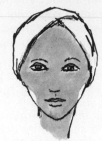

hollow cheeks

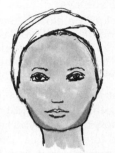

square jaw

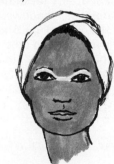

close-set eyes

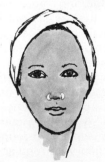

thin nose

THIN FACE. Blend a darker shade across the jawline to cut length and therefore increase width.

HOLLOW CHEEKS. Apply a lighter shade to hollows.

DOUBLE CHIN. Conceal it with a darker tone.

PROTRUDING CHIN. Blend a darker shade over and under the chin.

RECEDING CHIN. Blend a lighter shade over and under the chin.

SQUARE JAW. Use a darker shade on the extreme sides of face and jawbone.

LOW FOREHEAD. Play it up with a lighter shade.

HIGH FOREHEAD. De-emphasize it with a darker shade.

DEEP-SET EYES. Apply a lighter shade on the upper lid area, carrying it clear up to the eyebrows.

CLOSE-SET EYES. Blend a light shade under the brows and at the bridge of the nose.

DARK CIRCLES UNDER THE EYES. Use a lighter shade, preferably a heavier foundation cream, a stick cover-up, or one of the special lighteners designed to hide shadows.

PUFFINESS UNDER THE EYES. Conceal it with a darker shade.

BROAD NOSE. Highlight the middle of the nose by blending a line of light foundation down the center. Tone down broad nostrils with a darker shade on the side of the nose.

LONG NOSE. Blend a darker shade under the tip of the nose and at the edge of the nostrils.

THIN NOSE. Create width with a lighter shade over the sides of the nostrils. Cut length with a darker shade at the tip of the nose.

HOOKED NOSE. Use a darker shade down the center of the nose (in the hooked portion).

the skin a fresh, even tone and smooth texture and increases the clinging power of other makeup. Some are medicated to counteract oiliness and blemishes; others are moisturized to keep skin soft.

Which type of foundation? Foundations come in many forms and have varying degrees of covering power. Some are opaque enough to hide minor blemishes and skin discolorations. Others are so sheer that they provide a natural ''no-makeup'' look whereby variations in skin coloring show through but the skin is given a subtle, translucent smoothness. You will probably need to experiment a little to find the type and brand that best suits you. There are three basic types:

LIQUID FOUNDATIONS. Whether in aerosol, roll-on, or plain bottle, these are easy to apply and look the most natural. They are excellent for all skin types. Different brands vary greatly in oil content and covering power. Ask the advice of a cosmetics saleswoman and test carefully.

To apply liquid foundation, place a dot of it on your chin and blend it across the jaw, using your fingertips. Then put a dot or two on each cheek and blend well along previously applied color. Be sure to carry the foundation all the way out to your ears. Repeat with another dot for the nose and mouth area, and finish with a dot or two for the forehead. Use upward and outward movements, being sure that the foundation covers the entire face. When using an aerosol foundation, press the actuator button very lightly. Because the foundation has been whipped into an especially light, spreadable form, you need only the tiniest puff for complete coverage. Work foundation gently into any tiny lines around the eyes and mouth, spreading the lines smooth so that they take up the color. Use any base remaining on your fingers to blend color down under the chin and jaw so that the color fades out gradually. Many women like to use a foundation over the entire throat area. This is fine *if* it doesn't rub off on dress and coat collars.

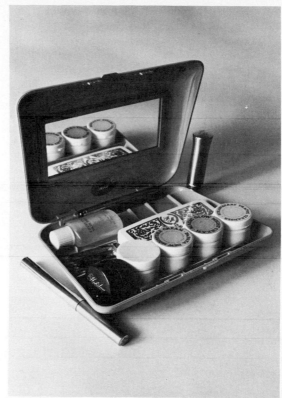

Courtesy of Mel Dixon, Harper's Bazaar

A makeup kit for desk drawer or locker is handy for quick makeup changes or repairs. Whenever possible, redo makeup completely during the day.

CREAM FOUNDATIONS. These come in tubes, sticks, cream cakes, or jars and usually provide heavier coverage that is better for nighttime. They are good for concealing dark circles and blending in skin discolorations. Some girls use them under liquid foundation during the day to cover trouble spots. Cream foundations are especially good for very dry skin. They must be applied carefully and sparingly to avoid a ''make up'' look. Cream foundations are applied with the fingertips in the same manner as liquid bases.

DRY CAKE FOUNDATIONS. These are applied with a wet sponge. They have good covering power

71

but are apt to look artificial in daylight. Because of their drying effect, they are best suited to oily skins.

Cake foundations should be used very lightly and sparingly. Be sure that the sponge is kept clean and allowed to dry thoroughly. A damp sponge in a closed compact is an ideal breeding ground for bacteria.

No matter which type of base you choose, inspect your face carefully to see that you have created a smooth, even finish. There should be no puddles or streaks of color, and the foundation should be blended so smoothly that no one can tell what is natural and what is bottle-bestowed.

The reflection of her skin tone on the sheet of white paper will help this girl determine her basic coloring.

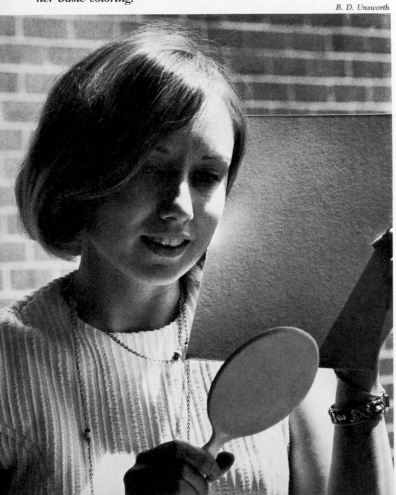

Which shade? There are four major skin shades: pink (red tones), cream (neutral tones), bronze-olive (golden yellow tones) and brown (ranging from dusky tan through red-browns to nearly black). If you are in doubt about your coloring, stand before a bright sunlit window and hold a sheet of white paper next to your cheek. When you look in a hand mirror, you should see a reflection of your skin tone on the paper. If your skin is light, search for any pink or olive tones. If you can't see either of these tones, your skin shade is probably cream. If your skin is brown, look also for other undertones—pink or red tones, yellow tones, or blue-black tones.

Once you have decided on the proper color family, you will want to choose a shade in that family that matches the deepest tones of your skin color. Be careful not to select too dark a shade, because this will be hard to blend into your natural coloring at the neckline, and nothing looks more phony than a pink or tan face perched like a lollipop on a white neck. Too light a shade looks chalky. In choosing a foundation, it is usually best to consult a reliable cosmetics saleswoman. She will probably test the shade on the back of your hand. The color in the bottle is so concentrated that it looks much darker than when it is a gossamer film on your skin. If your complexion is sallow or dull, the cosmetician may suggest a pinkish shade to add life to your skin. If, on the other hand, your complexion is more ruddy than you wish, she may suggest an ivory shade to tone it down.

❦ All-In-One Makeups

There are several products that combine foundation and powder together as an all-in-one makeup. Some come in cake form, others in a tube. The cake forms do not usually give as much covering power or hold up as long as a regular base plus powder. Most tube forms are comparable to a regular base with powder. One of the chief virtues of these products is that they are quick and easy to use. They are best for oily or normal young skin that does not need much makeup and is not lined or wrinkled.

❀ Blushers

Blushers come in both cream and powder forms and provide a becoming rosy bloom that perks up coloring. The chief virtue of blushers is that they are easy to use, blend in very well, and give a softer look than is possible with rouge. This makes them particularly effective for brightening a smile and correcting sallow complexions. Blusher (in a subtle tint) can even help create a healthy outdoor glow. Dust it on forehead, chin, and cheekbones—wherever the sun would add natural color. Blushers can also be used for camouflage, although foundations are preferable because they are longer-lasting. Because blusher provides a darker tone, you can use it to shadow imperfections—for example, on the corners of a square jaw.

Powder types are brushed on after makeup is complete; cream blusher is finger-blended over foundation before powdering. Apply sparingly and lightly. You can always reapply if more color is desired.

Which shade? Choose the blusher color that closely matches any red tints in your coloring—pink for those with pink undertones, peach for those with bronze-olive undertones, a brownish shade for those with brown undertones. Those with other skin types can use either pink or peach, depending upon their clothes. In general, peach looks better with orange, yellow, yellow-green, tan, or red outfits while pink is preferable for the blues, blue-greens, pinks, rosy reds, purples, and grays.

❀ Rouge

Not every face needs rouge. Many girls skip rouge for daytime wear or use a blusher, which gives softer, less conspicuous color. In the evening, however, when artificial lights tend to draw color from complexions, a touch of rouge lends a flattering bloom.

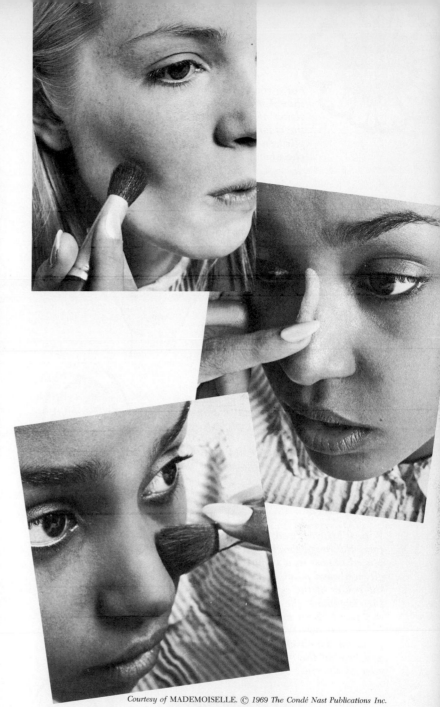

Courtesy of MADEMOISELLE. © 1969 The Condé Nast Publications Inc.

The girl at the top is playing up the interesting contours of her cheeks with blusher. The girl in the middle is camouflaging a broad nose by highlighting the bridge with light foundation and (in the bottom picture) by applying blusher at the sides.

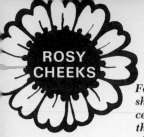

For a round face, rouge should start under the center of the eye, and the color should be applied on and below the cheekbone.

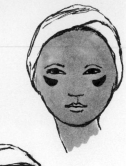

With a square face, the rouge should start under the center of the eye, on the cheekbone, and blend it out as far as the end of the eyebrow.

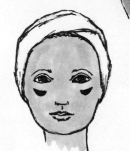

For an oblong face, the rouge should be placed lower on the cheek, even with the outside of the iris; it should extend almost to the edge of the face.

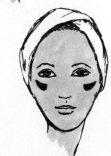

With a heart-shaped face, the rouge should be placed almost in a triangle, with one point under the center of the eye on the cheekbone, the second point about an inch below that and the third point on the cheekbone, just beyond the outer edge of the eye.

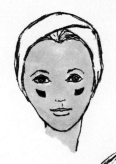

For a diamond-shaped face, the rouge should start under the center of the eye and extend along the cheekbone no farther than the outside of the eye.

The secret of success with rouge is to apply it *very sparingly.* There are four types—cream, gel, liquid, and cake. Cream or gel rouge gives the most natural effect and can be blended easily. Use the merest touch of rouge. Better too little than too much—you can always add more. Blend thoroughly until only the faintest suggestion of color remains. Liquid rouge is slightly more difficult to use because it must be applied quickly before the color sets. For dry or normal skin, cream, gel, or liquid rouge is most satisfactory. These types are usually applied directly after foundation and before powder. Cake rouge, on the other hand, is applied after powder, and, to soften its appearance, should be followed by an additional fluff of powder over the rouge. Dry rouge is less lasting than the other varieties and is slightly more difficult to blend for a natural effect.

Which shade of rouge? The shade you choose will depend on your coloring. The lighter your skin, the lighter your rouge should be. Remember that rouge defeats its purpose if it is obvious. If your skin has cream, olive, or brown tones, you will probably look best in a coral or orange-red rouge; pink-toned complexions need a soft pink rouge.

Placement of rouge. Rouge does two things: it shapes a face and gives it additional color. Where you place your rouge is most important. If you have an *oval face,* smile at yourself in the mirror and place your rouge in a wing-shaped triangle from the top of the most prominent part of your cheek out along the cheekbones. Start the color under the center of the eyes, and let it fade out gently toward the temples.

A *broad face* can be made to seem more oval if you apply rouge fairly high on the cheekbones. Start under the center of the eyes and do not extend the color too far out on the cheeks.

A *long, thin face* can gain width if you place rouge a bit lower on the cheekbones and extend the color outward toward the hairline. Start the rouge on a line with the outer rim of the iris.

74

Never rouge in an obvious little circle or bring rouge closer to the nose than a point directly under the center of the eyes. Rouge should go no lower than the tip of the nose or it will create shadows that make your face sag. If you have shadowy circles under your eyes, they will be less obvious if you blend a little rouge over the edge of the circles, as a slight extension of the regular rouge area.

❦ Powder

Powder provides the smooth matte finish that gives your makeup a soft, glowing unity. Some girls with complexions that need little makeup skip powder for daytime wear. They prefer the fresh, dewy look of foundation alone.

Your powder shade should match your foundation unless it is one of the translucent or transparent types that provides a matte finish without adding color. Always use a clean disposable puff or cotton to *press* powder gently all over your face, fluffing rather than rubbing the powder on. Brush all excess from your brows and lashes and from around your nose.

Tip: After your makeup is complete, you can set it by patting very lightly with cotton that has been wrung out in cold water. This helps keep makeup intact longer.

❦ Lipstick

Use lipstick in an artful way to make the most of your mouth—to shape it, to emphasize the beauty of your lips, and to pick up the color of your costume.

Which shade? All lipstick colors fall into three basic categories: the blue-reds (from pale candy pinks to deep wines), the true reds, and the coral-orange reds (from pale peach to russet-brown red). The blue-red shades are best for pink complexions; the coral-orange shades enhance olive complexions. True reds and corals or pinks with brown undertones go well with brown complexions. Almost any shade can safely be worn with a cream complexion. The

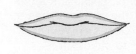

THIN LIPS. *Outline with a darker shade and fill in with a brighter color, carrying it to the outer edges of your lips. Don't exceed the rim of your lips or the profile will look phony.*

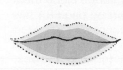

FULL LIPS. *To make them look thinner, bring foundation up over the lip edge and keep the lip outline just slightly inside natural borders. Use a lighter shade to outline and fill in with a darker one. Choose subtle shades. Extreme colors— either very light or very dark—exaggerate the lip shade. So, too, do shimmering iridescent and glossy lipsticks.*

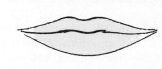

WIDE MOUTH. *Don't carry color into the corners; let it fade away gradually.*

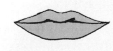

SMALL MOUTH. *Extend color as far as possible.*

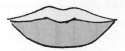

FULL LOWER LIP. *Color lower lip a slightly darker shade than the upper lip (keeping in the same color family, of course).*

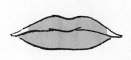

DROOPING CORNERS. *Let lipstick fade out before it reaches the corners of the upper lip, but extend color as far as possible into the corners of the lower lip.*

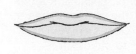

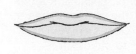

LOVELY LIPS

beiges are good on young girls who have a lot of natural color. If you have very fair coloring, keep to the lighter shades of lipstick. When you purchase a new lipstick, make sure the color does something for *you*. Just because it's the most ballyhooed shade of the moment, has a catchy name, or looks marvelous on your best friend isn't reason enough to choose it.

The most important consideration in deciding which lipstick to wear is how well it goes with your outfit. Your colors must match or at least harmonize. This usually necessitates owning at least three lipstick shades—one in each color category. You can often blend them to suit your needs. The chart on page 84 has been devised to help you choose coordinated makeup for each outfit. In general, costume colors with yellow in them (greens, browns, oranges) harmonize best with orange or true-red lipsticks. Clothes in blues (blue-greens, purples, maroons, pinks) look good with blue-red cosmetics. Costumes in off-red colors (orange, coral, rose) are tricky and should be matched as closely as possible to avoid color clashes.

Paint yourself a pretty mouth. Unless you use a colorless lip gloss or a near-natural shade that blends in with your own lip coloring, you must do a perfect job of outlining your lips. If lipstick is smeary or frayed, your whole expression

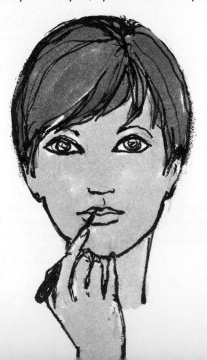

seems awry. If you haven't yet experimented with a lip-liner pencil or a lipstick brush, you owe it to your pretty smile to give them a try. Their benefits: they create a cleaner, neater lip outline and are less likely to cause skid marks because their slender girth allows you to control where you're going much better than a thick stick does. You may find your hand has better control when using a brush if you rest your curled little finger on your chin.

Just a reminder—before applying lipstick, make sure the remains of the last job have been thoroughly wiped away and that your lips are free from cream or moisture so that new lipstick has a clean, dry surface to cling to. Always blot your lips first to be safe.

If you use a lip-liner pencil, shape your lip outline with it, then fill in with your lipstick. When using a brush, put plenty of lipstick on the bristles so that you can make an even line. Then, keeping your lips closed and relaxed, draw a firm outline of half your upper lip. Repeat on the other side. Then do your lower lip. Now retrace the complete lip line with the mouth open and the lips stretched taut so that all lip creases will be filled and a sharper line will be achieved. Fill in with your lipstick, carrying color back deep enough so that no boundary line is visible.

Lipstick should always be applied to both lips. When color is merely put on the upper lip and then the lips are pressed together to transfer color to the lower lip, wearing quality is reduced because too little stain is left. Also, the bottom lip will not be shaped correctly.

A trick that many models use to make their lipstick last longer is to powder lightly over and around their lips before applying color. This helps lipstick set better and keeps color from creeping or smearing. Lipstick is allowed to set for a few minutes and then blotted gently with tissue. This is followed with another dusting of powder, another application of color, a few moments' wait, and a final light blotting. Try this method next time you're invited out to dinner—it keeps lipstick on *you,* instead of on silver and glassware. When you blot your lips, use gentle pressure. Biting down hard removes too much color. Of course, you never blot iridescent lipsticks—blotting removes the shine.

If your lipstick tends to change color, try using moisturizer and tinted foundation under your lipstick or one of the stick foundations made for this purpose.

Correcting your lip line. If you want to do a little revamping of your lip line—and a very little is all that you can get away with—you must proceed with caution. Lips painted out beyond their borders don't fool anybody, neither do Cupid's bows, pointed upper lips, or exaggerated lower lips. See the chart on lip lines on page 75.

❧ *Accentuating Eyes*

Eye makeup provides an attractive frame for the eyes—making them seem larger, more radiant, more alluring. Girls with light brows and lashes achieve a particularly impressive improvement, and it is a great asset to those who wear glasses.

Eyebrow care. Eyebrows are the exclamation marks of the face. They add expression to the eyes and balance to the rest of your features. If they are too pale, the face takes on a blank look; too short, features look pinched; too long, eyes are overpowered. Well-tended brows do much for the beauty of the entire face.

KEEP EYEBROWS NEAT. Eyebrow beauty begins with brushing. It's amazing how well scrawny brows and straying hairs respond to regular brushing. A mascara brush is most satisfactory, but even a hairbrush will do. Brush hairs in toward the center of the face—opposite from the way they grow—then straight up, and smooth them into place by running a comb or finger over the top edge of the arch. Every time you comb your hair take a moment to comb brow stragglers into line. Shaggy, untidy brows can make the whole face seem to droop.

SHAPING EYEBROWS. The most flattering shape for your eyebrows is usually the one Mother Nature designed for you. Artificial upslants,

high, surprised-looking arches, and long, thin, penciled tails merely look peculiar. The natural arch usually needs a bit of sharpening and refining, however, to make it most attractive.

Tweeze only the stragglers that blur the clean outline of your brows, plucking only stray hairs at the bridge of the nose and *beneath* the arch. Please don't tweeze above the arch or pluck any but the lowest stragglers from beneath the inner third of the brow. The brow bone protrudes there and looks peculiar if it is bared. By all means don't tweeze eyebrows into a thin, unnatural line. Some girls who have gone wild with their tweezing have come to rue the day. After they saw what they had done and how unattractive it looked, they were horrified to find that the plucked hairs didn't grow back. This occasionally happens, particularly with girls in their teens.

Your eyebrow should begin just above the inner corner of the eye. (The space between the eyes should be the width of an eye.) If your eyes are very close-set, brows may be plucked just a tiny bit farther out—no more than one-eighth of an inch—to add width.

What is the proper length for your eyebrows? Try this: Hold a pencil against your face with one end at the side of the base of your nose and the other end at the outer corner of your

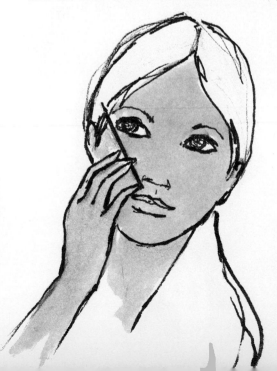

eye. To be in balance with the rest of your features, the tip of the eyebrow should extend just to the line formed by the pencil. If your face is round or pear-shaped, the outer tips of the brows should point out toward the hairline. A long or oval face is flattered by eyebrows that arch down at the tips so that the curve will soften the lines of the face.

To keep eyebrows smoothly tapered, tweezing should be done at least once a week—or, better yet, whenever you spot a stray. Plucking will be quick and painless if you apply a bit of face cream to the brows before you begin. Hold the skin taut with one hand and use tweezers to grasp the hair as near as possible to the root. A quick pull in the direction the hair is growing, and out it comes! Finish with a wipe of alcohol to guard against possible infection.

INTENSIFYING EYEBROWS. Many of us weren't born with dark, dramatic eyebrows, but thanks to a bit of eyebrow powder or pencil, we can all arch a brow effectively. Unless you have

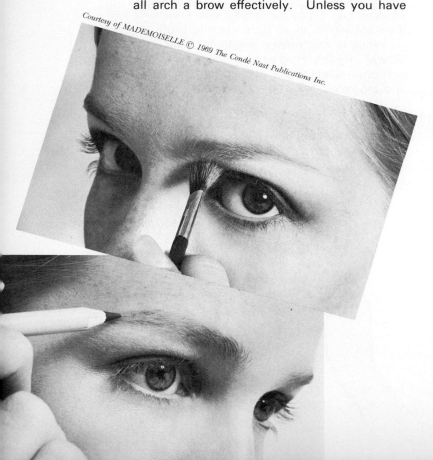

Courtesy of MADEMOISELLE © 1969 The Condé Nast Publications Inc.

jet black hair, avoid a black shade. With other hair colors black tends to look unnatural. Brunettes and darker blondes should use charcoal gray or brown; light blondes and redheads should choose a light brown or auburn shade.

Eyebrow powder produces a softer, more natural effect than pencil and is better for darkening brows, while pencil is helpful for filling in sparse brows. Powder forms should be brushed on lightly in the direction brow hairs are growing. Eyebrow pencil should be applied in tiny, featherlike strokes to the hairs of the brow—never drawn in a straight line. Each line should be in the same direction as the hair is growing. Color should be sketched in lightly, as though each hair were being touched up. Do not apply pencil to the skin unless brows are extremely sparse or do not extend far enough. Soften the appearance by rubbing the darkened brow gently with your fingertip to avoid a hard, crayoned line; then blot with facial tissue. If you have lengthened your brows, check your profile to be sure that the line is not too long or too obvious.

Eyeshadow. Eyeshadow should be applied subtly and carefully. The effect should be only the slightest suggestion of color. Only the added beauty of your eyes should be apparent—not the makeup.

Soft blues and greens are generally the most flattering shades; lavender adds depth to blue eyes; taupe is often attractive on brown skins. You'll want to experiment to see which colors flatter your particular eye coloring and the costume you plan to wear. Experiment, too, with application techniques. Makeup fashions are changeable, and the fact that a new technique is touted in beauty articles doesn't guarantee that it is automatically flattering to everyone. Test carefully to find the best ways to enhance your eyes.

Generally the most flattering method is to apply a colorful eye shadow—just the tiniest smidgen—lightly to the center of the upper lid, close to the lashline. Smooth the color gently along the lashes to the outer corner of the lid, concentrating the color in the outer corners, where the natural shadows appear. Blend the shadow lightly up toward the eyebrow, stopping at the crease of the lid. The color should gradually fade off into nothingness. To make your eyes seem brighter, try blending a muted brown shade from the crease up along the bony ridge of the eye socket so that it covers just a little of the bone and fades out toward the temple. You might also try a bit of white shadow just beneath the arch of the brow to create an illusion of greater space and make the eyes seem larger.

After applying cream or stick eyeshadow, set the color with a fluff of face powder. This helps prevent color from collecting in the creases. Women who have this trouble may do better with powdered eyeshadow. Powdered eyeshadow should be applied to a clean, dry lid. Any oily residue should first be thoroughly removed or powdered over lightly.

Eyeshadow is not flattering to all women. It should be skipped by those who have naturally shadowed lids, darkly circled eyes, very little space between eyes and eyebrows, heavily lidded eyes, or a wrinkled eye area.

Eyeliner. Cleverly applied eyeliner can make your lashes seem more luxuriant and your eyes larger and more interestingly shaped. To achieve this, eyelining must look as natural as possible. The aim is a delicate tracing of color that appears to be part of your lashes. Your liner color should match your lashes (it should not be darker) so that it blends in inconspicuously.

Eyeliners come in pencil, cake, cream, and liquid forms. Pencils are easier to work with; liquid and cream liners provide more intense color; and cake types provide a softer matte finish. Brush-on types require a hand that is both steady and practiced. Eyeliner pencil should be well sharpened. If the pencil seems too hard, it can be softened by holding the tip under hot water.

To apply an eyeliner, draw a line (or a series of tiny dots for a more natural effect) across the upper lid *as close to the lashes as possible* so it will look like part of the lashes. Start about

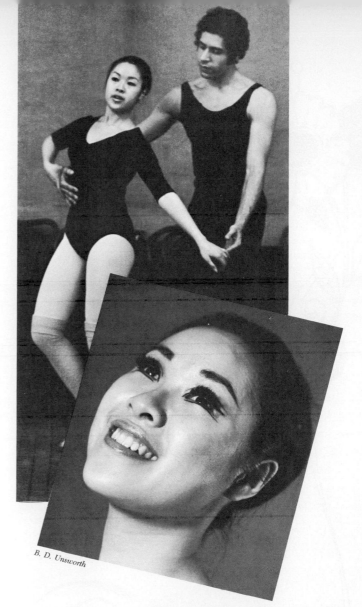

B. D. Unsworth

Stage makeup is fine for performers seen at a distance, but up close under the bright lights in an office it looks overdone.

one quarter of the way in from the inner corner and carry it to the outer corner or ever so slightly beyond the outer corner. Obvious corner extensions are passé. If your eyes are small or deep-set, be sure your line is very fine, a mere thread done in a light brown or gray shade.

Many experts advise against outlining the lower lids because the eyes then tend to seem smaller. If you wish to line your lower lids, use

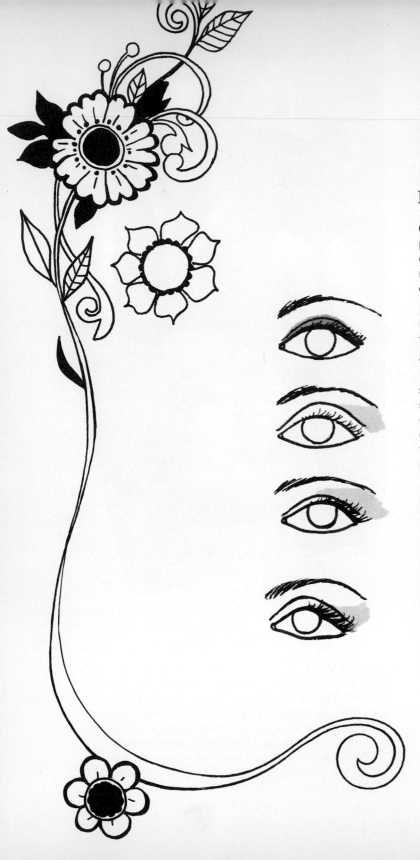

FOR MORE BEAUTIFUL EYES

Camouflage with eye makeup. With a little practice, you can soon make any special camouflage techniques you need simply another routine part of your makeup procedure. The extra beautifying effect is worth the effort.

PROTRUDING EYES. The lid will seem to recede if darker shadow (preferably brown) is applied from the lashes to the crease and if white is used just beneath the brow. Use an eyeliner.

DEEP-SET EYES. To bring out the eyes, use light shadow (white or bone if your lids are naturally shadowed) from lashes to bony ridge. A bit of darker shadow can be used at the outer edge of the bony ridge with possibly white just under the brow. Eyelines should be omitted or kept as thin as possible.

CLOSE-SET EYES. Start eyeshadow, liner, and mascara at the center of the lid, concentrating the color toward the outer corners. Blend eye shadow out toward the temples.

DROOPY EYES. Outer corners that tip downward can be given a more wide-awake appearance if the eyeline is very thin at the inner corner but widens toward the outer corner and if mascara is concentrated on the outer lashes. If shadow is used, the color should be concentrated on the outer half of the lid, widening toward the outer corner and sweeping up toward the brow tip. Use an eyelash curler for extra upturn.

80

a series of tiny dots or a very soft line, prefer-ably using a pencil in a light shade. Start the liner under the iris and keep close in among the lash roots. Don't join the lower line to the up-per one or your eyes will seem smaller.

In making eyelines, accuracy counts. All allure vanishes when there are smudged edges or incorrectly drawn lines. Before a public appearance, plenty of private practice is advis-able. Remember that the idea is to draw at-tention to the eye, not to the makeup. Eyelines defeat this purpose unless they are applied with great caution.

Fashions in eye makeup change from sea-son to season. Keep abreast of what's new and try the new techniques, but evaluate them carefully. Unfortunately manufacturers are sometimes guilty of starting a new fad merely to promote a new product. Be sure a new style flatters you.

Curling eyelashes. Lashes seem longer if they are curved upward. You can do this with gentle pressure when you apply mascara, or you can use an eyelash curler. Only the upper lashes should be curled. Regular brushing will coax lashes to curl naturally, and will also promote thicker growth. Women who wear glasses find that the annoyance of having lashes bat against lenses is lessened if they use a curler regularly.

Mascara. Darkening eyelashes with mascara provides a flattering frame for the eyes, making them look larger and more radiant. Blondes and redheads with very light lashes find that mascara is one of their most important beauty aids. But even the darkest lashes have light tips and seem longer and more luxuriant when mascara is added. If your lashes are short, you can lengthen them with one of the products that add lash-like fibers to your own lashes.

Black or brownish-black mascara is best for most women, but brown will give a more natural effect for those with very light lashes.

Mascara comes as a cake, cream, or a liquid in a tube with a roll-on or brush-on applicator. A tip to make mascara cling longer: start with dry, clean lashes and give them a preliminary light dusting with face powder. Apply mascara

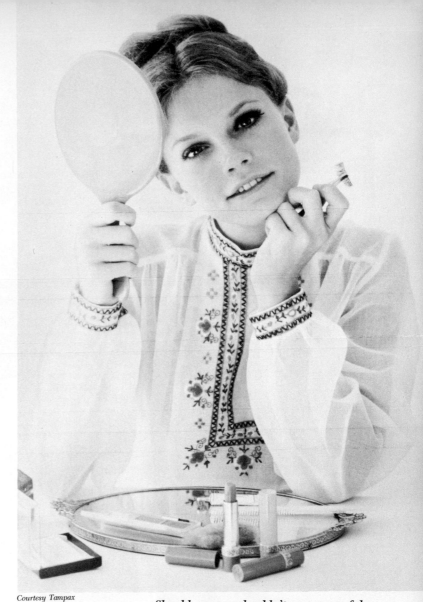

Courtesy Tampax

Should you or shouldn't you wear false eyelashes? Often they make you look more glamorous, but at work they can look extremely artificial and, consequently, be inappropriate.

with upward and outward strokes along the entire length of the lashes, from roots to tips, concentrating color on the outer lashes. If you use cake mascara, remember that the brush should not be too wet or it will pick up so much mascara that the lashes will look blobby and artificial. Lashes should not stick to-gether—each hair must be separate. If the

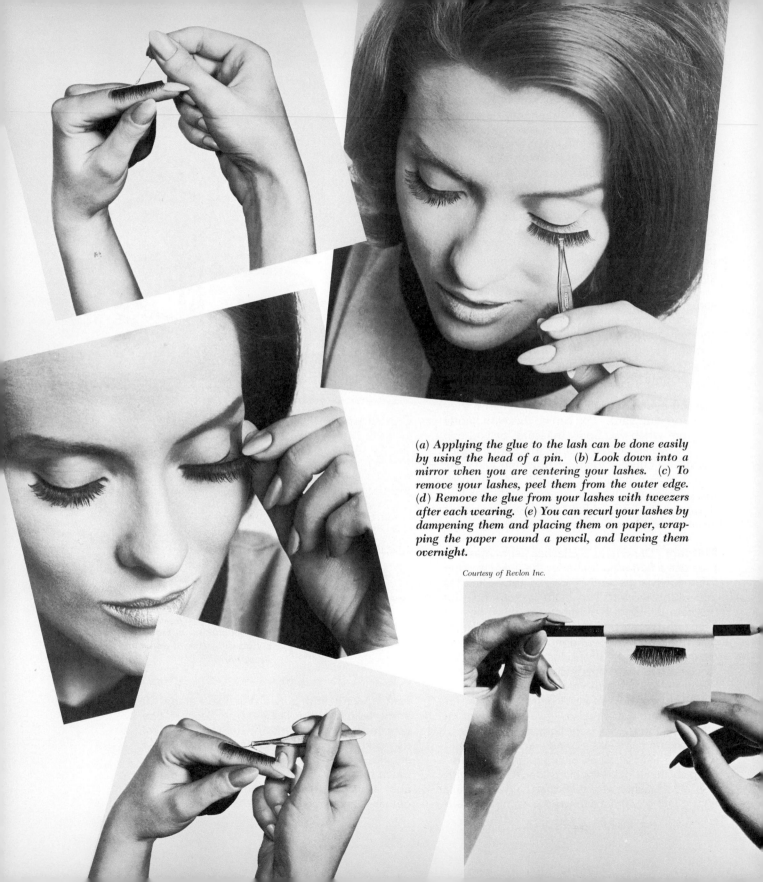

(a) Applying the glue to the lash can be done easily by using the head of a pin. (b) Look down into a mirror when you are centering your lashes. (c) To remove your lashes, peel them from the outer edge. (d) Remove the glue from your lashes with tweezers after each wearing. (e) You can recurl your lashes by dampening them and placing them on paper, wrapping the paper around a pencil, and leaving them overnight.

Courtesy of Revlon Inc.

lashes do become matted or beaded, remove the excess by combing or by brushing with a clean brush (rinse the brush well, shake dry). Apply mascara only to the upper lashes; mascara used on lower lashes is likely to flake off. Some girls find a second coat beneficial. Wait until the first coat has dried before applying a second. Clean the brush thoroughly after each use. And remember not to rub your eyes!

False eyelashes. If your lashes aren't worth fluttering, you might want to try false eyelashes. They're fun for evening and parties, although not usually appropriate for business.

You can buy full-width lashes in varying thicknesses or half lashes that go on just the outer corners of the lid. To look most natural the lashes should be about as long or only slightly longer than your own and should be shorter at the corners than at the center. In many large stores a cosmetician will fit them for you. If this service is not available to you, check the width of the strip by holding it against your eye. The lashes should begin and end where yours do. Cut off any extra width at the outer edge of the lash strip.

False lashes are applied after eye makeup is complete. Always handle eyelashes delicately, holding the base strip rather than the individual hairs. To apply (a) put the lash adhesive on the head of a pin and spread this along the base of the lashes. Then look downward into a hand mirror that is flat on a table and, holding the lash strip with tweezers, (b) center it close to the roots of your own lashes. Carefully press the strip into place. To make the strip secure, you can gently roll the skin of the lid over the lash base with your finger. Blend false lashes into your own with a dry mascara brush. (c) Touch up the eyeline if necessary.

To remove lashes, (d) grasp the outer corner of the lash base and gently peel it from your lid. After each wearing, (e) use tweezers to pull the glue off the base. Then clean the lashes with a mascara brush dipped in warm water and recurl them while damp by placing the lashes on paper and (f) wrapping them

around a rounded pencil. An elastic band will hold them until dry. If new lashes seem a bit stiff, you can soften them by dipping them in warm water and recurling them.

Always store false eyelashes in their case to preserve the curve of the lash base.

Beautiful eyes are healthy eyes. Your eyes deserve every bit of pampering you can give them. Business girls who spend much of their day typing, proofreading, or scanning mail are particularly susceptible to eye troubles. Try to work in good light—and this applies at home as well. When you are reading or doing close work, give your eyes a restful change by occasionally looking up and as far off as possible. For the sake of your eyes, don't let yourself be lured into reading on buses or bouncy trains. If your eyes feel strained from too much reading, dust, or sun glare, bathe them or treat them to eye drops.

One of the best refreshers for tired eyes is "looking at black." Close your eyes and let yourself relax as you imagine you are in a completely darkened room that has walls draped with black velvet. See only black—deep, rich black—for two or three minutes. When you open your eyes, they'll feel much fresher.

❀ A Smooth Finish

No makeup is complete until it has passed a careful final inspection. What might get by when viewed across a dressing table often shows up at closer range. Take a moment to check with your hand mirror. Is the foundation even and well blended? Do you have a chin line of foundation? Is there any excess powder? Do rouge and eye makeup look natural? Does your lipstick pass the profile test? A few moments' final check is a valuable investment in beauty, poise, and self-assurance. When you know your makeup is perfect, you can forget about it. Then you can concentrate on enjoying yourself and being charming to everyone else.

MATCH YOUR MAKEUP

Costume color	Lipstick and nail polish color	Eye makeup colors		
		BLUE OR GRAY EYES	GREEN OR HAZEL EYES	BROWN EYES
Black, white, gray, beige, navy	Any shade	Blue, gray	Green, gray	Gray, blue-green, turquoise
Pink, red, orange	Closely matching shade	Blue, gray, turquoise	Blue-green, turquoise, blue	Turquoise, gray, blue
Blues, purple, rose, lavender, maroon	Blue-red (pinks)	Blue, lavender, violet, gray	Blue, lavender, violet, gray	Blue, lavender, violet, gray
Greens, emerald, olive, forest	Yellow-reds (peach, orange, coral)	Blue-green, green	Green, blue-green	Green
Yellows, tans, corals	Yellow-reds (peach, orange, coral)	Turquoise, blue-green	Blue-green, turquoise	Blue-green, green
Blue-greens, aqua, teal	Red-red, blue-red, or yellow-red (depending on accessory color)	Turquoise, blue-green	Blue-green, turquoise, green	Blue-green, turquoise
Browns, russets, coppers	Yellow-reds, red-red	Turquoise, blue-green	Green, blue-green, brown	Brown, blue-green

❦ Watch the Styles

Fashions in makeup come and go. As with clothing, what is loudly proclaimed as *the* look one year may be completely rejected in a year or two. The girl who took pride in perfecting a certain eye makeup technique may find a few seasons later that the same look is obviously dated. Keep your ideas on makeup flexible. Learn all you can about new cosmetics, new shades, and new application techniques. Test each trend carefully, modify it to your own personal needs and adopt only what is truly flattering.

---

1 *Stand in good light while you examine your face closely. Based on what you have learned, decide what type skin you have.*

2 *Visit a cosmetic counter and study the various products available to decide which would be suitable for your particular skin. Find the items necessary for a complete cleansing, lubricating (if needed), and stimulating routine. As soon as your budget permits, purchase any of the essentials you lack so that you can soon enjoy the benefits a complete skin care program brings. Follow your beauty routine carefully. Treatment products must be used regularly to bring results. The cream that sits unused on a dressing table can't help anyone.*

3 *Pamper yourself with a complete beauty facial. Give yourself the "works" and see what a wonderful lift it adds to your appearance—and your morale.*

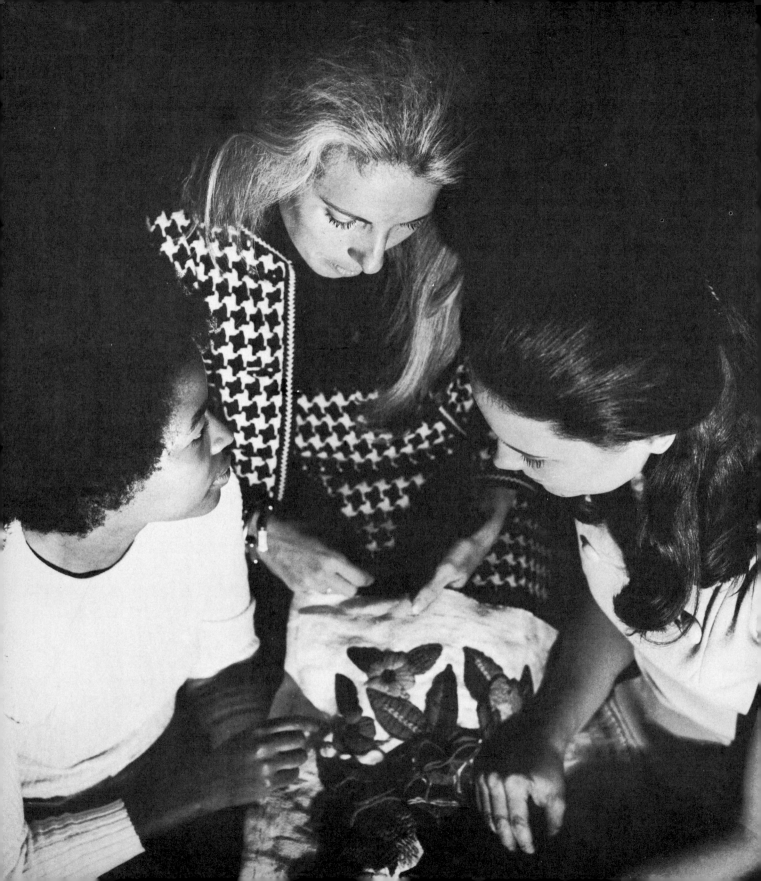

BEAUTIFUL
HAIR

Your hair is probably your most important beauty asset. Hair care and styling offer so many opportunities for changing and revitalizing appearance that every girl owes it to her good looks to become skilled in these techniques. And a flattering, fashionable hairdo sets you off as a clever girl with plenty of grooming *savoir faire.*

Hair is not attractive unless it is clean. When hair becomes dull and clings together in sticky strands, no hair style will look pretty. A regular shampoo schedule is the answer. How often should you shampoo? Often enough to keep hair clean and sparkling, which is probably about once a week. Every girl has to make her own decision on this because, depending on the oiliness of her hair and the amount of soot and dirt it's exposed to, washing time can vary from every four or five days to every ten days. Even if your hair is very dry, it isn't wise to put off a shampoo longer. Dirt will clog up the pores and prevent the oil glands from functioning properly. Bear in mind that in summer, when you perspire freely, hair must be washed more frequently to prevent a sour, dirty-hair odor.

Before your shampoo, brush your hair vigorously to loosen scalp scale and to sweep out loose hair and dirt. Then wash your brushes and combs, including those in your purse. Why is it that some girls who are otherwise respectably groomed carry revoltingly filthy combs? For the sake of your grooming reputation, as well as hair health, keep your brushes and combs sparkling clean. A quick method to clean them is to soak them in sudsy ammonia and warm water while you shampoo.

Then give the combs a quick run through the brushes, rinse, and shake out. When you dry your brush, stand it up on end with the handle in a glass or jar and the bristles exposed to the air. This prevents any weight on wet bristles, which might weaken them, and allows water to drain away from the base of the brush so that the bristles won't be loosened. Don't dry your brushes on radiators; the heat may warp them.

When you shampoo, wash your hair twice with shampoo and rinse it until it squeaks. Rinse thoroughly, for any soapy residue will dull hair. Choose a shampoo that is suited to your hair condition and that will work effectively in the water you use. Consult labels and experiment until you find the products that work best for you.

You can be sure all soap film is removed if you finish with a lemon juice rinse (especially good for blondes) or a vinegar rinse (for brunettes and redheads). The commerical rinses that highlight your natural hair color and provide added sheen are also good.

If your hair is dry or tends to take off in all directions after a shampoo, or if your permanent is new and a little hard to handle, try a cream rinse. Cream rinses counteract the static electricity that causes hair to stand on end. They also contain hair-conditioning ingredients that make hair softer and more manageable, making them especially good for extremely curly hair.

❦ Working Up a Shine

The secret of soft, glossy locks is just this: healthy hair. Your hair can look its prettiest only when it is kept in top condition. A nutritious diet and sufficient sleep again play a big part here, and daily massage and hairbrush sessions help keep hair healthy, bright, and gleaming. They improve circulation in the scalp, stimulating the blood to speed up its beauty work and helping to regulate the supply of natural hair oils.

Whether your hair is dry, normal, or oily, brushing is important. If your hair is oily, you won't want to brush too vigorously. Firm but gentle lifting strokes will give your scalp the stimulation it requires. Concentrate on hair more than scalp. At first your hair may seem to become more oily, because the oil is being spread throughout the hair instead of being allowed to remain on the scalp where it clogs the pores. However, brushing will, in time, help to correct this over-oily condition. To prevent the spread of oil through your hair, you can work a piece of cheesecloth over and down through the bristles of your brush. Then, as you brush, dirt and oil will cling to the cloth.

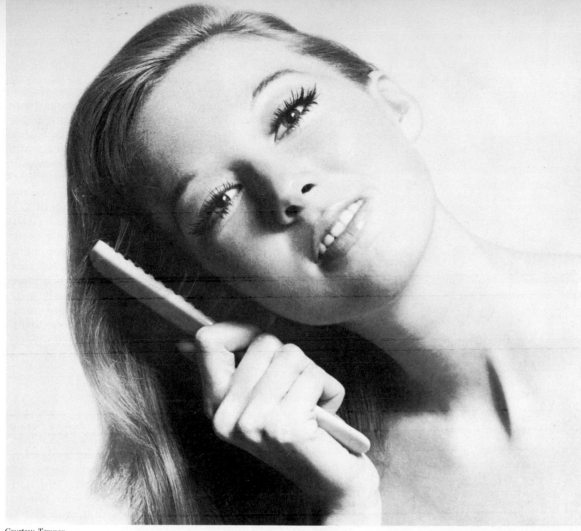

Shift the cheesecloth frequently so that a clean section can be used.

A brush with natural bristles is generally recommended by hair specialists. The irregular shape of the natural bristle provides more surface to clean and polish the hair, and natural bristles have a more gentle effect. Nylon bristles are sharp and may cut delicate hair.

Do you know how to brush your hair? Ridiculous as the question may seem, many people don't know how. They merely glide a brush lightly over the top of the hair, which does little good. You should touch your scalp as you brush. Use long, firm strokes, sweeping the hair up from the roots and out to the very tips. Don't snap the brush at the finish of each stroke because this can cause split ends. Lean forward, holding your head down, and brush the back hair forward over your head. Then brush the side and top hair up, opposite to the way it normally lies. Don't bother counting strokes. Just do a good job, and keep at it until your scalp tingles all over. Incidentally, brushing is an excellent beauty treatment for your complexion as well.

You'll probably notice that your brush picks up considerable dirt in the process. To avoid merely transferring dirt from one section of your hair to another, wipe the bristles at intervals on a lintless cloth or tissue. Rinse your brush off whenever it becomes soiled, and give it a thorough washing before each shampoo.

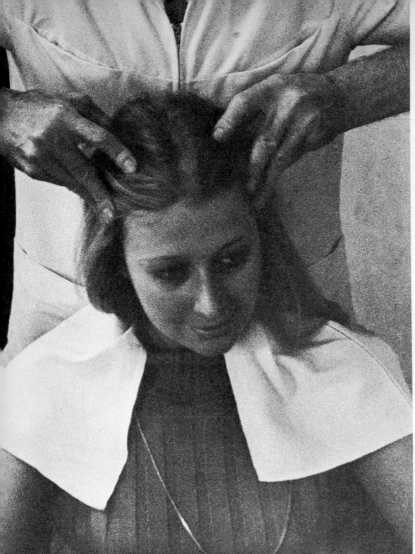

To duplicate the benefits of a professional massage, rotate your fingers in back-to-front spirals, moving the scalp. Daily massage beautifies hair and complexion.

❦ Make Massage a Habit

A young typist with gorgeous hair says she wakes up her scalp each morning by giving it a good massage. Smart gal! Morning may be too hectic a time for most girls, but perhaps in the evening you can manage three or four minutes for massage while you're reading or watching television. A massage does wonders to stimulate your scalp as well as to promote

general relaxation and relieve nervous tension. Put your fingers under your hair now and rotate your scalp. Does your scalp feel lose and move easily? It should. When you massage, use both hands, one on each side of your head, and work with the pads of your fingers so that your nails won't scratch. Begin at the nape of your neck and slowly rotate your fingers, moving the scalp as you do. Then slide your fingers to a new position and rotate the scalp again. Gradually work forward up over your head to your front hairline. Then, starting behind your ears, spiral up and forward along the sides of your head. Remember that your fingers should move the scalp; they should not merely slide over the surface. Keep repeating these back-to-front spiraling patterns all over your head, giving special attention to your hairline. Feels marvelous, doesn't it?

❦ Hair Problems

Dry hair. Dry hair is lusterless, brittle, often hard to manage. Among the causes: poor diet, too much sun, salt water, swimming pool chemicals, a poor permanent, use of coloring products, illness—or just plain neglect. To help avoid trouble, always rinse your hair after a swim. Dry hair usually responds well if it is given proper care. A preshampoo conditioning treatment is very helpful. There are several excellent commercial conditioners, but good results can also be obtained with a traditional preshampoo hot-oil treatment. This involves warming a few tablespoons of cooking oil (vegetable oil—never mineral oil) and rubbing it well into your hair and scalp. Then a towel wrung out in very hot water can be wrapped around your head in a turban and left on for fifteen or twenty minutes to spread the oil evenly. Reheat the towel whenever it cools (or use a dry towel and sit under a dryer set for low heat). If time allows, you'll gain greater benefit by leaving the oil on for a couple of hours or, better yet, overnight. In this case, make yourself a turban of aluminum foil or cellophane wrap, and cover your pillow with a turkish towel. A hot oil treatment is often helpful in conditioning hair for a permanent. However, because some experts believe that an oil treatment just before a permanent may affect the way the permanent takes, the treatment should be given at least a week beforehand.

In addition to preshampoo treatments, there are postshampoo cream rinses and conditioners—some "instant" ones, requiring about five minutes; others requiring longer periods (and giving greater benefits). Never use lemon rinses, because they have a drying effect.

Dry hair, particularly, needs the extra stimulation of massage and hair brushing to stir up lazy oil glands. Brushing should be thorough but not too vigorous. Treat hair gently by using a wide-tooth comb and avoiding tight or sharp setting implements. If hair sprays dry or dull your hair, you may find a conditioning hairdressing more satisfactory for disciplining hair because it will add sheen as well as body.

Oily hair. Even fairly soon after a shampoo, oily hair may become drab and stringy. Frequent washing is necessary to keep it pretty. Wash your hair in warm water—never hot—and rinse with cool water. Follow up with a lemon or vinegar rinse. To help tame down your overactive oil glands, make a habit of massaging your scalp *every* day. The extra stimulation will gradually help the scalp regulate oil production. Brushing is also helpful, but the brush must be kept clean. Look for shampoos and setting aids that are specially formulated for oily hair. Avoid those containing lanolin or other lubricants. For emergency cleanups between shampoos, you may want to try a powder-type dry shampoo that brushes out, taking unwanted oil with it. Some of the improved aerosol types are quite effective.

Dry shampoos are an excellent between— shampoos cleaner for girls with oily hair. The spray blots up oil without disturbing the set.

Courtesy of Phillip E. Pegler, Clairol

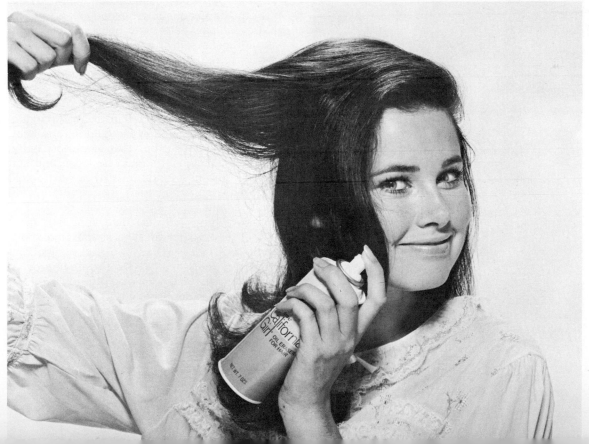

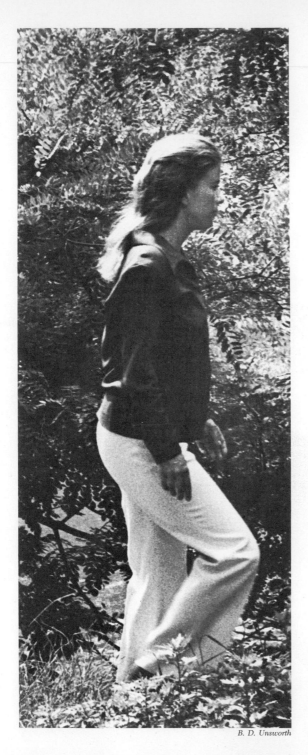

Simple hairstyles are most successful for oily hair. Fashion permitting, set hair on large rollers that give bulk rather than in small curls that encourage hair to separate into sections. Sun and air will help an oily condition. Avoid snug hats and scarves that block scalp ventilation, and don't wear hats of fur or other overly warm materials.

Limp, lifeless hair. Poor hair is usually the direct result of poor nourishment. This may be due to an inadequate diet or it may result from an illness, an operation, a severe shock, or nervous tension that saps strength and robs hair of the nutrition it needs. Perhaps you've noticed how an illness, particularly one accompanied by high fever, can cause hair to fall out. An intense mental or physical strain or shock will also take its toll. Good nutrition, plenty of brushing and massage, and the use of cream rinses and lubricating conditioners and dressings will gradually restore hair beauty.

Especially beneficial for limp hair are the special conditioners that improve the texture of hair and add body as they condition. These have the happy effect of bolstering your hair so that it behaves better and holds its set longer, yet still looks soft and lovely. Use narrow or medium-size rollers, rather than thick ones, and a hair spray in a hard-to-hold formula.

Fine hair. Fine hair is often sparse, fragile, and stubborn, developing definite flyaway tendencies in cold weather and hanging limp in heat. Try all the various props that give more body: a permanent (which should be loose and soft because fine hair tends to frizz), an extra-hold type of hair spray, a cream rinse, a setting with an extra-hold wave lotion (or stale beer). Frequent washing will also give your hair more bulk. Keep your hair style simple and short; length pulls out waves and makes fine hair harder to keep neat. The texture-improving conditioners are also very helpful for fine hair. They give it enough body and bulk to achieve better control without hiding its silky beauty. Use narrow or medium-sized rollers rather than thick ones.

Coarse hair. Coarse hair tends to become wiry and bushy. A good cut will help tame it, and a professional permanent will make it more manageable. Brushing is important. Use wave set or spray and extra large rollers.

Curly hair. Though the envy of girls whose hair is straight but limp, curly hair can be too much of a good thing. It limits hair styles, tangles easily, and may stubbornly corkscrew out of place between treatments or in damp weather. Routine care for curly hair calls for a good hairdressing and a cream rinse after each shampoo. Use very thick rollers and set your hair while it is wet. Comb it out *gently*—overworking it will undo the set. Guard your hair against dampness by wearing a showercap at bath time and a hat when it rains.

Usually short haircuts are the easiest way to manage curly hair; longer styles are likely to become bushy. Frequent professional shaping is essential, whether the style calls for straightening the hair or whether it retains the natural curl.

Many black girls choose a "natural" or Afro style, which can be very becoming. But camouflage techniques on pages 96–99 should be considered, and make sure you have the style shaped to suit your face and figure. Girls who are quite tall or heavy usually find other styles more flattering. If your hair is so curly that other styles are difficult to adopt and care for, straightening your hair may be the answer.

Straightening methods include homestyle electric combing, hot pressing, and straightening permanents. The permanents last until new hair grows in (about three or four months). Hot pressing is good from shampoo to shampoo. Electric combing lasts only a few days and gives out in dampness. Although hot pressing and straightening permanents can be done at home, both methods can damage hair. It's usually wiser to visit a trained beautician for these treatments.

Before any straightening permanent, be sure your hair is in peak condition. Dry, brittle hair is likely to break when straightened. Always insist on having a strand tested before the

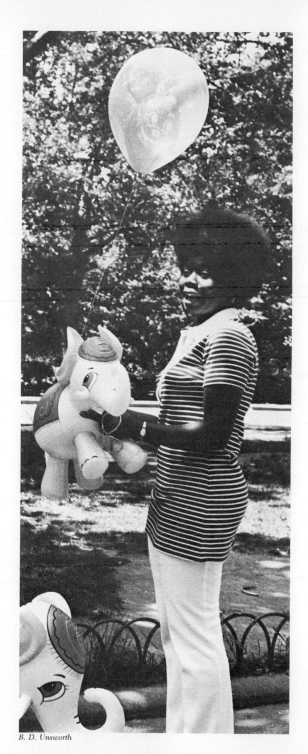

B. D. Unsworth

93

rest of your hair is done. This is particularly important for color-treated or kinky hair. Kinky hair is often so fragile that some hairdressers recommend that the strand test be given a week or more in advance to make sure there is no breakage. Straightening permanents are usually very drying and should be followed with plenty of gentle care, lubricating conditioners, and special shampoos, hair sprays, and setting products that are designed to help dry hair. Curling irons and electric combs should not be used after a straightening permanent.

Baldness. This is a problem that seems to be increasing among women. Some of the causes advanced by dermatologists include brushing hair with nylon-bristle brushes, which seem to tear and cut hair, wearing tight hats that restrict circulation, overteasing, and pulling hair into tight hairdos that tend to cut hair and cause it to break.

As mentioned before, an illness or shock of some sort to the nervous system may cause hair to fall out. It may take quite a while—months even—for the condition to correct itself. If it doesn't seem to be improving within a reasonable time, consult your physician. Stimulating circulation with massage is usually quite helpful, but vigorous brushing should be avoided.

Dandruff. Dandruff is *not* to be confused with the flaking off of dead scalp scales, which is a completely natural process. Real dandruff actually is rather rare. Nevertheless, we are occasionally bothered by an avalanche of white flakes on our shoulders and collars. The best remedy is to go to work with a hairbrush and massage—more stimulation is usually the best remedy. Shampoo more frequently, too. Special dandruff-removing shampoos and tonics often alleviate the situation, whether the dandruff is genuine or not.

Because dandruff can be spread from one person to another, never borrow or lend a comb, hat, or anything else that is used on your hair.

Sun damage. While sun is excellent for brightening blonde hair and for improving oily condi-

tions, it can play havoc with dry hair. A pretty sun hat or a gay scarf is the ounce of prevention that is worth many sessions with hot oil treatments and special conditioners. Once the damage is done, however, these treatments will gradually help hair regain its beauty. Also try cream rinses and after-shampoo conditioning treatments. They are very beneficial for damaged hair.

Split ends. Split ends are caused by anything that causes dryness—a permanent, too much sun, and so on. When hair is dry, it breaks more easily. Then, if pins or rollers are yanked out carelessly, the ends split. The only cure is to cut them off. Split ends should always be trimmed off before a new permanent. Always try to be gentle in handling your hair, and try to counteract the dryness before the ends split.

❦ Which Hair Style for You?

There are several factors that determine your best hair style—the shape of your face, the various features that should be emphasized or minimized, your figure, your personality, and the type of life you lead. As a business girl, you'll naturally need an easy-to-manage style that looks crisply neat and attractive. It should be fashionable but should not be overly dramatic or so ultrasophisticated that it looks out of place with your trimly tailored business clothes.

For business your hair should be kept fairly short, preferably above shoulder length. If your hair is long, it can be swirled into a neat chignon or caught up in a neat twist of curls or swirls. Long, flowing manes detract from the look of efficiency and sophisticated maturity that every business girl strives for.

Do you know how high your hairdo should be to balance your face most attractively? Here's a guide to help determine the approximate maximum height that is most flattering. Once again prop a book flat under your chin as you face your mirror; then measure with a ruler. The length from the outer corner of your eye to the book should equal the distance from the eye corner to the top of your hairdo.

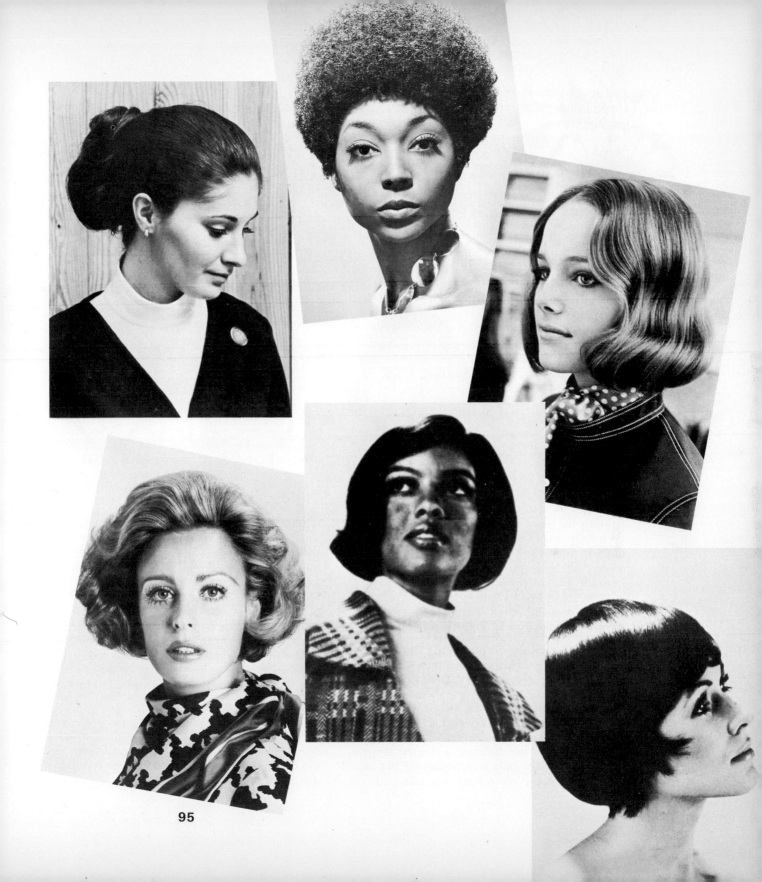

95

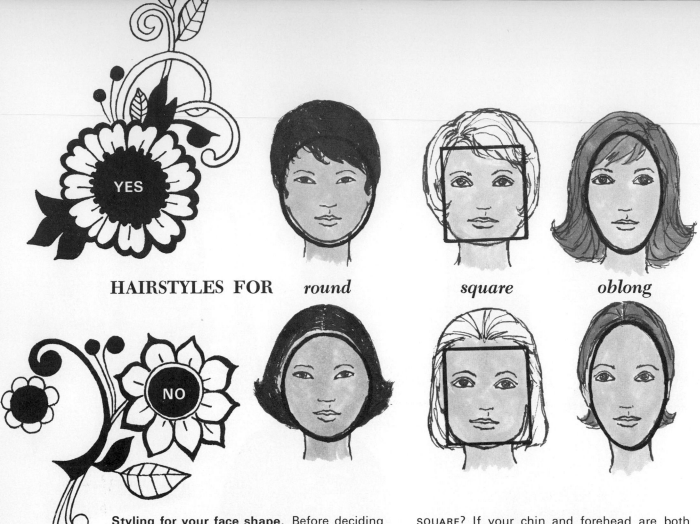

HAIRSTYLES FOR *round* *square* *oblong*

Styling for your face shape. Before deciding on a style, analyze your face to see if any camouflage tactics can be used to flatter your features. With hairdos, the idea is to create an illusion of width wherever the face is too narrow, to cover up any places that are too wide, or to disguise broadness by creating an illusion of slimness through adding height and length.

WELL ROUNDED? If you have full cheeks and a softly curved cherubic chin, your face may look almost round. To counteract this effect, you will want to keep hair fairly smooth at the sides, perhaps allowing a few curls to come forward over your cheeks. Soft curls and high waves at the top of the head will add height, and a little below-the ear fullness will give length. Because a center part is broadening, you will want to choose a more flattering side part.

SQUARE? If your chin and forehead are both broad, your face probably falls into the square category. Square faces have a look of strength about them, but they are usually most attractive when the sharp angles are softened by curving lines and the width is slimmed down. To achieve this effect, use either high top waves or a dipping side bang. Beware of flat center parts, straight-across bangs, or hair pulled back tightly at the forehead. You will probably look prettiest if your hair is shorter or longer than chin length, with a wave or curl coming in at the cheekbone.

LONG AND NARROW? Your aim is to cut the length of your face and to add fullness at the sides. Bangs are for you; brief, softly waved ones that dip to the side in an irregular line are especially good for shortening a high brow. Keep soft

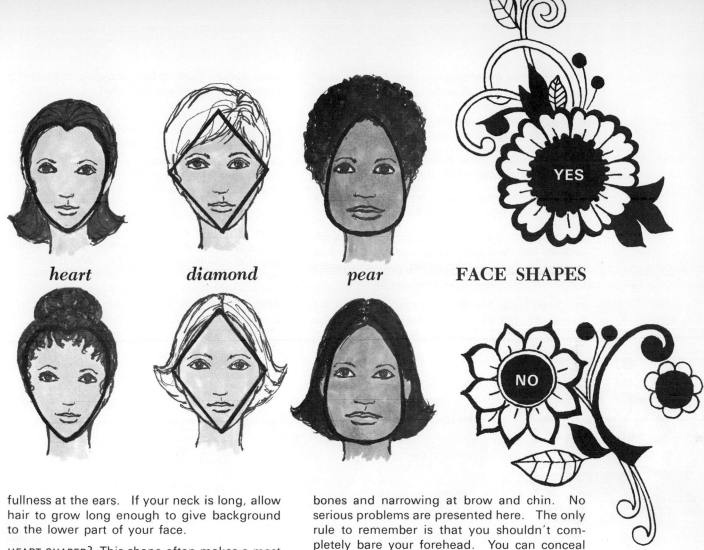

heart   *diamond*   *pear*   **FACE SHAPES**

fullness at the ears. If your neck is long, allow hair to grow long enough to give background to the lower part of your face.

HEART SHAPED? This shape often makes a most attractive face. If you have a pretty chin, perhaps you will want to play it up more by keeping your chin line clear. If, however, you wish to camouflage too pointed a chin, try soft curls below and behind the ears or a loose page-boy style. If you are lucky enough to have a widow's peak, which often accompanies a heart-shaped face, you can dramatize it by combing hair high or back to show off the hairline. You need only be wary of adding width at the temples. Keep temple hair smooth, perhaps allowing a soft, gentle, inward curve.

DIAMOND SHAPED? Many interesting faces have a diamond shape—wide through the cheek-bones and narrowing at brow and chin. No serious problems are presented here. The only rule to remember is that you shouldn't completely bare your forehead. You can conceal its narrowness with a short puffy bang that is wider than your forehead and perhaps flows into short curls at the temples to add fullness.

PEAR SHAPED? If your forehead is narrow and your jaw wide, you will want your hair to add width at the temples to balance your full chin. This is easy to achieve with a center part and curls at the temples, or use wide bangs to add breadth at the forehead. Although you will want to keep your hair smooth below the ears, you can try some of the dramatic, softly pulled-back Grecian styles with a cluster of curls at the back of the head. Short hairdos that flow up and back should also be flattering.

Consider the other angles. The front of your face is not the only view that you must consider when deciding on a hair style. Have you a special profile or figure problem? Your hair can help camouflage here, too.

HIGH FOREHEAD. Hide it behind soft bangs or hair that dips down over the brow.

LOW FOREHEAD. Add height by fluffing your hair up and back from your hairline.

GLASSES. Don't crowd your face with low bangs or with hair brought forward on your temples or cheeks, but you should let your hair partly cover the side pieces of your glasses.

RECEDING CHIN. Use fluffy bangs or waves at the forehead. Lift hair at the temples and let the sides sweep back softly, showing a flattering distance between ear and chin.

JUTTING CHIN. Avoid a flat line in back—no shingled styles. You will want to keep fullness at the lower part of your head and to use a soft puff above the forehead. Be cautious about trying bangs or any style that carries the hair down over the forehead.

PROMINENT NOSE. Keep hair interest back and away from the nose to provide balance. Use soft waves above the forehead to break a profile line that emphasizes the nose. Avoid a center part.

HEIGHT PROBLEMS. Check your coiffure in a full-length mirror before giving it your okay. If

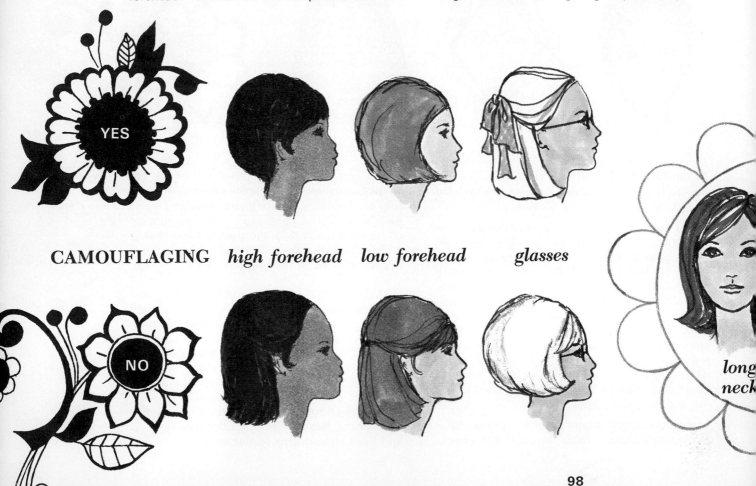

CAMOUFLAGING *high forehead* *low forehead* *glasses* *long neck*

98

you're tiny, steer clear of bushy styles or long hairdos and select fairly close-cropped coifs. Tall girls should avoid high top curls and cap cuts such as pixie or natural cuts that make their heads seem too skimpy for their tall frames.

FIGURE PROBLEMS. *Narrow shoulders and big hips* call for neither too wide nor too narrow a hair style. Either extreme is unbecoming. *Large head, small body?* Choose a neat cap cut. *Large bosom?* Keep hair short to medium in length; avoid long bobs.

NECK TROUBLES. If your neck is short, keep your hair short and curled up, especially in back at the nape of the neck, where you should be able to see at least the curve where the neck joins the shoulder. A good deal of the neck should show. If your neck is long, keep your back hair long enough to cover part of the neck and to fill in below the ears.

Next time you shampoo your hair, have a little fun experimenting with a variety of suds cap coiffures. While your hair is soapy, you can test the effect that will be created by a dip at the temple, a high-rising pouf, hair bulk at different heights along the side of your face, hair swirled forward onto the cheek or swept back behind the ears, and so on. Try the effect of various coiffure lines to see what they do for your features. Concern yourself only with the basic outline of the style, and check the profile and back views to determine what is most flattering.

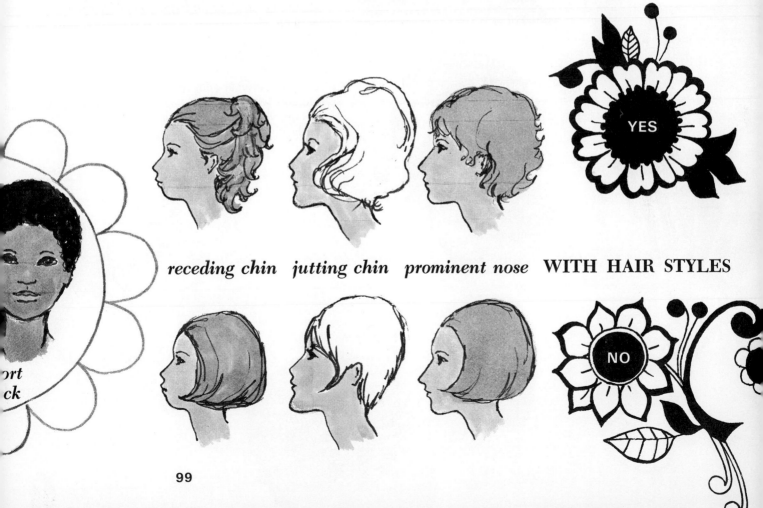

receding chin   jutting chin   prominent nose   WITH HAIR STYLES

YES

NO

99

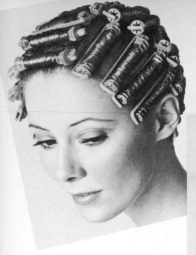

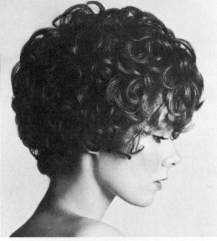

🌷 The Importance of Good Cut

A good cut is essential for hair to look its best. The most skillful setting can't compensate for a choppy cut. Cutting and thinning your own hair is an art you can't master until you grow eyes in the back of your head. Leave this to a hairdresser. He knows the intricacies of making your particular type and texture of hair look its best.

Even if you're letting your hair grow, it's a good idea to have your hair shaped every so often so that it keeps its good line. Each hair doesn't grow at the same rate, and the best cut can become straggly. Trimming is particularly important before you get a permanent. All split ends and remnants of an old permanent should be snipped off before a new permanent is given.

🌷 Long May It Wave

Unless you wear your hair poker-straight or are blessed with hair that has a natural tendency to curl, you will probably need to give your hair body in some way. Texture improvers, wave

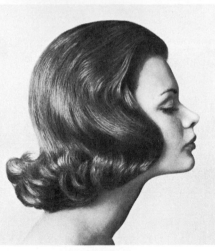

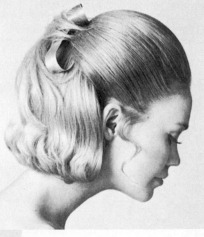

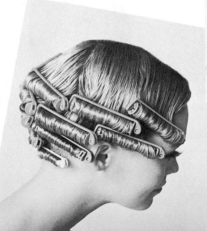

100

set products, and hair sprays give your set greater longevity, and a permanent is a great boon for locks that tend to go limp.

Many girls have become quite expert at using home permanents. There are many varieties available that can be suited to your hair texture, to the amount of curl desired, and to the time you have available. Whether you give yourself a permanent or go to a beauty salon, insist on a test curl first to be sure you will have no unpleasant reactions to the chemicals. Even if you have used the same brand before, take time for test curls. Your body changes continually, and you may have developed an allergy to some of the chemicals or, although extreme caution is taken by the manufacturers to keep each batch of wave lotion the same, some slight variance might affect you. Your hair is such an important beauty asset that you don't want to risk unhappy results. If you use a home permanent, never save leftover permanent waving lotion or neutralizer. Once opened, they deteriorate from exposure to the air.

The main purpose of a permanent is to give the hair body. Some women make the mistake of thinking that a tight frizzy permanent will last

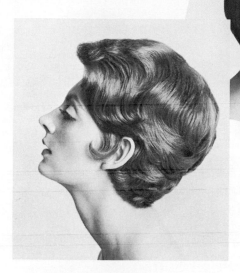

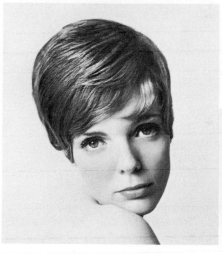

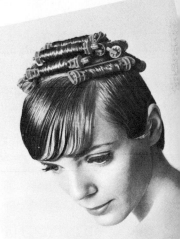

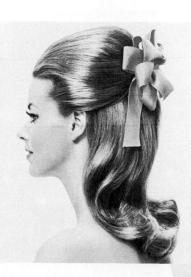

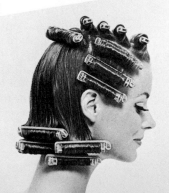

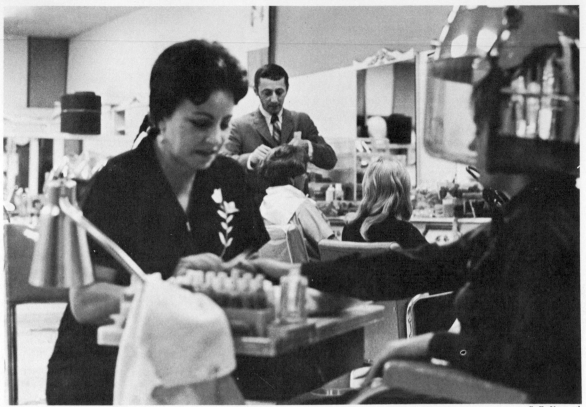

A trip to the beauty salon can be an inspiring and enlightening experience. Watch carefully how the operator sets your hair and later as he arranges your coiffure. You can often pick up tips to improve your own styling techniques.

longer. It never will look right, for by the time the kinkiness has worn off, the hair will be too long. Most hair still needs regular setting even with a permanent. A permanent merely makes the hair more curlable, but it is the set that creates the curl.

❦ The Smart Set

Save up your pennies so that every now and then you can treat yourself to a good-for-the-soul professional hair styling. Just the luxury of being prettied and pampered is enough to make any girl's spirits soar, but you can also

improve your own setting technique if you watch carefully and ask pertinent questions. Any hair stylist is willing to help you learn how to maintain the lovely coiffure he has created for you, so don't be afraid to ask for setting directions. Note particularly how and where your hairdresser places curls and the direction he pulls the hair before starting to wind it.

To locate a good hairdresser, ask friends whose hairstyles you admire which hairdresser they go to. Many good operators work in local shops, and once you've found one who understands you and your hair, you're in luck. Incidentally, when you go to a beauty salon, be punctual. Time is money to a beautician, and it isn't fair to keep him waiting.

It's helpful to have some idea—but a flexible one—of the type of coiffure you would like. You already know your face shape and

102

what styles are generally most flattering. Some girls bring pictures of the hairdos they like and ask their hairdresser if he can adapt one to their particular features. As a busy career girl, you will probably want a style that is easy to care for and, unless you can afford to have your hair set professionally every week, you should be sure that your stylist understands that you don't want anything too complicated.

When he sets your hair, he will probably give you a box of clips or rollers so that you can hand them to him one at a time as he works. Before you go under the dryer, select a magazine to read. (You will, of course, leave the magazine in the drying room when your hair is dry.) Usually there is a regulator for the heat of the dryer beside or behind your chair. Keep the heat set high as long as possible and stay under the dryer until an attendant comes for you. The person who bobs up every few minutes to ask if her hair isn't dry yet is a nuisance.

When your hair is being combed out, avoid unnecessary conversation so that your stylist can concentrate. Notice the tricks he uses in arranging your hair. First he brushes your hair back hard. This softens the curls and puts snap in your waves. Then he carefully arranges the curls where he wants them so that your coiffure takes on line and form. Does he use light, lifting strokes when he combs your hair, perhaps taking just a few strands at a time? Does he back-comb or tease your hair to give it more body? When he arranges a wave, does he clip it in place and then give it a wisp of hair spray to encourage it to stay put? Does he brush your hair over the side of his hand to create a flip or to turn ends under? Does each curl or wave section flow harmoniously into the allover pattern? Watch his techniques so that you can duplicate his results at home.

When it comes to tipping, your stylist should receive from 10 to 20 percent of your total bill, depending on what is customary in your area, and a smaller tip should go to the person who washed your hair. Slip the tip into a uniform pocket if they are busy with other clients. When the stylist is the owner of the shop, you are not expected to tip him.

❧ The At-Home Set

With a little experimentation—and a few tricks in her curler bag—any girl should be able to turn out near-professional results at home.

Rolling your own. Rollers are helpful in setting high, loose curls or deep, soft waves. They are particularly desirable for removing the kinkiness from hair that is too curly. Select the size roller for the size curl you want: the thicker the roller, the looser the curl. Probably you will need two or three sizes. Plan your setting pattern beforehand—where to use little ones (short ends, sides wherever a tighter curl might be wanted, or where more body or lift is required), and where to use big ones (top waves, long ends). Section off a strand no more than a half-inch thick and not quite as wide as the roller. Before you start rolling, stretch the hair straight up and a little back from the way you want the curl to go. The trick is to get all the ends folded neatly around the roller, so that there will be no bent or unset ends. If you have difficulty, cover the ends with an end paper or piece of tissue. Curls should be rolled evenly, in straight lines. Each roller should rest directly in the center of its section.

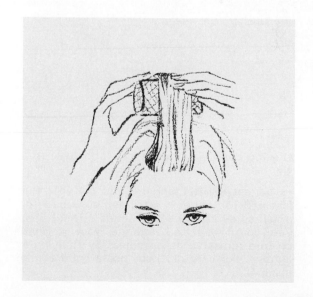

Pin curls. Pin curls don't provide as much lift and height as rollers, but with them you can create soft shadow waves as well as curls. To make a pin curl, block off a small lock of hair—no more than one inch square. Comb hair straight out or up, as the case may be, and place your forefinger directly in front of the strand, close to the scalp. (This curl will turn toward your face; for curls that turn away from your face, place your finger behind the strand.) Then wind the lock of hair around your finger smoothly and firmly. Slip the curl off your finger, carefully tucking in the ends so that there will be no frizzy tips. Secure the curl with a curl clip.

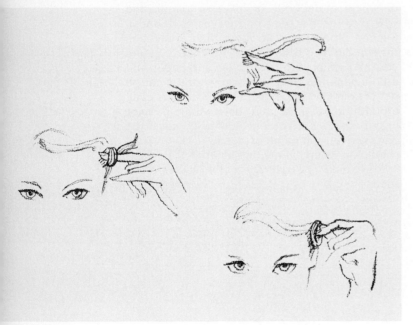

Curling cues. Try these ideas for a successful set.

• Your set will last longer if you wet your hair first and use either a wave set, stale beer, or a hair spray as you set the curls. Then, after you comb out and arrange your finished coiffure, preserve its prettiness by spraying it lightly. For very dry hair, use a hairdressing instead.

• When using rollers, crown hair will flow smoothly into back hair with no high-low dividing line if, for the last curls across the crown, the hair is pulled back at a 45-degree angle instead of straight up before winding.

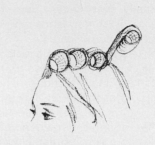

• If your hairdo tends to "break" between roller sections, make an uneven zigzag line when sectioning hair as you set it. Be sure a wound-up roller rests directly in the center of its section. Adjoining rollers can be clipped together.

• The placement of your finished pin curl and the direction in which it is wound determine the way your hair will go when it is combed out. For instance, if you want your hair to have a lift at the sides, pull the hair high before you start to wind and place the finished curl higher than its roots. Wind curls toward your face if you want your hair to come toward your cheeks. Wind curls toward the back of your head if you want a swept-back look.

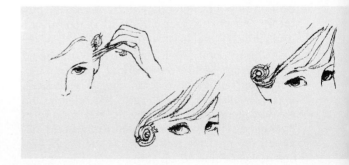

• To make a wave, arrange your pin curls in neat, even rows and alternate the direction in which the curls of each row are wound (one row all wound forward, the next row backward, and so on).

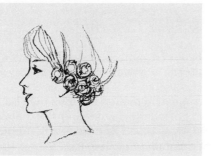

• Two or more rows of pin curls will produce a softer, fluffier effect than one row.

• If bangs are to be swept to the side, you can give them direction and height by combing them down on your forehead in the direction desired and applying tape to the ends. Instead of sticking it tight at this point, move the tape upward enough to create a curve in the bangs and then attach the tape firmly.

• Another trick for giving a soft lift to straight bangs is to pin a rolled facial tissue at your hairline and comb wet bangs over and under the tissue. Then pin the hair to the underside of the tissue to create a roll. This gives softer, fluffier bangs and avoids the childish, straight-across Dutch boy look.

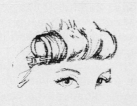

• Cheek curls can be set with transparent tape if your hair is coarse or curls easily. Set the curl in the desired position and secure it with tape until your hair dries. The same technique can be used with flat bangs.

• Hair worn short and straight in back will cling smoothly to the nape of the neck if a strip of tape is placed across these ends when the hair is set.

• If you put your hair up at bedtime, cover your curls with a kerchief or a frilly night cap to keep them in place while you sleep.

Tricks for emergencies. If your flip suddenly flops or if you were just too sleepy to put up your hair the night before, a set of heat-up

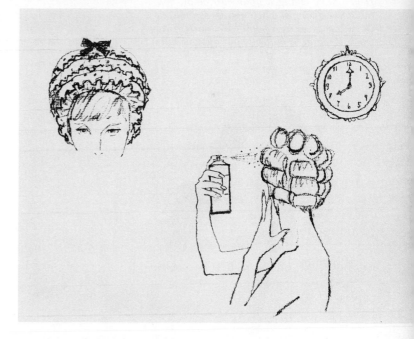

curlers (either electric or a hot-water variety) are handy for reviving your hairdo. Curling irons are also helpful. In lieu of these, try this quick pickup. Whip your hair up in rollers and spray thoroughly with hair spray. (Always hold the can 10 to 12 inches away so that you get a finely dispersed mist.) In about twenty minutes your hair should be dry, ready to comb into a pretty style.

Have a stubborn roller separation that won't blend in when you comb out your set? Teasing sometimes helps. Teasing will also give a sagging coiffure the extra lift and shape it needs. To do this, take a good-sized section of hair, hold it up or out from the head, and use gentle, light strokes to comb it, layer by layer, back from the tips toward the scalp. To prevent "ratting," work in a definite pattern from front of head to back. Lay each teased strand forward as you finish. Then after all strands are teased, smooth hair gently into place by brushing lightly over the top, starting with the lowest or last-teased section and working forward.

If you have changed your hair color, you have to be careful when you go swimming in the ocean or in a pool. You must rinse the salt water or chlorine out of your hair quickly.

Another trick for adding height is the lift-and-spray technique. First fluff hair as high as you want it. Then spray lightly and, before the spray dries, pick up small strands of hair with a rattail comb or pencil and lift again.

❦ Hair Coloring

Every brunette occasionally gets a yen to be a blonde and every blonde probably wonders how she would look as a brunette or a redhead. Appealing though the idea may be, any girl who is considering changing her hair color should learn as much as possible about how it will look on her and how it will affect her hair before she takes the drastic step.

Few girls realize what they are getting into in the way of expense and time when they decide to change hair color. Dyeing should be done by a professional. It must be done well or not at all. Unless directions are followed carefully, the hair can come out streaky or, worse yet, badly damaged and weakened. Dyeing is expensive and takes a great deal of time, and once you've started, you have to keep at it. Giveaway roots of another color just won't do. In addition, special aftercare is necessary so that the hair doesn't streak or become brassy or change color unattractively. Girls with dyed hair must be wary of the sun. Special hairdressings help; they should be reapplied frequently—every hour or so. After a swim, salt water or chlorine must be rinsed out immediately. You will also need special shampoos designed for color-treated hair and regular conditioning treatments. Dyeing is very drying, and hair becomes brittle and strawlike unless tended carefully. As you can see, there are likely to be many extra expenses involved, and these should be taken into account before you begin.

If you want to liven up your hair color, why not experiment with improving your natural color? Blondes who want a bit of brightening will find that Grandma's suggestion of a lemon juice rinse still is a valid beautifier. Temporary color rinses and shampoos are easy to use and

106

will add a little temporary color. Semipermanent ones add more color. Most varieties can be washed out with your next shampoo; others last through several shampoos. These products usually add sparkle and color highlights that dramatize your natural color rather than produce a drastic change of color. If your hair lacks oil, it's not advisable to use a color rinse too often. Both commercial rinses and lemon juice tend to have a drying effect.

If you do decide to change your hair color, heed the advice of the experts and go to a slightly lighter rather than a darker shade. A darker shade will look artificial and will not flatter your complexion. Occasionally a young girl—even a teen-ager—finds that her hair is turning gray. There's nothing more striking than a young face with lovely white hair, but if she is bothered by the change and wants to hide her gray hairs for a while, she should choose a color that is a shade *lighter* than the predominant color.

A note of caution: A skin patch test should be given before a hair dye is used to be sure you are not allergic to the ingredients. This patch test should be repeated *each* time you use it, because some people tend to develop a sensitivity later on.

❦ Wigs—Instant Hairdos

A flattering wig is an investment in fun. When your own hair droops, your spirits needn't. When you own a pretty wig, you're ready for any interesting or last-minute invitation. Some wigs can match your hair so perfectly that no one is the wiser. Others can create a new you—with a different length hair or a style your own hair just wouldn't adapt to. You may even try a different color. If you've thought about changing your hair color, you may find a wig is a better answer. You can enjoy the fun of a new hair color without the fuss, involved upkeep, and irrevocability of dyeing or bleaching. Best of all, you can be sure the results will be good before you commit yourself, because you can see how you will look.

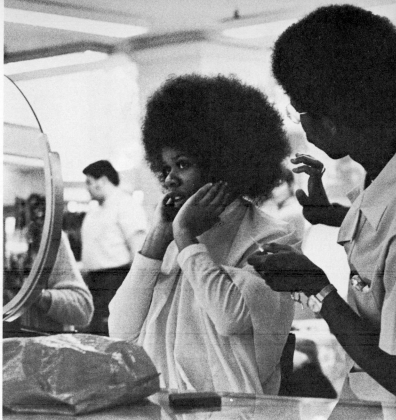

B. D. Unsworth

Wigs are available in a large variety of colors, styles, and prices. Most of them need some trimming and styling to make them suit your individual face and head contours.

Wigs come in both real hair (usually expensive) and synthetics such as Dynel and Kanekelon, which look amazingly real and are not expensive. The price usually depends on the quality and the length of the hair. The longer the hair, the more expensive the wig. In wigs of real hair, the type of hair is also a factor. Asian hair is less expensive than European hair, but it is also darker and coarser and lacks the color variations that are available in European hair. Some wigs are hand-knotted, others machine-made. Wigs of real hair usually must be professionally cleaned. Most synthetic hairpieces can be handwashed in gentle suds. (Check when you buy.) Also synthetic varieties are nonallergenic, nonflammable, good about humidity, and unaffected by sun. Furthermore, they won't retain odors.

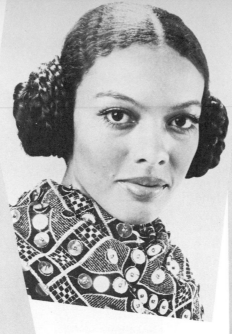

Add-on hairpieces and wigs—with or without parts—help busy girls present a well-groomed appearance on short notice.

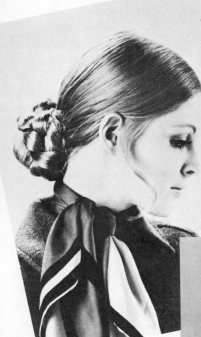

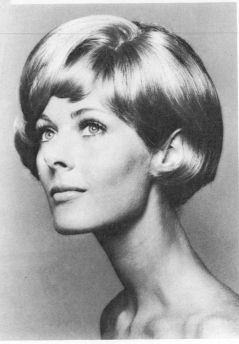

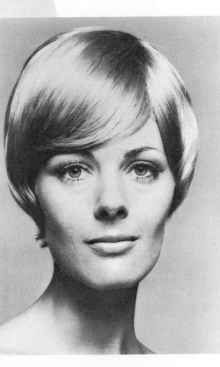

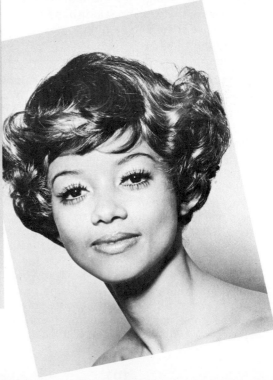

When you're buying a wig, try it on first. Buying by mail order is risky. Even though the stretch bases adjust to the shape of your head, they should be tried on. Some styles are bigger and deeper than others. If you have a large head, you must be particularly careful; too small a wig may have a bathing-cap tightness that won't be comfortable for long periods. A wig that fits properly should be almost unnoticeable to its wearer.

Check a wig you are considering to see how the hair has been attached to the base. It should swirl smoothly, the way natural hair grows; otherwise it won't be as easy to shape and style. To test this, spin the hairpiece in your hand and see if the hair swings freely as a unit with no stubborn wayward locks.

Don't be surprised if your wig needs a second cutting. No, the strands don't grow, but they may stretch a bit from brushing.

Any wig should be pampered to keep it at its best. After taking it off, brush or comb it so that it will be ready for the next wearing. Store it carefully (plastic head forms are a help for storing and for at-home stylings) and give it room to breathe. Wig boxes shouldn't be airtight. A chiffon scarf makes a good wrapping. For traveling, a simply styled wig can usually be stuffed with tissue paper and popped into a plastic bag. It will survive the trip handsomely. If you travel a great deal, you may want to try one of the wigs that holds its style even through washing. These are quite easy to maintain.

Keep synthetic wigs away from sources of heat. Very high temperatures can cause the set to "melt."

If your hairpiece seems to be suffering from static and fly-away jitters, the cure is cold air. Just put it in the refrigerator overnight and it should regain its neatness. Special sprays are available, but they should be used sparingly because the more you spray, the more often cleaning is necessary.

1 *Be on the alert for hairdo ideas that you can try. As you watch TV or look through magazines, study the hairstyles you see. Look closely at girls you meet—particularly those whose hair texture and face shape are similar to yours—to find flattering lines you might adapt.*

2 *Conduct a hairstyling session for yourself. See how your hair looks with different parts—a center part, various side parts, or a diagonal part. Then experiment with various hairdos. Can you wear your hair pulled back smoothly or do you need a softer, fluffier frame at the top? At the sides? How about bangs? If your hair is long, fold it up to see how you'd look in a short cut. Brush your hair forward at temples and ears, then backwards. Experiment with many styles and study your face and profile to see which are the most flattering.*

3 *When you have settled on a flattering hairstyle, play with it a bit to see if your everyday wear-to-work version can perhaps be glamorized for evening wear.*

109

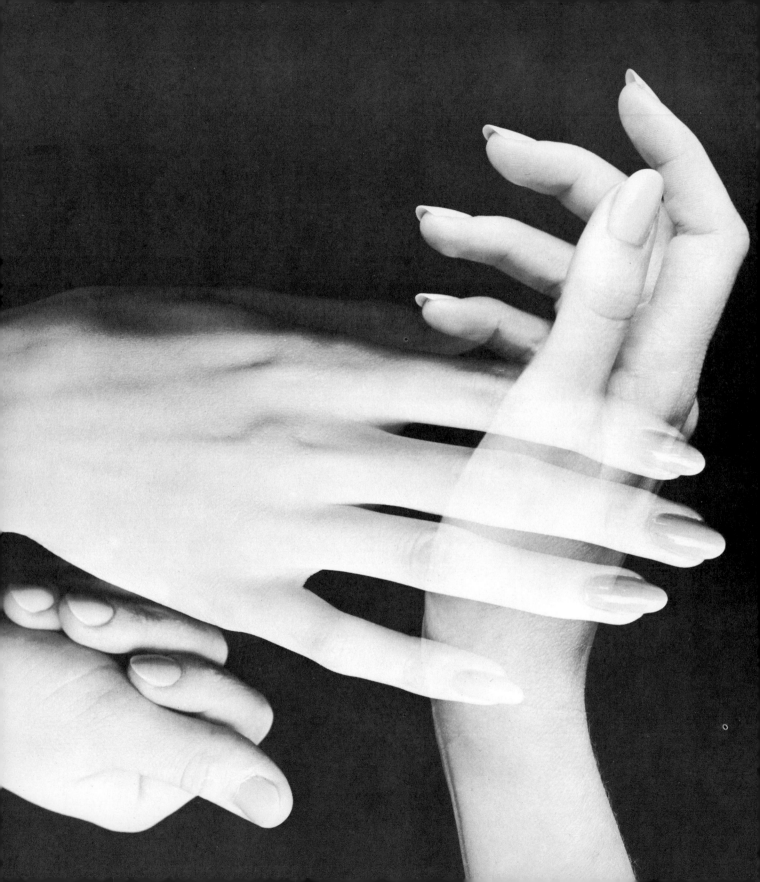

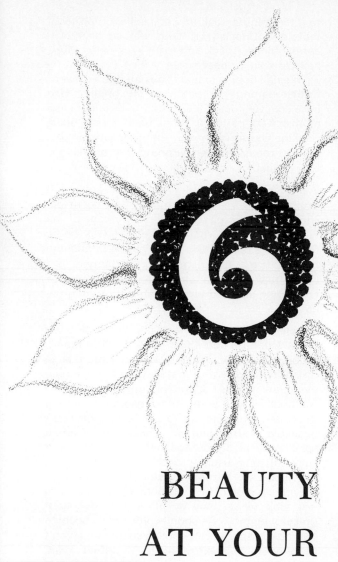

BEAUTY AT YOUR FINGERTIPS

For hands to have the smooth, clear loveliness that poets extol and the unchipped, color-coordinated nails that fashion decrees, frequent attention is required. But this attention is well repaid. A business girl's hands are always on display—as she types, files, operates a machine, or takes dictation. Graceful, impeccably groomed hands are a great asset to personal charm. A little attention several times a day is the best way to keep your hands smooth and soft. In fact, every hand washing can be a beauty treatment if you push the cuticle back with your towel as you dry. If your hands or nails become stained from carbons and mimeograph inks, use the special cleansers that are designed to tackle these stains gently and efficiently. When you wash your hands, scrape your nails along your palm to force the soapy lather under the nails and clean away germ-breeding dirt. After you dry your hands (thoroughly, of course), apply hand lotion if your skin is rough. Rub it well into your cuticles to prevent hangnails. Many career girls keep a small bottle of lotion in a desk drawer. Nightly use of a hand cream prevents troubles as well as curing them. Creams are more effective than lotions because the heavy consistency of the cream allows greater concentration of lubricants. While you're at it, rub a little cream on your elbows to keep them soft and attractive. As a special nighttime treatment for chapped skin, slather hand cream on thickly and don plastic gloves or an old pair of white gloves. Leave them on overnight, and your hands will be soft and lovely again by morning. But it's best to avoid chapped skin, if possible. One measure is to wear rubber gloves during washing and cleaning chores. Fabric-lined types are the most comfortable and don't cause hands to perspire. Teach your fingers to be nimble inside gloves. If a surgeon can perform a delicate operation while wearing gloves, any girl should be able to use them when she does her hand laundry or the dishes. Another hint: cream applied before tackling a dirty job prevents grime from being ground in, makes it easy to wash off. Also, in nippy weather put your gloves on before you go out the door. Don't risk chapping. If you have trouble with perspiring hands, you should rub in a little antiperspirant.

❦ Nail Problems

With a little extra care and forethought, you can eliminate most of your nail problems and make your nails healthier, stronger, and more attractive.

Weak nails. If your nails break easily, look to your diet. Foods rich in calcium (milk and milk products) and protein (meat, eggs, fish) help strengthen new nail growth. Many girls find gelatin, with its high protein content, helpful in improving nails—drink a tablespoonful of *unflavored* gelatin dissolved in a glass of fruit juice daily. (Don't be too impatient to see results. Only new growth can benefit, and it takes about four months for nails to grow out from roots to tips.)

Nail breakage can also result from an illness or run-down physical condition. The nail that was formed while you were sick or weak may be inferior, and this weak spot will show up months later when the nail grows out.

If your nails peel, dryness may be the cause. Skip nail polish for a while, because it tends to be drying. Wear rubber gloves for water chores such as laundry and dish washing, especially when you must use strong cleansers or scouring powders. When your nails seem dry or brittle, use a rich hand cream or nail cream nightly and occasionally treat your nails to a ten-minute soak in warm olive oil or vegetable oil. Check your filing method also. Incorrect filing—back and forth—can also cause nails to split or peel.

If a nail begins to tear, you can often prevent further damage by patching the break. Use base coat to glue on a tiny snip of tissue or wisp of absorbent cotton that has been spread apart until the fibers are gauzy. Then top with polish. Special repair kits for patching nail breaks are also available.

White spots or ridges. These marks can result from internal upsets but more often occur because of a blow or pressure on the base of the nail when this portion of the nail was being formed—a reason to be very gentle in pushing back cuticle. They cannot be eliminated, but if you feel they are unsightly, they could, of course, be covered with polish until they grow out.

Nibbled nails. If you are a nail nibbler, do make a determined effort to stop. Nail biting, though a difficult habit to break, subtracts so much from poise and maturity that you should overcome it as soon as possible. How? Methods vary. Some girls resort to painting their nails with one of the vile-tasting products available at drug stores. These are designed specifically to discourage nail biting (or finger sucking!) and usually work well. Other girls find success in merely fortifying themselves with the anticipation of how attractive their new nails will look when they've all grown out to a graceful length. As soon as your nails become passable, apply a pretty polish so that you won't be tempted to destroy the lovely effect. Bad habits are easier to break if you distract yourself from the habit. To discourage nail biting, keep your hands busy in another way—perhaps consciously try out attractive hand positions (possibly one that involves holding one hand in the other so that neither is available for nibbling). If you yearn to munch, try carrot sticks or celery for more rewarding fare. Before you know it, you'll be proudly displaying ten pretty nails and will no longer be embarrassed when people look at your hands.

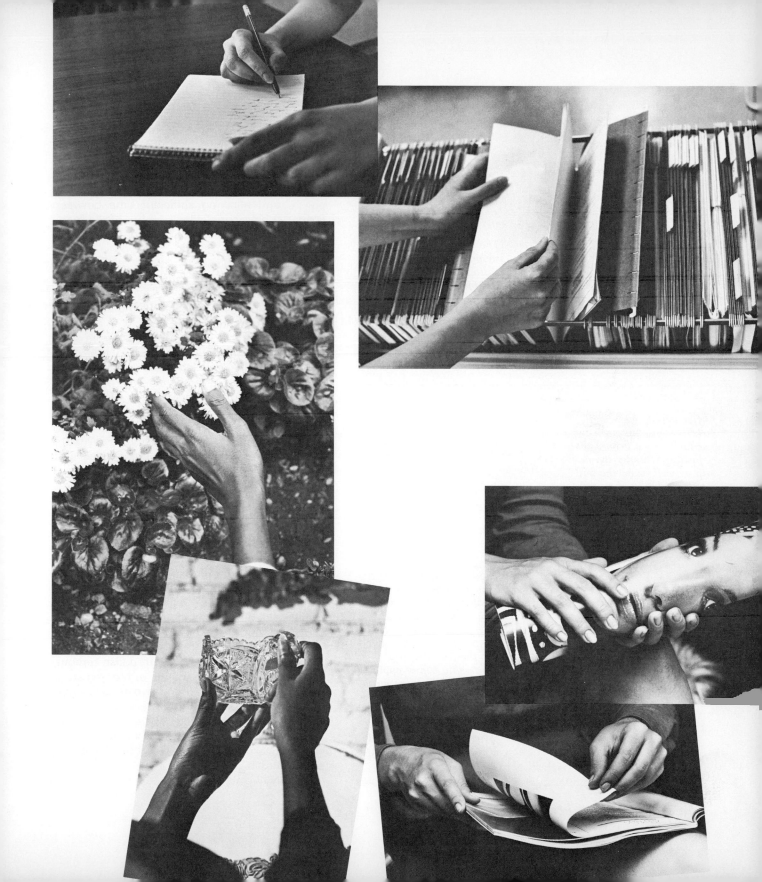

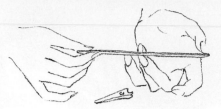

File nails in one direction only—from sides to center. Do not file deeply into corners or make extreme points. Keep nails in a graceful, oval shape.

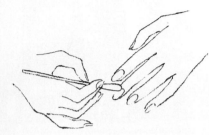

Then soak fingers in warm, soapy water. Push the cuticle back gently with the towel when you dry. Dip a cotton-tipped stick in cuticle remover or cuticle oil and push the cuticle back gently. Never cut the cuticle.

After wiping each nail with remover to clean the surface, apply a base coat, brushing it under the nail tip as well as on the nail itself to double the protection.

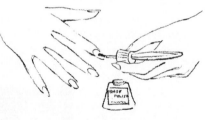

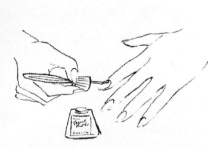

Apply two coats of polish. There should be just enough enamel on the brush to create an even flow onto the nail and give good coverage. Redip the brush for each nail. Let the first coat dry thoroughly before applying the second. As you finish each nail, wipe a hairline of polish from the edge of the tip to bevel the edge. When polish is dry, apply a protective top coat.

❧ Give Yourself a Manicure

You can easily give yourself a manicure that will rival a professional's if you follow the same procedures a manicurist does. This means using a base and a top coat (unless these are "built in" your polish), applying two coats of polish, and allowing sufficient time between coats. A manicurist allows an hour for a manicure alone, plus *plenty* of time for final drying. A good manicure should give you a week's worth of lovely nails—actually a timesaver when compared to the short lifespan of a halfway, slapdash job.

After you have removed all the old polish, follow the steps described here.

File nails in one direction only—from sides to center, not back and forth. Do not file deep into corners (leave at least one-sixteenth of an inch at each side) or make extreme points, but keep nails in rounded, oval shape. This makes them stronger and gives them a more graceful appearance. Hold the file so that it slants under the nail. Holding the file straight against the edge of the nail can cause tips to peel into layers.

Soak fingers in warm, soapy water and dry them thoroughly, pushing the cuticle back gently with the towel as you dry. Dip a cotton-tipped orangewood stick in cuticle remover or cuticle oil and apply it to the cuticle of all nails. Then gently push back the cuticle of each nail—never press hard. Snip off any stubborn hangnails but do not cut the cuticle. Cutting merely encourages the cuticle to grow back thicker and more ragged. Wash off the cuticle remover. (Never leave cuticle remover on for more than ten minutes.)

After wiping each nail with polish remover to clean the surface of any oil, dirt, or moisture, apply a base coat, carrying it over and under the nail tip to double the protection. Do your most difficult hand first (right hand for the right-handed, left for the left-handed). Allow the coat to dry thoroughly—until it is slick to a light touch.

Apply two coats of polish, doing your fingers

114

in the same order as with the base coat. There should be just enough enamel on the brush to create an even flow onto the nail and give good coverage. Redip the brush for each nail. Let the first coat dry thoroughly before applying the second. As you finish each nail, wipe a hairline of polish from the edge of the tip. This bevels the edge and makes the polish less likely to chip. When nail polish is thoroughly dry, clean up any smears, using a cotton-tipped orangewood stick dipped in polish remover. Then apply the top coat to the nails, bringing it over and under the edge of the nail to provide extra protection where polish is most likely to chip.

When you are finished, wipe the neck of each bottle with remover. This dissolves any hardened bits that might prevent caps from fitting tightly and postpones the inevitable thickening of the enamel. Nail polish that has thickened can be restored by adding a few drops of the *same* manufacturer's solvent. Never use remover for this purpose.

After a manicure it is important to keep those lovely nails from hard labor for at least an hour. Actually, nail polish takes several hours to harden completely, so you will want to guard your nails in every way possible. A good time to polish your nails is shortly before bedtime so that they have time to harden undisturbed. If you *must* work during the drying time, protect your manicure by being extra careful. The sprays that encourage quick drying of polish are helpful when you are in a hurry.

❦ Camouflage for Lovelier Nails

Occasionally a girl has nails so unattractively shaped that she doesn't want to call attention to them with nail polish. She can resort to colorless polish or to one of the lighter shades, but if she uses a few tricks in applying her nail enamel, an oval illusion can often be created. Round or square nails, which give the hand a stubby look, can be disguised if you don't carry polish all the way to the sides of the nails. If your nails fan out toward the tips, keep the polish away from the sides at the tips of your nails.

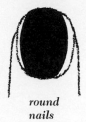 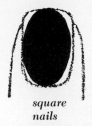 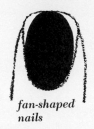

round nails   *square nails*   *fan-shaped nails*

Colored nail polish does tend to make fingers look longer. But if your nails are very short or bitten off, polish is a lost cause. Medium-length nails are best—short enough for efficiency yet long enough to form a gracefully tapered fingertip. Long claws make bosses and dates shudder. The soft colors that are currently fashionable are flattering to most hands. Dark or bright nail polish colors should be avoided by girls with heavily veined or bony hands. Dark colors attract attention to a problem that is best played down. Nail polish color must be coordinated with the rest of your outfit. It must match, or at least harmonize with, your lipstick. When your nails are a luscious pink shade and you suddenly decide to wear the dress with the orange trim, take time out to whisk a coat of "Pale Pumpkin" polish over the offending pink color. An extra coat or two of nail enamel will not do any harm, and it actually will make your polish more chip-resistant.

❦ Why Manicures Don't Last

If even a complete manicure—base coat, two coats of polish, and a top coat—doesn't hold up for you, do a little detective work to discover the cause of the problem. If nail enamel chips, the trouble may be due to:

• A film of oil or moisture on the nail when the first coat was applied. (Always wipe each nail with polish remover just before applying the base coat—no matter how clean your nails seem.)
• Polish that is too thin.
• Forced drying (putting your nails under cold water, blowing on them, or holding them before a fan or heater)

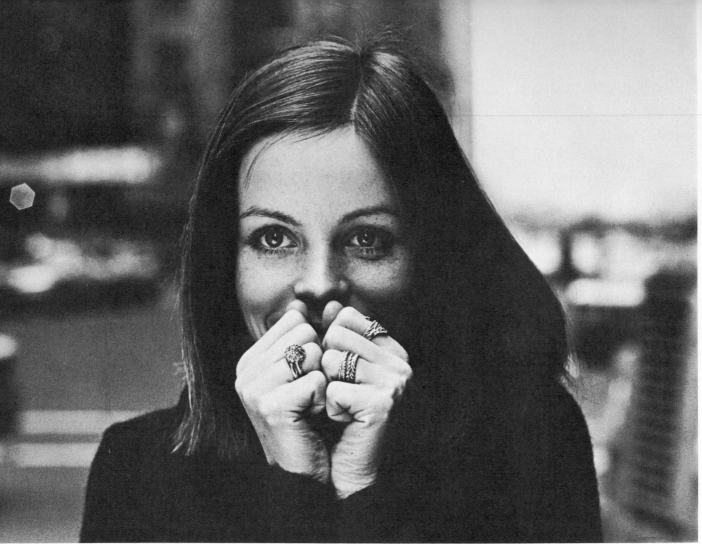

If nail polish peels, it is usually due to:

- A film of oil or moisture on nails.
- Enamel that is too thick.
- Application of a fresh coat before the preceding one has had time to dry properly.

The chief menace to manicures is, of course, rough treatment. Using nails as tools—to dial phone numbers, to pry open bobby pins, to slit letters—is murder for manicures. Make it a habit to use the balls of your fingers rather than your nails whenever possible. Harsh detergents, abrasive cleansers, and scouring pads also do damage. Wear rubber gloves for such cleaning chores.

Chipped or ragged polish can cancel out an otherwise well-groomed appearance. When you wear polish, it must be kept in perfect condition. Should a chip suddenly occur, remove the polish and do the nail again. When such accidents happen during office hours, a bottle of neutral-toned polish and some remover kept in your desk drawer will come to the rescue. Apply a new coat of polish to all nails, and once again your grooming rating rises. The place for such repairs is, of course, the ladies' room—never an office desk. The time—during your break or lunch hour. No boss will appreciate even the most perfect grooming if it is maintained at the expense of business time.

❦ *Rings on Her Fingers*

When your hands are smooth and well cared for, and your nails are shapely and beautifully manicured, the finishing touch to call attention to their loveliness is the right ring. Other than an engagement and wedding ring, which carry their own special aura, there are many types of rings that can add drama to your appearance.

Before you make a selection, consider the color of your skin and the type of metal that looks best against it. Gold ranges from white through yellow and pink tones; silver is beautiful against a glowing tan; and copper is dramatic for peach-toned skin. Because copper is generally casual, it is less versatile than other metals, however. Jewels, both real and fake, come in an astounding range of colors and shades; they, too, should complement your skin tone and should coordinate with the color and degree of formality of your outfit. In choosing stones, remember that strong colors are best on well-shaped hands with good skin color, because they call attention to any imperfections.

Consider, the overall size of the ring against the size of your hand and the length and shape of your fingers. As a rule, it is better to keep your ring in proportion to your hand rather than having it appear to weigh your finger down. Finally, select your ring to harmonize with or complement specific clothes. Not every ring can be worn day in and day out with every outfit.

1 *Give yourself a complete manicure, following all the steps a professional manicurist would use.*

2 *Start a hand care campaign today, devoting special attention to cuticle and nail health and to healing any roughened or chapped skin.*

3 *Are you remembering to lead with your wrists to make hand movements more graceful? Stand in front of a mirror and practice the hand-yourself-the-pencil exercise that was described on page 22. Let all your hand gestures be gentle curving motions.*

4 *The way in which a person shakes hands is sometimes taken as an indication of his personality. Make a conscious effort whenever you shake hands to use a firm but delicate touch.*

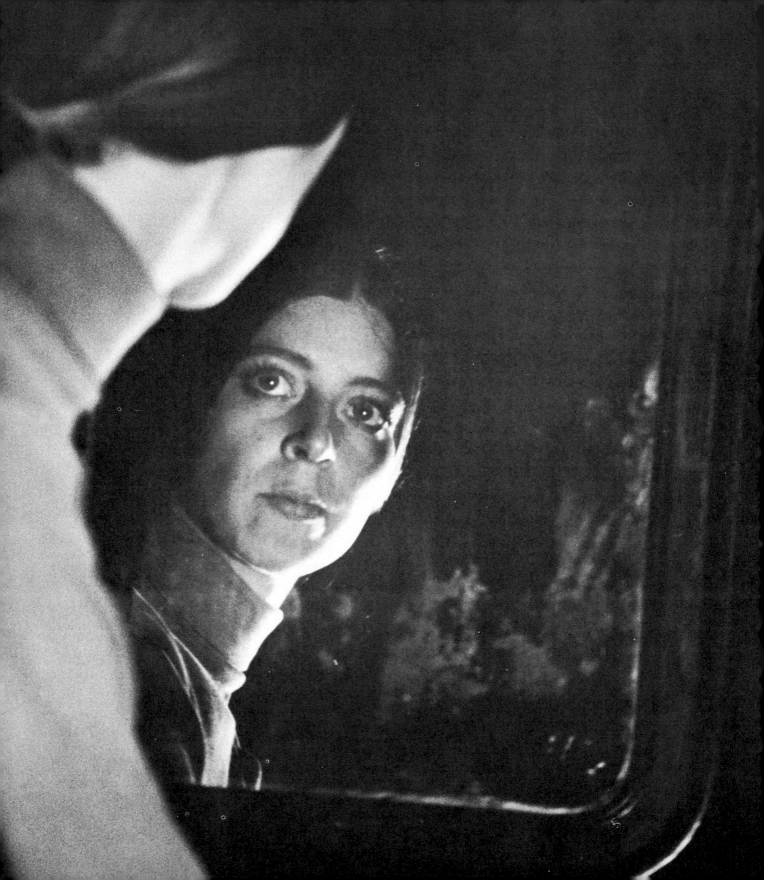

MORE THAN SKIN DEEP

The beauty of perfect features and a lovely body is only one type of beauty. More important in the impression we make on others is the beauty that comes from a likable personality. A face that glows with the warmth of a kindly, sparkling personality has a vivacious quality that is far more attractive than mere beauty.

Let the face you show the world advertise you as someone who is nice to know and fun to be with—but even more important, as someone who has the capacity to become a lifelong friend. Remember that too much reserve, whether it stems from innate modesty or a bad case of self-consciousness, detracts from charm because it puts people off. However, attractive facial expressions, particularly when they reflect sincere reactions, can make any girl stand out from the crowd as effectively as though she carried her own spotlight around with her. It's amazing how quickly a warm smile and sparkling eyes can charm friend and stranger alike.

This inner beauty that shines out through the surface is the kind that most quickly draws others to us. It is also the kind that anyone can develop. Rather than resulting from the luck of having had handsome grandparents, it comes from the humor, enthusiasm, kindly warmth and consideration, imagination, and individuality that you project.

Developing your personality to its fullest potential is extremely rewarding. It attracts friends, but, even more important, is the effect, on your confidence, your feeling about yourself, and your capacity to enjoy others.

❦ Beauty from the Inside Out

To help polish up your personality, consider the following qualities and what you might do to develop your own charm potential.

Humor. The gay, clever remark, the light mischievous touch—these make a person fun to be with. Some people have such a practiced sense of humor that gaiety comes easily to them. Others need to remind themselves to look for fun. Have you noticed how your own cleverness increases when you're with an amusing friend? You catch the same mood and are

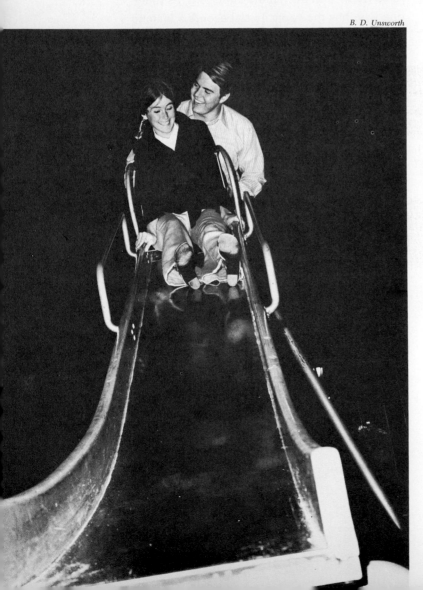

B. D. Unsworth

inspired to respond with humor that you might not bother to use with a more sober person. Humor, like playing the piano, improves with practice. The girl who feels hers could do with some improvement should analyze the humor of acquaintances she admires, should make a point of reading amusing writers, and should be on the lookout for things in her daily life that strike her as funny. It's surprising how many humorous little incidents we notice once we look for them. Often we're just too busy or don't bother to notice these small bits of humor but they make good anecdotes to pass on to others—and in the meantime provide a bit of lift for our own spirits. Look around for the humor in life and you'll easily find it.

Sometimes one of the best places to look for humor is in yourself. Learn to laugh at the silly things you do. Maybe they are a little embarrassing, but often they can be funny, too. A professor of psychology used to say, ''If your blunder won't make any difference three years from now, don't worry about it.'' Most of your goofs, horrendous as they seem at the moment, won't make much difference even three months from now. You're the only one who will remember them. And unless something can be done to make up for an error, you might as well just laugh it off and chalk it up to experience.

Imagination. Like humor, imagination sets a person off as being more interesting and clever than the rest. Like humor, it also improves with practice. The most creative people have developed the habit of wondering about the things they see and, instead of stopping there, they go on to plan what could be done to improve a situation or make something more attractive. Become an analyzer as well as a keen observer of life and stir up your ideas to meet the challenges.

Enthusiasm. Genuinely shared enthusiasm is a delight. It gives a glow to its possessor and creates a warm bond with others. When you enjoy something, let your enthusiasm show.

Some girls naturally bubble over; others are more subdued in their appreciation. You needn't worry if the milder form is more natural for you. Enthusiasm must be genuine to ring true.

Some girls find it hard to be enthusiastic because they are born worriers or because they are so dragged down by the rigors of life. The cure: set about eliminating as many of the worries as possible, concentrate on the things you do enjoy, and try to look for pleasure in little things you do. Find pleasure in the look of a neatly typed letter, rather than distaste for the carbon that smudges your fingers. Enjoy the fun of a barbeque and overlook the bothersome flies.

Warmth and thoughtfulness. Warmth and thoughtfulness go hand in hand, and both easily come to the girl who is enthusiastic about her life and friends. She's engrossed in her pursuits and cares so much about her friends that she can't help expressing her warmth and thoughtfulness in almost everything she does. She knows that it's worthwhile to take the time to do an unexpected favor for someone, to pay a well-deserved compliment, or to ask about something that interests the other person. These are the friendly actions that bring people closer together and help them share in life more fully.

Individuality. In all you do—in the way you dress, the way you style your hair, the way you act—develop an individuality. Let it be *your* type of humor, *your* creative touch, *your* enthusiasm—not a cookie-cutter copy of the rest of your crowd, or even of your best friend. Develop your own flair, the personal style that brings out the best of the real you.

Analyze what your proper role is and stick to it. Perhaps nothing definite may come to mind immediately, but keep looking. You want to develop a style that satisfies your best standards. Study those you admire most—favorite friends, teachers, even historical figures and fictional characters. Some of their greatness will surely rub off on you as you gain inspiration

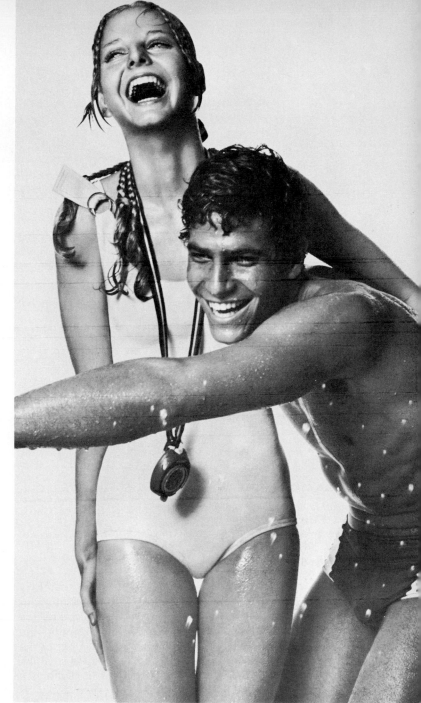

Courtesy of Harper's Bazaar

A sparkling personality is a lot more important in winning friends, both male and female, than beauty is. And enthusiasm is a big part of a sparkling personality.

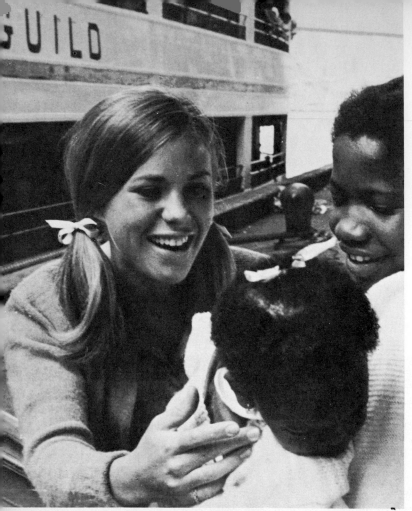

GUILD

You can have a good time by helping others. This girl is working on a hospital ship sponsored by the St. John's Guild of New York. A ship makes getting shots and taking pills seem almost like fun.

Courtesy of St. John's Guild

and ideas. In your investigation sift carefully what you can and cannot incorporate into your own behavior. Such analysis helps you decide if you can be cute successfully, can be the clown, really are the all-girl-athlete type, or the dainty hot-house flower. From earliest childhood some girls have a definite role, such as a natural regal dignity, that leaves no doubt as to the manner in which they should act; they just can behave no other way. Others have only a hazy idea, but at least they do know how they can't act without the taint of phoniness.

Your personality will grow and change as you are exposed to more of life, but always try to project the best of your own individuality.

❦ Be Happy

The happy person is a more desirable companion than the gloomy one. Try to keep yourself in a good mood and you'll find it easier to be good-natured in your relationships with others. Here are some hints for increasing your happiness and helping prevent the petty annoyances that can be depressing.

• Accept others as they are and don't compare yourself with them. Concentrate instead on appreciating them as they are and on making the most of what you have.

• Veer away from petty criticism. Don't let mistakes, mixups, unintentionally tactless remarks, bad weather, or other mishaps spoil your days. The girl who can make fun out of a rainy picnic will endear herself to all her friends.

• Use your senses to the fullest. Many a day that's drab for others will be a pleasure to you because you've trained yourself to enjoy details they're not aware of at all. By using your eyes, your ears, and your other senses carefully you can add to your enjoyment of life. You will be aware of the beauty of cloud formations, the playful glee of youngsters, the delicate lacy pattern of leafless branches, or the bracing aroma of good coffee. Don't overlook your share of the beauty that is available for us all to enjoy.

• Develop your interests. Become engrossed in a hobby or join an amateur musical group. Work backstage in a little theater, do volunteer work for a hospital, political candidate, or charity organization, take evening courses in subjects that interest you, learn new sports—the possibilities are many. Such activities help you to grow and to develop appreciation of new and different things. Often they also bring you into contact with new people and help you make more friends.

• Weed out any strangling self-pity ruthlessly. A certain masochistic pleasure can be derived from picturing ourselves as "poor little me." Sometimes we tend to flaunt our difficulties almost proudly, and often we use them as excuses for inertia and lack of effort. All of us have limitations of some sort. It's how we surmount these limitations that reveals our strength and character.

❦ *Let Your Charm Show*

Have you ever met someone who seemed rather cold at first but turned out to be a wonderful person once you got to know her? Most people are a bit hesitant to make friendly overtures unless they are fairly sure they'll be well received. A forbidding exterior scares them off and a deadpan gives no clue as to what to expect. Let your smile, your laugh, the look in your eyes, even your gestures and movements express your good feelings so that others will know how nice you really are.

The sparkle that popular girls possess is the result of cultivating the art of expressing their emotions. As any good actor knows, developing an expressive manner is an art. The accomplished actor uses facial expressions and gestures with restraint. His actions are subtle, natural outcroppings of the personality he is portraying. So, too, must yours be. They must be natural and must express *sincere* feelings or they will seem false or comical.

Cultivate a smile. An easy, natural smile is the most important facial expression anyone

Gloria O. Smith, "Miss Black America," has no problem letting her charm show. She has been a great morale booster to American troops whom she has entertained on a U.S.O. tour of Vietnam.

Black Star

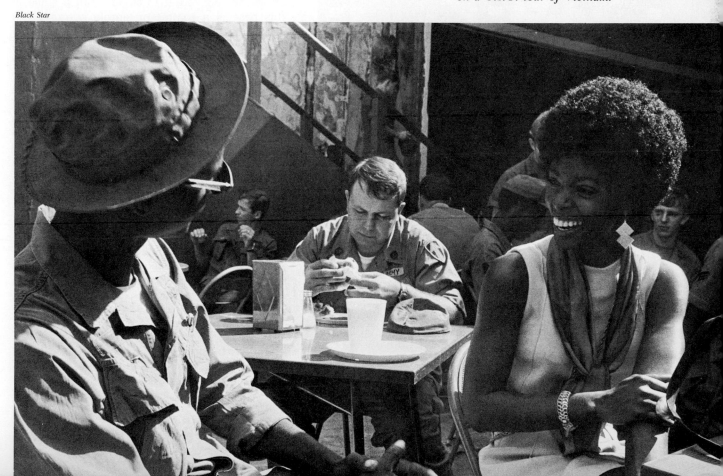

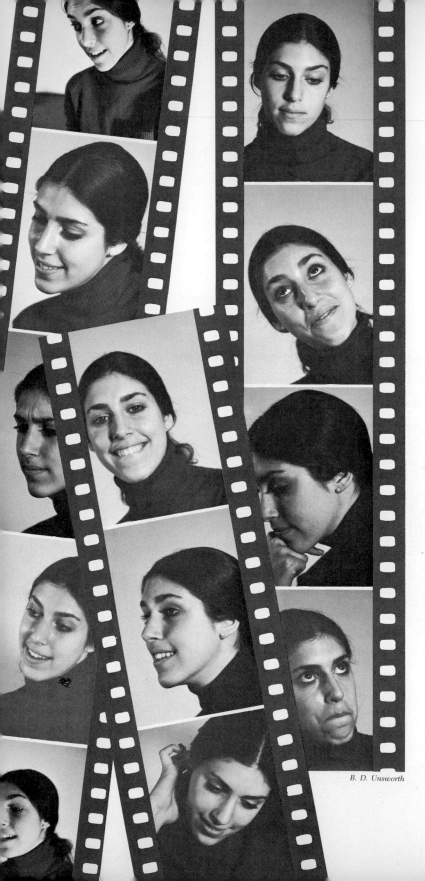

B. D. Unsworth

can have. When you have made a happy smile a habit, you have a beauty asset that will keep your face pleasant and youthful no matter how many gray hairs the years bring. Just as good posture is a matter of good habits, a cheerful expression is often merely a habit of remembering to smile. Although we may feel quite pleased with our world, we are sometimes just so naturally lazy that we allow our faces to remain blank. How much prettier is the girl who lets her pleasant feelings light up her face!

Conversely, when your spirits are low, do your best not to advertise it by your expression. This only spreads your gloom and can often increase it. Unhappy expressions are too costly to tolerate; if they become habits, they can actually distort features.

Sometimes nervousness causes our faces to remain blank, such as when we must speak before a group. We are so involved with the effort that we forget to smile. But a smile in this case is a matter of simple courtesy. It shows your listeners that you appreciate their attention. Needless to say, they will be more impressed by what you say if you back up your words with a gracious, friendly manner.

Whenever you feel self-conscious, take a deep breath to relax and then make yourself smile pleasantly. Just this small act of bravado helps conquer nervousness, makes you feel more self-confident. It also goes a long way toward hiding your insecurity. No need to tell you that a smile is contagious. Perhaps you can promote an epidemic!

Let your eyes sparkle. When you enjoy something, show it. Let your eyes radiate your delight. A sparkling expression is something you can develop if it doesn't already come naturally. Eyes can dramatize feelings with great effectiveness and subtlety. Let the sparkle in your eyes proclaim you as someone who's fun to be with.

Listen with your face. Some of the most successful conversationalists are the best listeners. Your face can often say more than words in encouraging a speaker. Let your features and expressions respond to his words and reflect his feelings. Show that you are concentrating on what he is saying by letting your eyes follow his. Blink occasionally to avoid staring. Nod slightly when you agree with a particular point. Even without saying a word, you will seem to speak volumes with great eloquence and understanding.

Mix with moderation. Any recipe for developing facial vivaciousness should include the caution "don't overdo it." Excessive mugging, screaming enthusiasm, and clownish behavior are childish. Any facial expressions you adopt must be an outgrowth of *your* personality. The too-cute wrinkling of the nose or the affected sidelong glance can be deadly if practiced by the wrong type. In everything you do, you want to express the mature warmth and kindness of a poised, cultivated young woman.

Check your unconscious expressions. Many people are unaware that they possess unpleasant facial expressions that give a wrong impression. Such things as frowning while concentrating, biting your lips, drumming your fingers, screwing up your face, or otherwise distorting your features unconsciously can make you seem unpleasant. Check yourself frequently for a day or two to be sure no bad habits have crept into your expressions.

1 *For one whole day see how many sincere compliments you can pay.*

2 *Act out the following situations, remembering to use your eyes as well as your mouth to reveal your feelings. Talk aloud and make up the dialogue as you go along.*
   a *You are greeting a good friend you haven't seen in some time.*
   b *Someone has just surprised you with an unexpected gift.*
   c *You are showing a friend a little baby robin that fell from its nest.*
   d *You are describing something beautiful you have recently seen or heard.*

3 *Demonstrate different expressions by acting pleased, angry, surprised, pained, sympathetic, humorously aloof, disappointed, impressed to a "Wow!" degree, and so on. Add your own ideas to the list.*

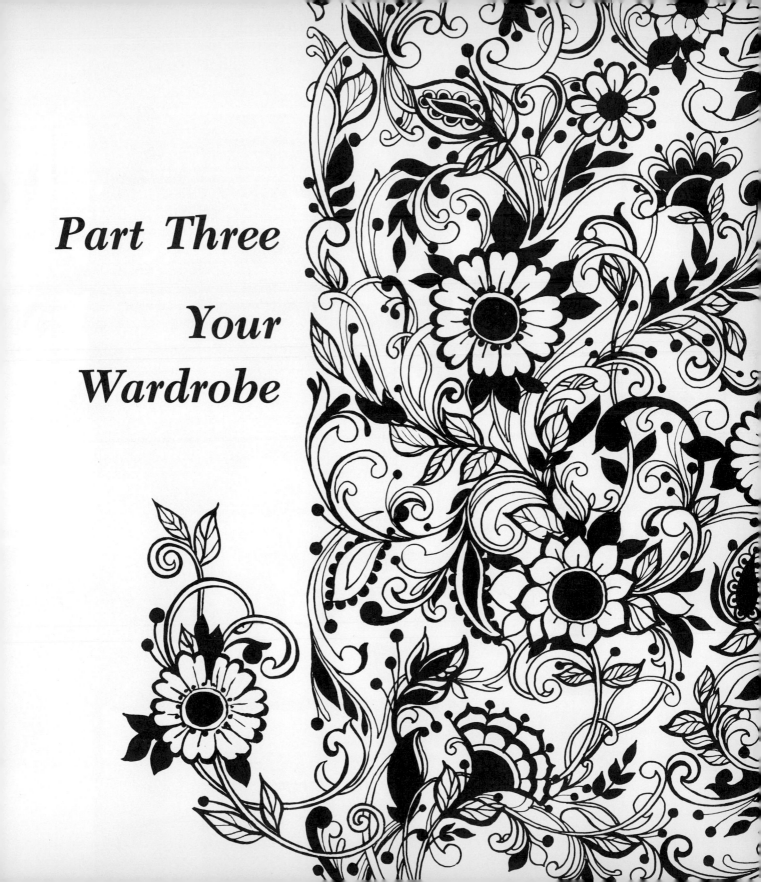

Part Three

Your Wardrobe

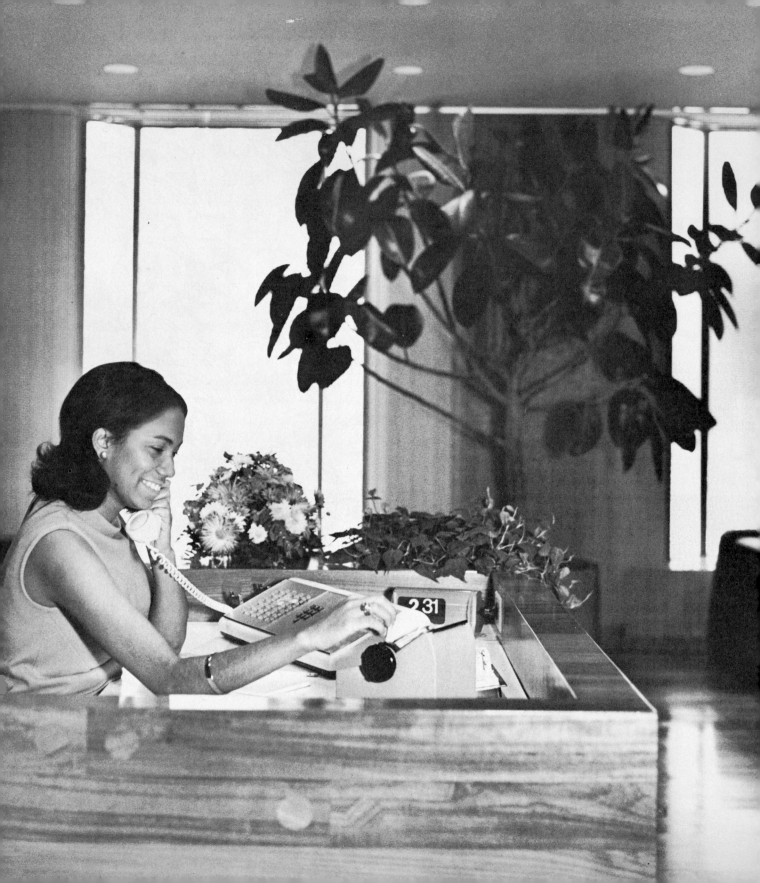

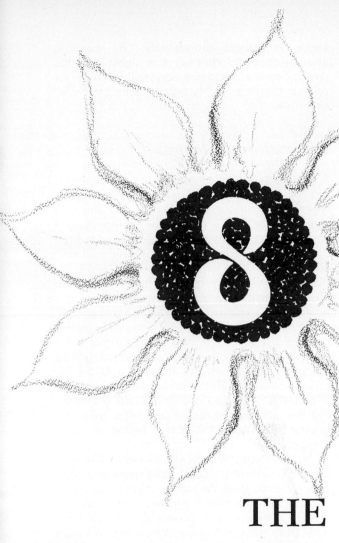

THE
WELL-GROOMED
LOOK

Who's the girl with the crisp, fresh look? You, we hope. In the business world you're not just under obligation to do a good, conscientious piece of work. Part of the bargain is that you look decorative while you're doing it. Companies often spend large sums of money to make their reception rooms and offices into glamorous settings, and they expect their employees to help further the effect by always appearing perfectly and tastefully groomed.

Of what worth are the potted philodendrons, the lavish draperies, and the modern furnishings if the customer is confronted with the sleepy-head who staggers in, featuring curlers and kerchief, or the gumchewer in the grimy blouse with a button missing? The customer won't be taken in by the elegant props. People, not props, produce the services and products he buys. After all, the company *is* the people who work for it. Their appearance reflects strongly on its reputation.

Not only the big brass and the board of directors are concerned about employees making a good impression. Your own particular boss is also mighty interested. Your good grooming is evidence that he knows how to pick a smart girl—that he's a pretty clever fellow. He may be only third assistant to the purchasing agent, but if he can choose an attractive and charming girl friday who's efficient as well, his prestige has leaped several notches. Needless to say, when he can take pride in you, the benefits are sure to bounce back your way.

Priceless as the well-groomed look is, it can be had for the taking. We all know the requirements of good grooming, but most haphazardly-strung-together characters feel they can occasionally get away with breaking the rules. "Nobody will notice that tiny rip," they tell themselves. Or, "I'm too tired to set my hair; it will just have to do." How they kid themselves! Everybody else is tired and busy, too, when it comes to an unpleasant chore, but smart girls make themselves do it. Men, particularly, have a keen eye for this type of neglect. The boss may not notice whether a girl wears the green suit with the gold scarf or the gold dress with the green scarf, but just let the hem sag or the spaghetti sauce splatter and his

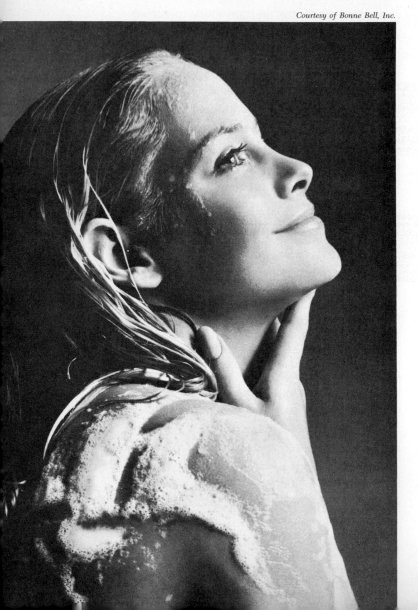

Courtesy of Bonne Bell, Inc.

eagle eye focuses immediately. He sees you on rainy days and after big date nights, and this day-in-day-out exposure crystallizes into an opinion that is a mighty potent factor at promotion time.

❦ Sweet and Clean

A daily bath or shower is the first line of defense against causing offense. A bath should be a thorough scrub session, yes, but it needn't be put on a par with a chore like hosing down a truck. Treat yourself to some of the bubble bath or bath oil preparations that leave your skin soft and silky and help waft tensions and troubles away with their relaxing fragrance. Give special attention to your elbows and feet, particularly the backs of your heels. A wet pumice stone can be used to rub off any unbecoming calluses. If you wish, dab on cologne or toilet water when you're finished. Apply cologne to the pulse spots—wrists, the inside of the elbows, the back of the knees—for the most effectiveness. If you're office-bound, please let this be only a discreet touch of a light fragrance. Anything too strong or too heady is inappropriate.

After a bath, ensure all-day daintiness with a good deodorant. Some girls mistakenly feel that it's enough to *be* clean. Unfortunately, a bath is no safeguard against future perspiration. Worst of all, the person who offends with body odor is usually completely unaware of the problem. Every girl owes it to herself to use a good deodorant *each day* throughout the year. Nervousness, hurry, tension, wearing heavy clothing indoors in winter, or the shock of cold when we go outdoors can cause perspiration troubles. Some girls find a deodorant loses its effectiveness through regular usage and that they have better protection by alternating brands.

If perspiration is a problem, choose a deodorant that is also an antiperspirant. Roll-ons or creams give the best protection. Some brands also come in an extra-strength version for those who perspire excessively. To be most

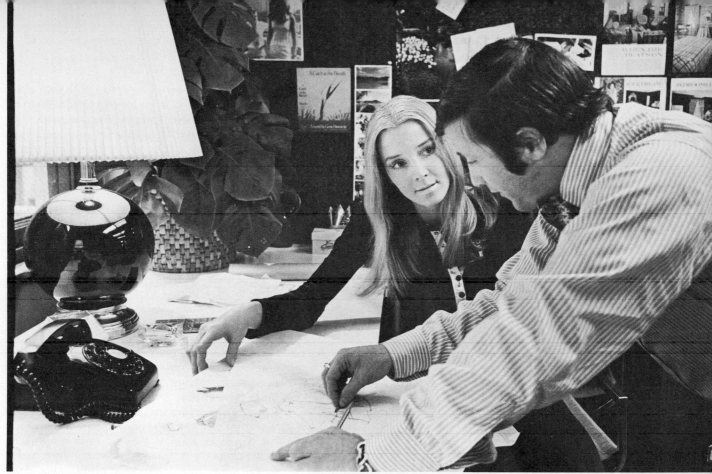

effective, antiperspirants should be applied to clean skin that has been thoroughly rinsed (remaining soap may interfere with the action of the chemicals). Use a generous amount, cover the entire armpit area, and go up onto the shoulder muscle. Cover an area as wide as a dress shield. Some girls need the protective build-up of two applications a day—one following a bedtime bath and a second the next morning. If nothing seems to control perspiration sufficiently, you might ask your doctor for a prescription antiperspirant.

Perspiration stains on clothing can be avoided by using dress shields, which should, of course, be laundered after each wearing.

A shaggy-dog look can spoil the appearance of the prettiest legs. If the hair on your legs is dark enough to be seen through your nylons, take a few minutes to defuzz them at bathtime.

In an office you often have to work closely with other people, so you must be careful of body odors.

Water-softened hair is easier to shave. If you use a safety razor, apply a shaving cream or rub the soap cake right on your wet skin to form an easy-gliding surface for your razor. If you use an electric razor, be sure your skin is thoroughly dry. Depilatories also do a thorough job. The new growth comes in just about as quickly after their use, but it is less stubbly than shaved hair.

Underarms must also be kept hair-free. Underarm hair not only looks unsightly, but it also tends to hold perspiration odor. During hot, sleeveless-dress weather, underarms must be shaved every two or three days, sometimes oftener. A daisy-fresh appearance can be shattered by whiskery underarms.

131

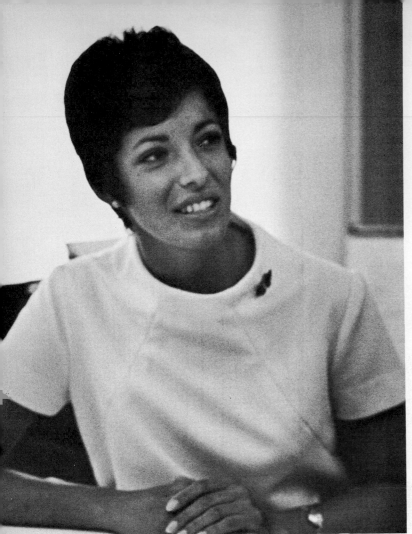

Employers appreciate the girl who manages to look neat and fresh all day, even in the midst of a hectic whirl.

While we're on the subject of cleanliness, let's not forget your teeth. Far too many people brush their teeth when they get up in the morning and neglect the toothbrush the rest of the day. Actually, the best time to brush is right after each meal, so that you brush away food particles that create mouth acids and cause cavities. You'll be able to do this if you keep a brush and a small tube of toothpaste in your desk at work.

An electric toothbrush and an electric jet water sprayer for teeth are marvelous for doing a thorough job at home. But at home or at work, dental floss is very helpful in dislodging food that has been caught between teeth. As you run the waxy floss between your teeth, you remove particles your toothbrush can't reach. Cleaning your teeth properly also helps keep your breath fresh. And when you have a hamburger with onions for lunch, you won't have to advertise the fact to the rest of the staff if you keep a package of breath-sweetening tablets or a small bottle of mouthwash in your desk drawer.

❧ Lovely All Day

Many a girl starts the day looking neat and fresh, but six carbons and three rush jobs later, her careful grooming may have wilted unbecomingly. The girl who's always well groomed is vaguely aware of her appearance at all times. Not that she's the constant primper (who drives everyone to distraction), but she takes enough pride in her appearance to scrub her hands as soon as they become smudgy, to clean spills on clothing right away, and always to be sure that she'd look presentable if an important visitor should arrive. Her grooming does no sorrowful "P.M. fade," because she occasionally checks her hair and quickly attends to any straggly ends. Whenever necessary, she cleans smudges off shoes, realigns a slipping scarf, smoothes a curling collar, tucks shirttails in securely, and checks face and fingernails for telltale grime. When good grooming is an automatic part of your life, you keep your morning freshness all day.

❧ Menstrual Care

During your menstrual period it is more important than ever to guard your daintiness. Despite the old wives' tales that are sometimes still whispered around, a daily bath does no harm during menstruation. In fact, it's more necessary than ever. Menstrual flow develops an unpleasant odor when it comes in contact with the air, and most girls also perspire more during this period. Change pads or tampons frequently, pay extra attention to cleanliness, use a deodorant powder on pads, and you can cross off any worries about embarrassing moments or offending odors.

Some girls notice that a day or two before menstruation they may feel more tense, more tired, perhaps slightly depressed. This is a perfectly normal reaction—as is the fact that your breasts and abdomen seem to swell and become tender at this time. Don't let it get you down. Take your mind off yourself and try to do things you enjoy. A little more rest and a little more exercise will probably help. Incidentally, many girls ask if they can go swimming during their periods, if they should wash their hair, if they can go horseback riding, biking, skiing. The answer to all these questions is yes. By all means keep up the activities you participate in regularly. The one precaution is that you do not allow yourself to become chilled. Avoid swimming in cold water and lying around in a wet suit—not the best of practices at any time.

If you are bothered by menstrual cramps, here are two exercises that should help alleviate them.

• Lie flat on your back on the floor. Breathe deeply, expanding your abdomen as much as possible while you breathe in and contracting it as you exhale.
• While lying on your back on the floor, bring your knees up close to your chest and hold them there. This stretches the opening of the vagina and promotes relaxation.

❦ Clothing Care

A girl can be wearing a dress that's straight out of *Vogue* and recently bore a three-figure price tag, but if it's wrinkled or stained by perspiration or if there's hair and dandruff on her shoulders, she might as well be wearing the $5.98 number from the bargain basement. No outfit can look smart unless it is kept in good condition.

Dresses, separates, suits, coats. Brush them after each wearing before you put them away, and give them a quick check for any spots, rips, or loose buttons. Give special scrutiny to elbows, underarms, neckline, cuffs, and hems. While you're wearing the outfit, you often fail to notice these areas. (Plastic cuff-protectors will help keep long sleeves from becoming soiled while you work.) If a dress needs pressing, keep it at one end of your closet—away from clothes that are ready to wear—until you have a chance to press it. Incidentally, many

Courtesy of Bonne Bell, Inc.

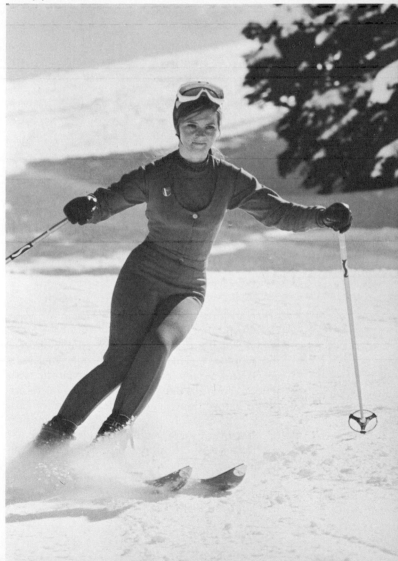

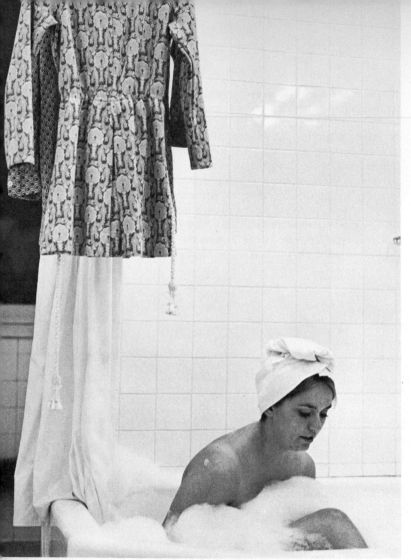

B. D. Unsworth

pressing jobs can be avoided if you hang your clothes in the bathroom while you take your shower or bath and let the hot steam remove the wrinkles. This works especially well with wools and crepes, but you must be careful with rayons, because they may shrink. Never steam moiré, lamé, heavy satin, taffeta, faille, or brocade. Instead, give them a very light pressing on the wrong side, using a cloth that is just slightly moist. Cottons and other washable fabrics can often be made quite presentable without ironing if you pat the wrinkled areas lightly with a wet washcloth and hang them in the open until they are dry.

Whenever possible, give your clothes an airing after they are worn. Hang them inside out and air them outdoors if you can. If not, hang them before an open window. Whenever you hang colored outfits in a sunny spot, it's especially important to turn them inside out to protect them from fading. This is also a good precaution to take when drying laundry.

Stain removal. When you iron clothes, be on the lookout for any stains you may have missed. Never press over a spot, because heat often sets the stain. Keep a bottle of cleaning fluid and other cleaning essentials on hand. If you can't remove the spot yourself, take the garment to a cleaner as soon as possible. If you know what caused the stain, tell him so that he won't have to experiment needlessly.

GREASY STAINS. To remove a stain made by butter, grease, mimeograph ink, wax, or other greasy materials, first wash the fabric as usual. Then work detergent into the stain and rinse with warm water; dry. Next sponge the stain with grease solvent and dry. If the garment is not washable, use only the grease solvent treatment, repeating until the stain is gone.

NONGREASY STAINS. Nongreasy stains can be caused by alcoholic beverages, antiperspirants and deodorants, candy, catsup, cocoa, coffee or tea, egg, ink, perfume, or a scorch. Sponge or soak the stain with cool water. Work detergent into the stain and rinse. If the stain persists, use bleach. If the garment can't be washed, sponge the stain with cool water. For a stubborn stain, work detergent in, soak for at least a half hour, and then rinse.

COMBINATION STAINS. Some stains contain both greasy and nongreasy substances. Chocolate candy, coffee or tea with cream, gravy, ice cream, mayonnaise, and milk all cause combination stains. For a washable fabric, sponge or soak the stain with cool water. Work detergent in, rinse thoroughly, and dry. Then sponge the stain with grease solvent and dry. Finally, try bleach. For a nonwashable fabric, sponge the stain with cool water. Then work detergent in and rinse; dry. Sponge the stain with grease solvent and dry.

SPECIAL STAINS. Here are some tips for removing a variety of special stains.

• Blood is easier to remove if you put a few drops of ammonia on the stain first. Then soak in cold water and wash in warm water. Don't use hot water first; this will set the stains.
• Regular carbon paper calls for working detergent into the stain and rinsing well. Put a few drops of ammonia on the stain and then repeat the detergent treatment. For duplicating carbon paper, begin by sponging the stain with diluted alcohol. Then use the detergent treatment and wash and rinse well.
• Correction fluid is a job for the cleaner.
• Cosmetics can usually be removed from washable fabrics by working up thick suds from undiluted liquid detergent or soap and rinsing well. If the fabric is nonwashable, sponge with grease solvent before you try the suds treatment.
• Ballpoint ink usually comes out with a washing, but if not, try bleach.
• Fruit juices call for immediate rinsing, then treatment like other nongreasy stains.
• Mud can be brushed off if you let it dry.
• Nail polish can be removed with pure acetone (not nail polish remover), but don't use this method on silk or synthetic fibers.
• Perspiration stains call for a thorough washing or sponging with detergent and warm water. Color can generally be restored with ammonia and a rinse, but if the stain is old, apply vinegar instead of ammonia.
• Rust stains should be spread over a pan of boiling water. Squeeze lemon juice on the stains and then dry the fabric in the sun. Rinse thoroughly. Try a commercial rust remover for stubborn stains.
• Soft drinks are no problem. Rinse the spot immediately, then treat as a nongreasy stain.

You can cut down on cleaning bills if you run a cloth dampened with cleaning fluid around a collar before you press it. This is particularly important with coats, because the collar is on display every time you let your coat drop behind you over the back of a chair.

Storing clothes. Although sweaters and unlined loose-weave knits should be stored flat, double-knit suits and dresses can be hung. It's advisable, however to guard against shoulder ridges by using padded hangers or broad wooden ones. If you haven't any such hangers, pad your own by wrapping them with old nylons or thick cloth. Then cover them with a pretty fabric to liven up your closet.

A good way to keep the vinyl items in your wardrobe (coats, boots, hats, bags) clean is by using a detergent spray cleaner. It's fast and easy.

Courtesy of Texize Chemicals, Inc.

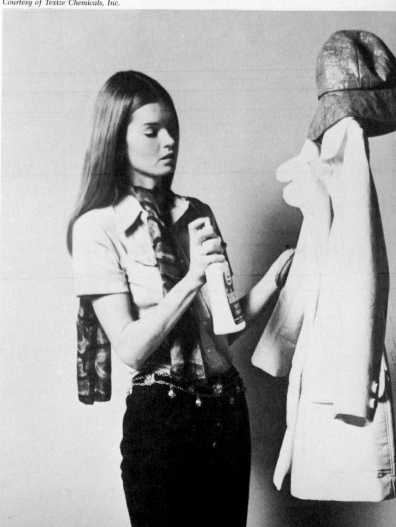

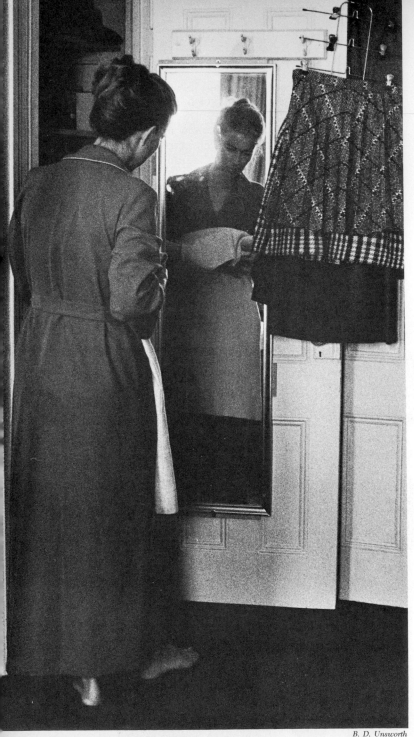

B. D. Unsworth

Your clothes will look their best if you hang them up right after you've worn them. Make sure the necklines are buttoned to prevent rumpling.

Closing dresses and blouses at the neckline before putting them in the closet allows them to hang smoothly and prevents collars from being rumpled. For further protection, use rod spacers to keep hangers from bunching, or try to maintain a two-inch space between hangers so that clothes won't be crushed. If your closet is crowded, see what you can do to create more room. Perhaps you can convert part of it into a double-decker section for skirts, blouses, and jackets by using two clothes rods, one suspended under the other by chains. Another thought: Keep separates at one end and fit shelves or a cabinet beneath. Or consider multiple hangers for skirts, blouses, and sports clothes.

Perhaps you're holding on to items that should be kissed goodbye. Before and after each season, weed out the tired, shabby, or outdated items in your wardrobe—you'll look better, feel more stylish, and have more free hangers. If storage space is at a minimum, possibly out-of-season clothes can be stored at a dry cleaner's (sometimes a free service if clothes are cleaned there).

Hemlines. In these days of changing hemlines, it's important that you keep your dress length fashionable. If your legs aren't quite show-off caliber, you can probably get away with wearing your hems about an inch or two below current fashion. But consider your hemline not only when you're standing but also when you're sitting, bending, or reaching high. You may find that you're showing much more of yourself than you think, particularly if you're a hippy girl. The cut of your clothing and the kind of fabric may also affect how much the hemline hikes up when you sit or bend. If you have difficulty keeping your garters covered, try panty hose.

Keep in mind also that standards of modesty vary. Many a girl has a business wardrobe that is an inch or more longer than her other clothing because she knows that her employer or his clients are upset by shorter hemlines. She may feel that their standards are old-fashioned, but rather than offend the standards they were raised to respect, she considers it more gracious to compromise a little.

Underwear. One of the most important points to remember about underwear is that it should be kept under. It should be completely invisible. No panty wrinkles or garter bumps allowed. (Garter bumps can often be avoided by rehooking the front garter—or by reversing the button tape—so that the button is turned in, toward your leg.) At neckline, underarms, or hemline there should be no peekaboo bits of white. Slip and bra straps can be kept under control when you wear a wide-necked dress if you use a dimestore lingerie guard that pins into the shoulder seam. When you take the dress off, you can snap the guard around the hanger to prevent the dress from slipping off.

It goes without saying that lingerie must be clean and should also be neat. Nobody else may know if you haven't had a chance to mend the lace on the slip you're wearing—but *you* know and can't help feeling a bit sloppy because of it.

Bras and girdles should fit properly and should be of sufficiently recent vintage that they do a good job. If you wear sheer blouses or dresses, be sure your slip covers your bra and is opaque enough and long enough to avoid telltale shadows. Never wear a black or brightly colored bra or slip with *any* light-colored blouse or dress—it shows through and labels you as a person who is careless about her grooming.

Odds and ends. Drooping or dirty accessories can ruin your appearance. Keep them in good order at all times.

HATS. Every once in a while, take a good, critical look at your chapeaux. Sometimes a hat gets a little battered and bedraggled without your noticing it. Be sure all trims are crisp and neat. If there is a veil, is it perky? A quick revitalizing trick for veils if you're late some morning is to run the veil over a lighted bulb. It will come out smooth and crisp.

If you have trouble keeping your hats on in windy weather, sew a small comb to the inner band at the front of the hat. Anchor the comb

137

in your hair at the front, put a hatpin in the back, and you're ready for the strongest blow.

SHOES. Regular brushing and polishing is essential for a well-groomed look. Keep some shining-up equipment in your desk drawer. A soft cloth saturated with a neutral liquid wax is very good for this purpose. Paper towels make a good emergency suede cleaner. If suede becomes scuffed, it can usually be rejuvenated with one of the special suede sprays. In general, watch for run-down heels or tips. A trip to the shoe repair shop as soon as you notice

Saturday morning is a great time to take care of those necessary jobs such as getting your handbag repaired, or getting something you need for your home.

B. D. Unsworth

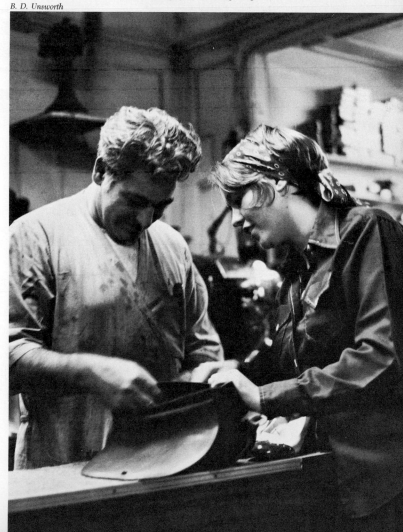

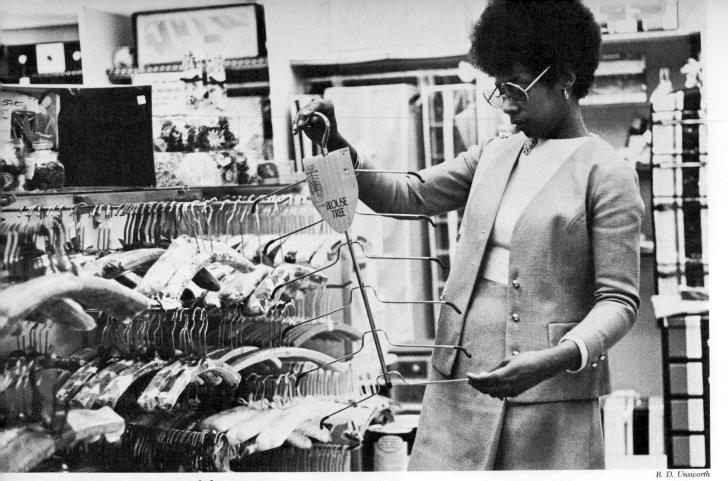

If your closets are overcrowded, you may be able to save some space by buying hangers that hold more than one item, while still keeping your clothes neat and wrinkle-free.

them can save you from having to buy new shoes. For the summertime problem of chafing from perspiration, put talcum in your shoes before putting them on. Air your shoes often and try to alternate pairs.

SHOE BOOTS. Wonderful for winter weather, they can save your shoe leather from wear and tear. They, too, need to be checked frequently for run-down heels and tips. Leather styles should be kept polished, just like shoes, as they will last longer under adverse conditions if you care for them well. You may want to keep a pair of shoes at the office for daily wear, or you can carry them in with you each day. There are many smart shoe bags available for this purpose.

PURSES. Shapely and unscuffed purses are a fashion must. Leather bags can be given new life with shoe cream polish in a neutral or matching shade. Plastics respond to soap and water. Suede requires brushing (in a circular pattern) with a suede brush. Fabric purses should be dry-cleaned. Occasionally turning bags inside out and brushing the linings removes the messy tobacco shreds, powder, dust, and who-knows-what that accumulates. When not in use, bags should be stuffed with tissue (so that they will retain their shape) and stored carefully in plastic bags to prevent scratches. Don't hang purses by the straps, as this will weaken the handles. To save space, a small bag can be stored in a larger one.

Occasionally take an inventory of the contents of your bag to see if anything can be discarded. Although men seem to have zillions of pockets, they don't appreciate your one lone carryall if it bulges or seems to overflow.

STOCKINGS. They should fit well without wrinkling or sagging. Any seams, ribs, or designs must lie straight, and there should, of course, be no runs, holes, or visible mends. Ankle smudges can sometimes be rubbed off with a *soft* eraser or a damp paper towel. Mud splashes usually cling to skin more than to hose and become almost unnoticeable if the stocking is removed and the leg is washed. Many girls keep an extra pair of nylons in their desks for emergencies.

If a snag or pull develops in an inconspicuous spot in a stocking, dab it with colorless nail polish to prevent major trouble. In a pinch, soap can be used as a temporary run stopper. Lightly apply a thick coating to the snag, and it will dry into a stiff protective crust. Later apply nail polish for more permanent protection.

ACCESSORIES. Your gloves, scarves, and jewelry should all be clean, neat, and fresh. Store them carefully to protect them from dust or wrinkling. Every now and then, go over your costume jewelry with a jeweler's rouge cloth or a silver polish cloth to remove tarnish and brighten the pieces up again.

❦ Morning Can Be Beautiful

Shortly before bus time Barbara reluctantly drags herself out of bed, grabs some cold cereal, and downs gulps of hot coffee as she slithers into the first blouse and skirt that seem to match. If time allows, she stuffs some jewelry into her pocket to be donned during her bus ride. Then a mad dash to the bus! By the time Barbara arrives at work, she may be fairly presentable, but her nerves are frazzled and her responses to the cheerful "good mornings" of the staff echo a bit hollowly. She realizes, too, that her appearance never has the carefully planned and coordinated look it could have.

When mornings become a hectic gray blur, no girl can look her best. The obvious solution is to get up a half hour earlier to allow enough

139

time for leisurely breakfasting and careful dressing—and, if necessary, for brightening drab spirits. But if this is too painful a prospect, you can save considerable time by planning the next day's outfit the night before. Switching handbags, laying out jewelry, hat, gloves, and special accessories, as well as all inner and outer clothing, makes dressing a speedy matter. It also allows time for experimenting with different accessories so that the same yellow scarf isn't always worn with the same brown dress. Of course, getting up just a little earlier is wise insurance—there's always the possibility that

B. D. Unsworth

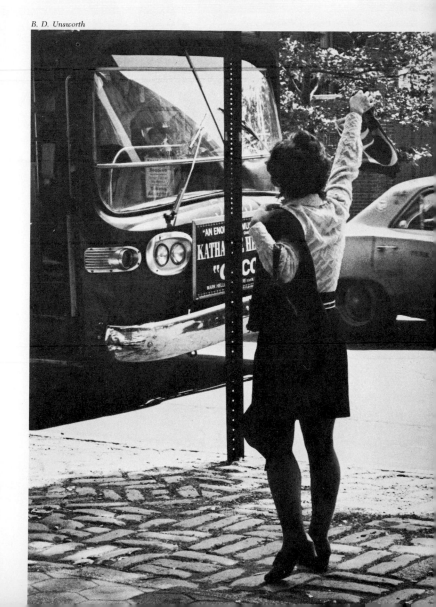

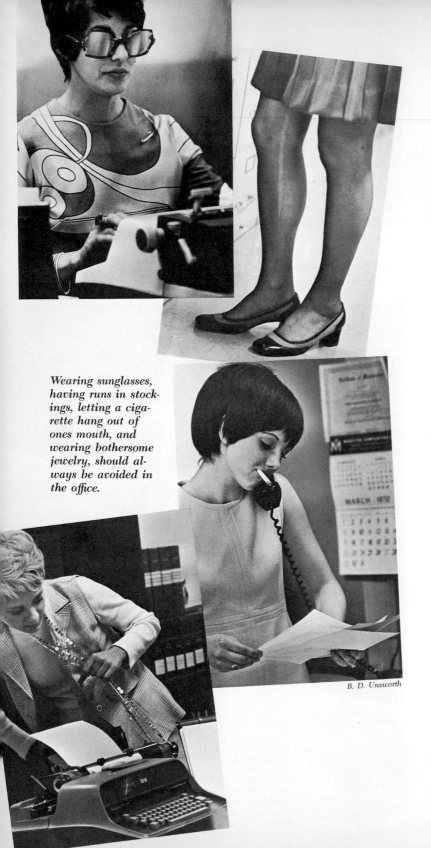

Wearing sunglasses, having runs in stockings, letting a cigarette hang out of ones mouth, and wearing bothersome jewelry, should always be avoided in the office.

B. D. Unsworth

there may be a downpour the day you'd planned to wear your new spring outfit!

❦ An Employer Speaks Out

An executive in a large plastics-manufacturing concern was asked for his opinions on what composed the well-groomed look for business girls. He was glad to have an opportunity to air his opinions because, as he said, far too many girls don't realize how important grooming is and how disturbing it is to employers to have shoddy-looking personnel around. ''We can't go up to a girl and tell her to do something about her hair or to go get a clean dress. We just look for some way to get rid of her as conveniently as possible.''

First on the executive's list came the request that clothes be neat and clean. ''A sloppy girl gets on my nerves. Some girls never notice annoying details like a skirt that's off center or a bow that's lopsided.'' Next he expounded on the need for tasteful and appropriate clothes. One of his pet peeves was outfits that were too dressy—necklines down to *there,* flashy fabrics, extreme styles, glittery jewelry. Another was distracting costumes—tight sweaters and skirts, form-hugging dresses, and short-short skirts. Also annoying were outfits that are too casual for office wear—bulky sports sweaters, casual flats, sporty school clothes, sunback dresses, jazzy hosiery—or other inappropriate items such as jangly jewelry or bulging handbags. Bare legs were also considered in poor taste. Now that air conditioning is so widely used in offices, there is no longer any excuse for stockingless legs. ''If a girl dresses like a businesswoman, she will be treated like one,'' he said.

Of course, your hair and makeup should be neat and appropriate, too. No extreme eye makeup or fingernails, either. But appropriate hairstyles are especially important. Stringy hairdos are strictly schoolgirl stuff. An employer is usually not too fussy about how you wear your hair as long as it's not terribly extreme and is clean, neat, and becoming.

A word to the wise: Don't do your prettying up at the desk and don't spend all day at it. An employer doesn't like to have to send the St. Bernards to get you out of the ladies' room. And a last vital point—when you stand up straight, you're helping yourself to appear better groomed.

❦ First Aid for Beauty

Every girl has a different idea of what grooming essentials she likes to keep in her desk drawer and carry in her purse cosmetic kit. The lists below are fairly typical and may give you some suggestions.

Some grooming needs for the desk drawer . . .

Cleansing lotion
Foundation
Rouge or blusher
Eye makeup
Hand lotion
Nail file
Nail polish remover
Colored nail polish
Colorless nail polish (run stopper)
Toothbrush, paste, and dental floss

Tiny sewing kit
Hair spray
Tissues
Cleaning fluid
Small clothes brush
Suede brush
Pair of stockings
Pair of clean white gloves
Compact rainwear
Collapsible umbrella
Shoe buffing cloth or shoeshine kit

and for the purse

Comb or brush
Bobby pins
Compact
Lipstick and brush
Nail file
Small safety pins (3–4)
Collapsible rain bonnet
Package of tissues
Breath sweetener
Needle and thread

---

1 Hold an inspection session of your entire wardrobe. Check carefully for any spots, split seams, loose or damaged buttons, weak straps, frayed edges, loose hems, soiled belts, dirty collars or trimming, wrinkles, and so on. Make a determined effort to see that anything wrong you discover is fixed as soon as possible.

2 What about your closet? Can you make it more tidy and efficient by rearranging shelves, adding shoe bags or other space savers, storing some garments elsewhere, if necessary, or trying some of the other suggestions in this chapter?

3 Take stock of your purse and your office beauty kit (if you are now employed) to see if there are any additional beauty or grooming aids that you might like to include.

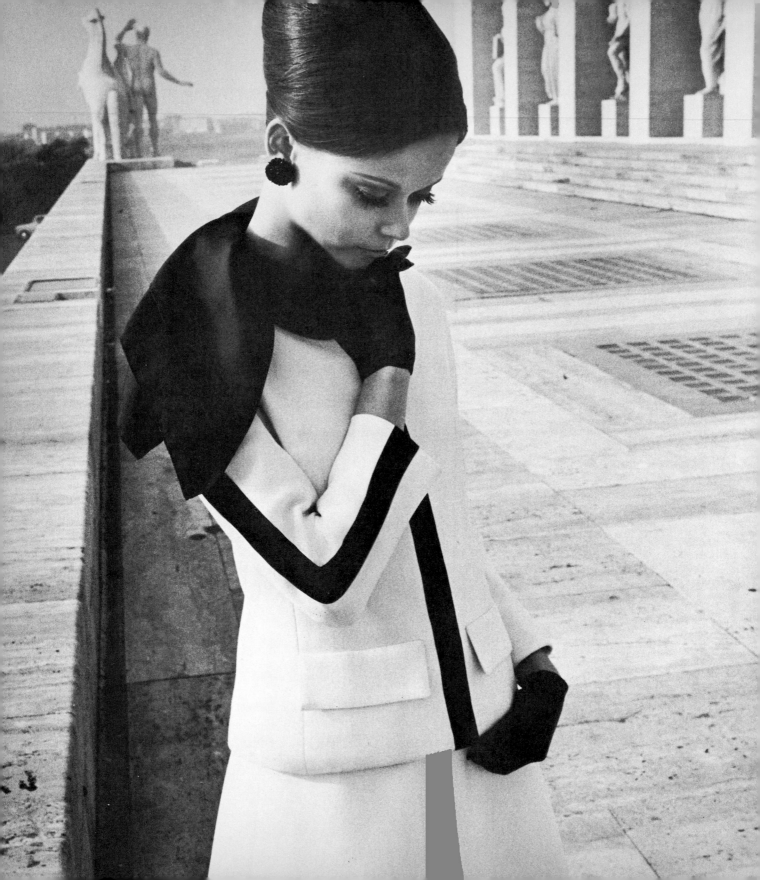

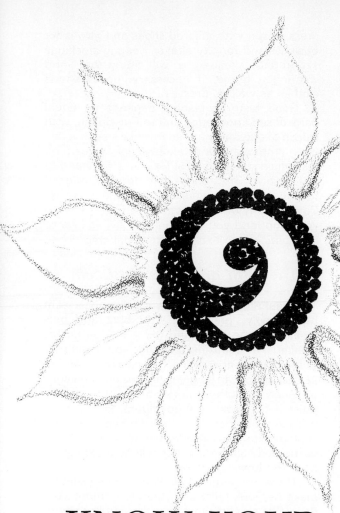

KNOW YOUR LINES

Rich or poor, fat or skinny, tall or short, we are all faced with the same problem—how to choose the clothes that are most flattering. If you are rich and willowy, with the preferred combination of horizontals and verticals, your task is, of course, considerably easier. But many girls who lack these plus qualities possess such a highly developed sense of fashion that they can give a look of chic and elegance to the simplest outfit.

Exquisite fashion sense is rarely inborn, but it *can* be acquired. Your taste can be sharpened by constant awareness and analysis of what *is* good fashion. Study the fashion magazines, the clothing ads, the window displays of the better shops, and the smartly dressed women you see. Scrutinize them carefully. Exposure to good fashion is an excellent teacher. Try to decide just what makes an ensemble outstanding. Is it the becoming design of the style, the beautiful coordination of color, or the clever use of accessories? Look for new features—a change in sleeve or collar, a jewelry fad, the set of the shoulders, a new silhouette shape. Consider what they would do for you. The girl who is on the watch for fashion smartness finds many ideas she can apply to her own wardrobe.

The essence of good taste is simplicity—simplicity with a flair, yes—but always refined, uncluttered simplicity. Tasteful attire is never ostentatious, never overdone, never offensively revealing in cut or fit, always appropriate. Good taste is conservative rather than spectacular. It lets you—not your clothes—be the star attraction.

In choosing a costume, the well-dressed woman considers what *lines* are flattering to her. Certain styles will dramatize your figure. Develop a clear, unclouded awareness of your good points and your bad points. Then select only those outfits with lines that do the most for you. Next, strive for a *coordinated look.* This depends on beautiful and discreet use of color and on a careful combination of clothing elements for each outfit. Dress, coat hat, jewelry, and shoes should all be equally casual or equally dressy and should all be in correct proportion to your figure and to each other. They should produce an attractive all-of-a-piece look. Third, the well-dressed woman is always *cued for the occasion.* Clothing must be appropriate—neither too casual nor too dressy. If you are in doubt about an occasion, wear an attractive go-everywhere dress rather than a party style that may seem overdone. In addition, your clothes should be *expressive of your personality.* What looks heavenly on one girl may be horrendous on another. Some girls (few) can wear ruffles and frills. Some girls (also few) can wear high-style exotic clothes. Discover what is right for you—the type of clothes that express the real YOU, the best you—and don't let yourself be hypnotized into buying something that is not your type. Of course, *fashionable timing* is essential—if you like a new fashion or new color and find it flattering, choose it at the upsurge of its popularity so that you can ride on its prestige. But be discriminating in your choice, and don't let fashion timeliness goad you into selecting something that isn't exactly right. The girl who throws caution to the wind and tackles an extreme or highly sophisticated fashion may find it more dramatic than she wishes. Keep pace with fashion as much as possible, always letting your own personality and physical enhancement be your first considerations. Naturally, no outfit is right unless it's a *good fit.* If it is to look smart, a dress must fit smoothly but not tightly, must set properly, and must be the proper length. Finally, being well dressed calls for *wearing all the essentials*—wearing a hat and gloves for church, wearing a trimly tailored

dress or suit with tailored shoes and gloves for business and for city affairs, wearing stockings year-round, wearing a well-fitting bra, and wearing a girdle, if necessary, under sports clothes as well as dresses.

Good taste in fashion depends on equal parts of self-knowledge and self-discipline, with a dash of originality added to make it completely YOU. Improve *your* self-knowledge by learning just which styles do most for you. Perhaps you will receive inspiration here for the original touches that give your fashions individuality. Combine this with unwavering self-control when you shop, and you will find your fashion sense blossoming into exquisite personal chic.

❦ The Slim and Shapely Look

The ideal American girl look is a slim one—slim but shapely, preferably with bust and hips measuring the same and the waist ten inches smaller. In choosing clothing, you should try to maintain—or create—this balance. An imperfect figure can be given an illusion of balance by wearing clothing lines and colors that disguise body flaws. A hippy figure, for example, will seem slimmer in the hips if you broaden the shoulder line and call attention to the upper part of the body so that the eye will be drawn away from the lower portions.

The average girl finds flattery in styles that make her look taller and, therefore, more slender. She should avoid lines that cut her height and add to her girth. All but the very tall and the very, very thin will find vertical lines most attractive.

❦ Fool the Eye

Camouflage in clothing is, as with cosmetics, a matter of attracting the eye to the best features and distracting the eye from any figure imperfections. Here are some of the tricks that can create desirable illusions.

• The eye will always be led along a line. In clothing a line can be formed by a row of buttons down the front of a dress, rows of tucking,

144

a band of colored trim, the bottom of a jacket, a neckline, the yoke of a blouse, a belt, a seam, fancy stitching, pockets, pleats, gathers, stripes or other patterns in the material, a necklace, or the angle of a hat. A line can be curved or straight. A line must never emphasize a figure fault. It must draw the eye away. The girl with a full bust, for instance, must not choose a blouse with a band of bright color across the yoke or with a breast-pocket trim. The stocky girl should avoid shortening horizontal lines such as those formed by hip patch pockets, a wide or contrasting belt, or a large brimmed hat.

• The eye will be attracted by the lightest or brightest color in a costume. A white collar or a bright jewelry accent will call attention to the face. A light skirt teamed with a dark blouse will draw the eye to the lower part of the body. For double-barrelled emphasis, use a lighter or brighter color to intensify a flattering line. The heavy-set girl who wears a black button-front dress will obtain a more slenderizing effect from white buttons than from dark ones.

• Light or bright colors make things look larger. Dark colors diminish. This is the reason a heavy woman appears slimmer in a navy dress than in a bright red dress. The foot seems smaller in a dark shoe than in a white shoe.

• By extending certain lines, balance can be given to a figure that is not in perfect proportion. If hips are too wide, puffy or cap sleeves will make shoulders seem broader and will thus make the hips appear narrower.

• The type of fabric can affect the illusion of size. A heavy-textured fabric such as a bulky tweed or a knit seems to increase size; so do shiny fabrics such as satin and glossy silks. A stout person will look more slender in a smooth-textured, dull-finished fabric.

• The fabric design can also affect size. Large prints or widely spaced prints, big plaids, and tablecloth checks are more enlarging than small overall prints, plaids, or checks. A stout person would do better to choose a tiny subdued print rather than a large splashy flower print. A petite girl will also look better in a small print, even though she has no need to create the illusion of slimness, because a large print may be too overwhelming.

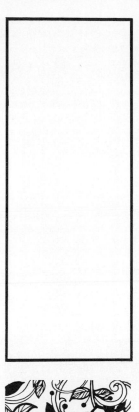

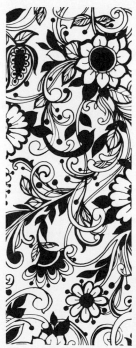
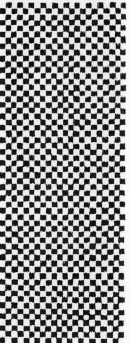

145

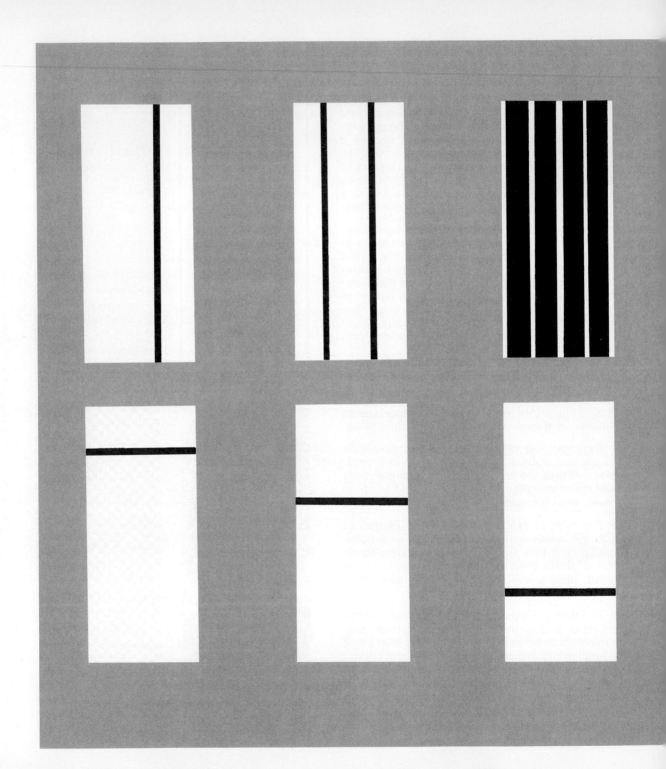

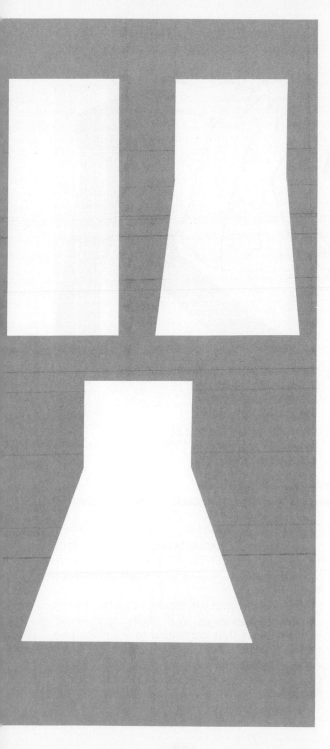

🌷 *Which Lines for You?*

The vertical line. A single vertical line is very slenderizing. It adds to height and whittles width, whether it is created by seaming, buttons, color, or trim—a flattering line for all but the very tall and very thin.

Not all vertical lines are slenderizing. Note on page 146 how much slimmer the shape with the single line looks. Multiple pleats and multiple vertical stripes, especially broad, vivid stripes can make a figure look heavier.

The horizontal line. A horizontal line, whether achieved by the lines of a jacket, by a seam, or by color, tends to cut height and to add width. How much your height is affected depends on where that horizontal line appears. Basically, the longer the unbroken area on the bottom half of your figure, the taller you seem. A high horizontal line, such as is found in an empire style, a bolero jacket, or yoke trimming, does not shorten you very much. A waist-length jacket, contrasting belt, or other line cutting your figure at the waist has more of a shortening effect, while a long jacket or overblouse or a tunic style shortens you much more.

The slender dress. A slender dress is sophisticated and adds height, but it is the hardest of the three basic styles to wear. It demands a perfect figure because of its stark outlines. Every so often, fashion imposes a Year of the Sheath, a lean year for all but lean females. Fuller figures should then look for peg-top skirts and gathers to give a little more ease to the silhouette. Narrow, straight skirts are not flattering to heavy or hippy figures.

The gentle flare. This easy silhouette is more feminine because of its soft, gently rounded lines. It is generally flattering. While it does not add as much height as the sheath style, its lines are subdued enough to still maintain a vertical look that does not diminish height.

The full flare. Notice the shortening effect of this silhouette. Its soft flaring lines are excellent for the tall or very thin figure. A short or round figure will look better in a more subdued flare.

SHORT

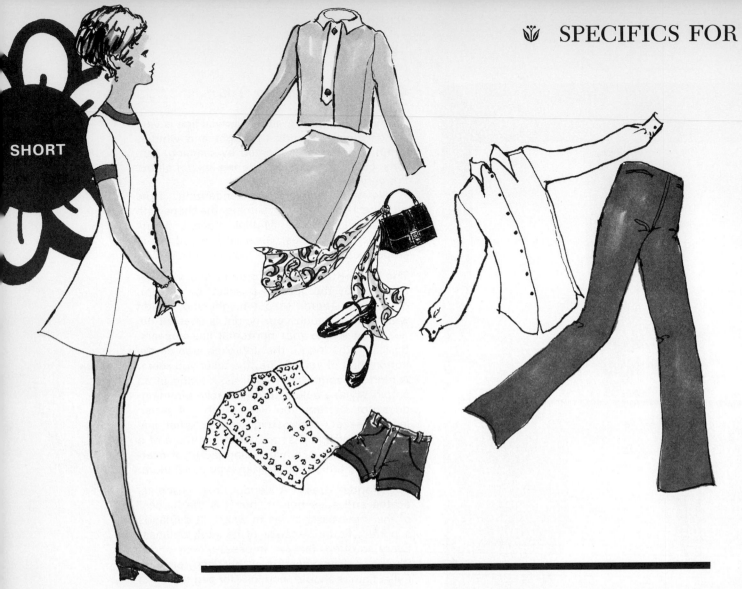

Under 5'4"? Here are the clothes that are right for you.

• Clothes and accessories that are in perfect proportion to your petite size.

• Vertical lines that are not cut by belts and trim. Belts should be narrow and preferably of the same fabric or at least of the same color as the rest of the outfit. The fitted, unbelted princess line and empire line are good for you. The shift is excellent.

• Skirts that are straight or gently flared. Too wide a flare is overpowering.

• One-color outfits.

• Waist-length jackets, boleros, short suit jackets.

• Short toppers, full-length coats (preferably fitted or boxy).

• Tapered or straight slacks, shorter shorts.

• Dainty accessories and shoes, gay small-brimmed hats that are scaled to your tiny size.

• Small collars and cuffs.

• Eye-catching details at neckline and shoulder area to draw interest to the upper part of your figure.

• Smallish prints and fabric designs.

148

your FIGURE TYPE

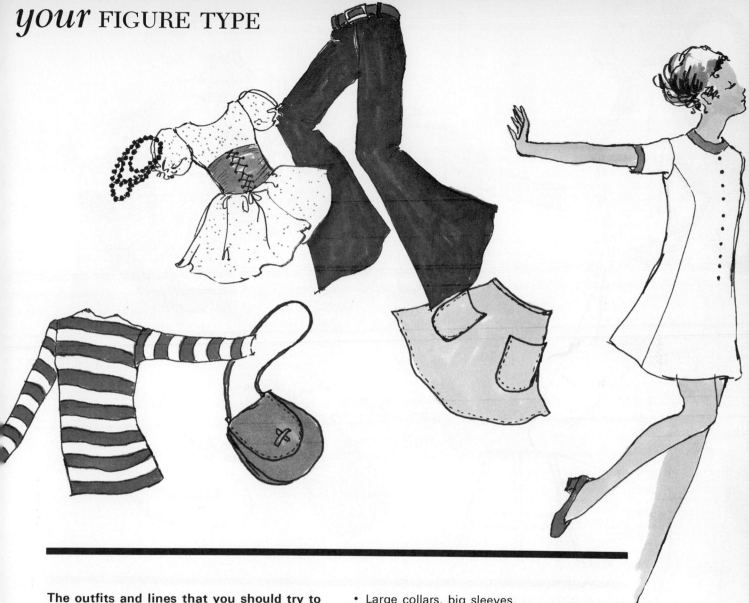

The outfits and lines that you should try to avoid are these:

• Anything that is not small-scaled, that cuts your height, or that appears to drag you down.

• Outfits with definite horizontal lines or accents—bands of contrasting color, yokes, contrasting belts.

• Long suit jackets, tunic styles.

• Three-quarter coats, very flared coats.

• Big skirt pockets, overly flared skirts, tiered skirts.

• Large collars, big sleeves.

• Wide belts and those with large buckles or heavy trim.

• Large purses, chunky jewelry, bib necklaces, big rings.

• Wide-legged slacks, hipsters, long shorts.

• Large bulky hats and wide-brimmed styles that produce a toadstool effect.

• Shoes with wide straps, wedge heels, or heavy design. Heels that are too high may be too much of a good thing. Medium-high heels prevent a walking-on-stilts look.

149

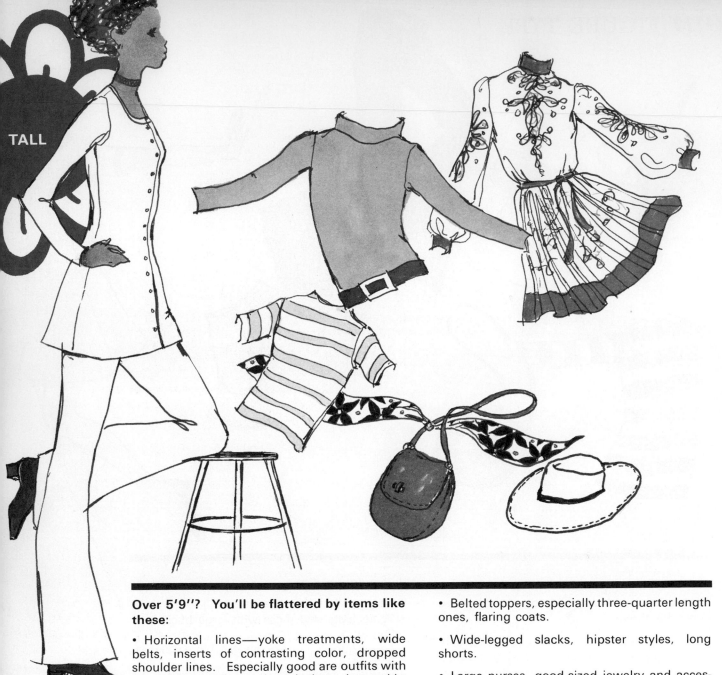

Over 5'9''? You'll be flattered by items like these:

• Horizontal lines—yoke treatments, wide belts, inserts of contrasting color, dropped shoulder lines. Especially good are outfits with low horizontal lines—long jackets, large skirt pockets, tiered skirts or those with horizontal trim, and tunic effects.

• Separates of different colors.

• Boxy jackets, tunics, and overblouses with slim skirts to break the line.

• Flared skirts.

• Belted toppers, especially three-quarter length ones, flaring coats.

• Wide-legged slacks, hipster styles, long shorts.

• Large purses, good-sized jewelry and accessories.

• Large flamboyant collars, big cuffs, interesting sleeves.

• Shoes with medium heels.

• Bold prints and plaids.

150

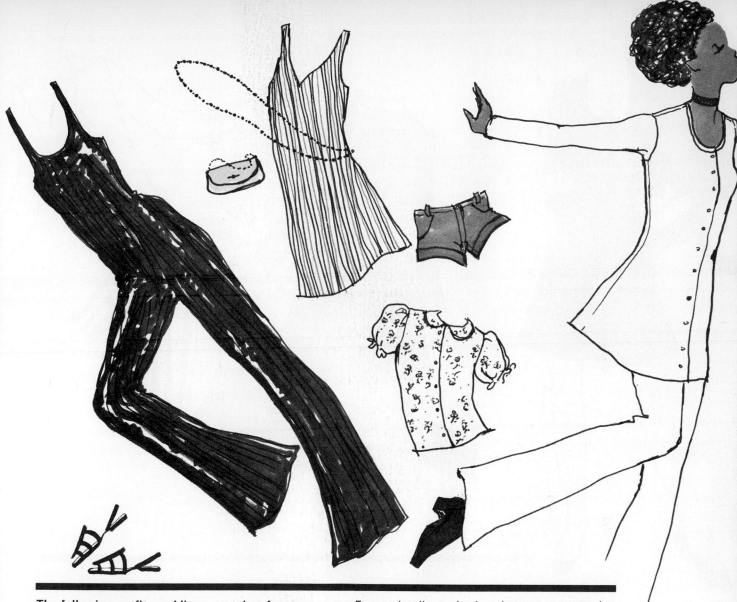

The following outfits and lines are taboo for you:

• Prominent vertical lines such as narrow sheath styles or dresses with a beltless waistline.

• Waistlines too short, hemlines too short or too long.

• Deep V necklines.

• Little-girl styles—you can carry the more sophisticated fashions.

• Severely man-tailored styles.

• Too many accessories—simplicity is striking for you.

• Fussy details and trimmings or accessories that are too cute.

• Slacks that aren't long enough, overly short shorts.

• Either very high heels or flats—both exaggerate height.

• Peaked hats or high-crowned styles—stick to low crowns and wide brims.

• Vertically striped fabrics, even in full-gathered styles—diagonal or horizontal treatments are more flattering to your figure.

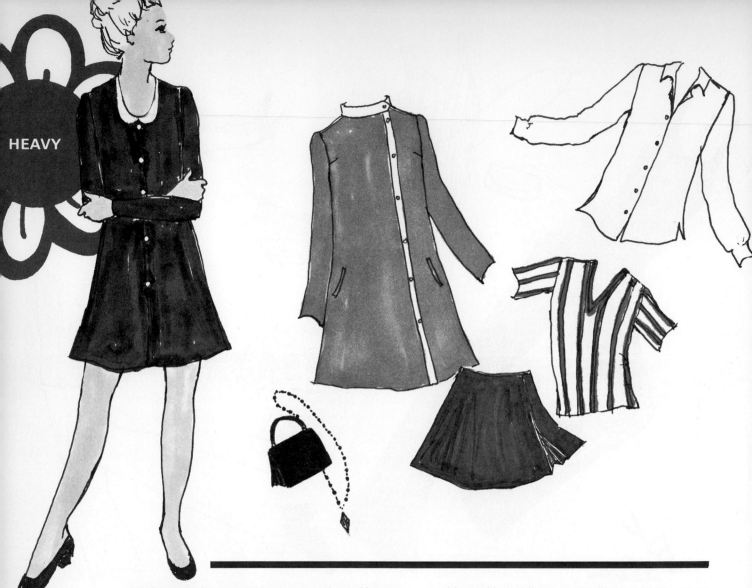

Full-figured? You'll look your best if your wardrobe includes:

• Vertical or diagonal slenderizing lines. Especially flattering is a vertical line that cuts you in a one-third, two-thirds ratio.

• A good foundation, preferably an all-in-one.

• Skirts that are not too straight. Gores or fullness at the side front will produce a more graceful effect. Modified peg-top styles are also good.

• Full-length coats that fit loosely, perhaps with modified back fullness.

• Hems an inch or so longer than current style.

• V- or U-necklines, collarless or with small lapels.

• Simple accessories.

• Self-belts or color-matching belts that are not too wide.

• Culottes for sports.

• Medium heels. High heels *only* if legs are slender.

• Simple hosiery in darker shades.

• Pretty, colorful hats with an upward tilt or with medium brims.

• Dark or subdued colors in shadowy patterns.

152

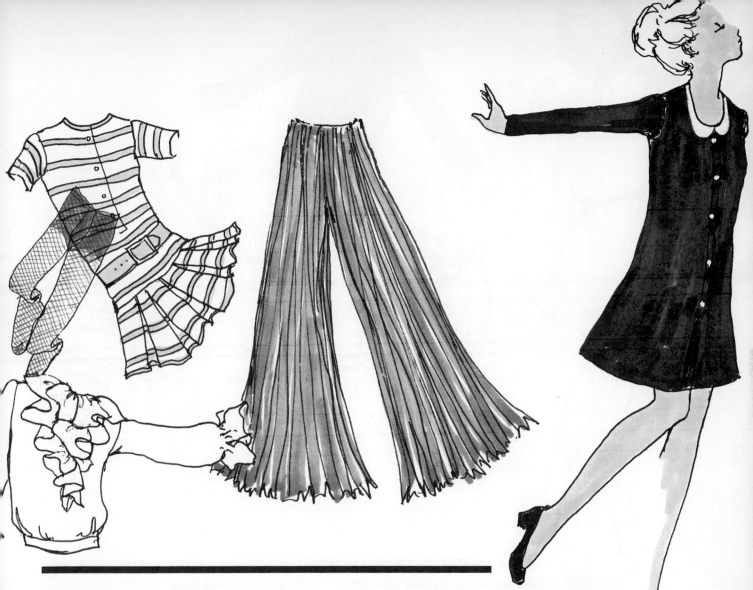

None of the following will be good for you:

- Horizontal lines in styling or fabric.
- Color contrasts that cut height. No two-tone suits or ensembles. Better yet, no suits.
- Clothes that are too tight.
- Straight skirts or very full skirts.
- Bateau or round necklines or any high-collar styles.
- Belted coats or short flared jackets that cut your figure.
- Too much jewelry. One important piece is best.

- Novelty belts, large buckles, wide belts.

- Ornate shoes.

- Light or brightly colored stockings, patterned or textured hose.

- Hats that are too small.

- Sleeveless, cap, or tight-sleeve styles unless arms are slender.

- Fabrics that cling to your figure (knits, jersey, chiffon), transparent fabrics, or stiff or bulky materials.

153

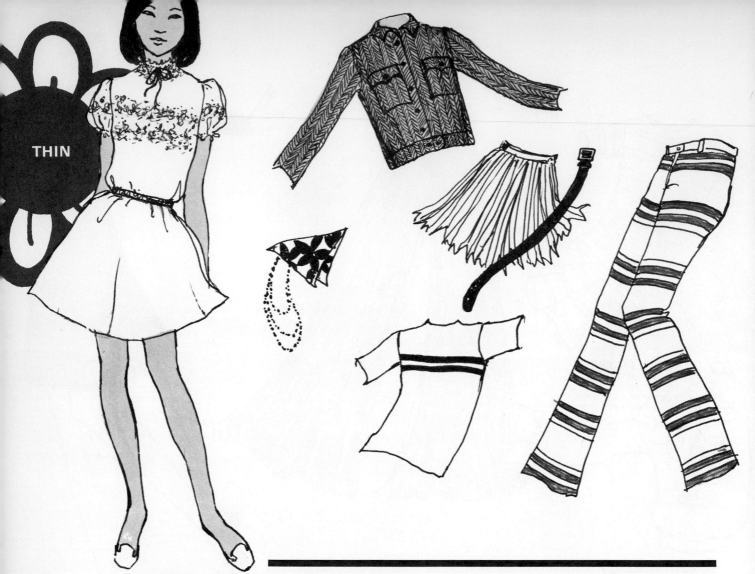

THIN

Too thin?   These are the styles that are right for you.

• Lines that are softly bloused or flaring.

• Skirts that are either gathered or pleated all around.   Wide, flaring skirts—if legs are not too thin.

• Suits that have a break in line, either a boxy jacket or a belted blousey style.

• Blouses and jackets with horizontal lines (stripes, yoke treatments, pockets, trims).

• Loose-fitting blouses that have tucking, gathers, or ruffled fronts.

• Coats that have fullness, or fitted styles with flared skirts.

• Wide contrasting belts.

• High necklines, turtlenecks, interesting collars, bow ties.

• Trimly fitted slacks, wide-legged or tapered; slim shorts.

• Bracelets, wrist-length or longer gloves, multistrand necklaces, scarves.

• Light-colored stockings, textured hosiery.

• Delicate shoes.

• Bright and light colors.   Prints are better than plain fabrics.

• Bulky fabrics (tweed, corduroy, loop knits or bulky knits), crisp fabrics (faille, starched cottons, taffeta), and shiny fabrics.

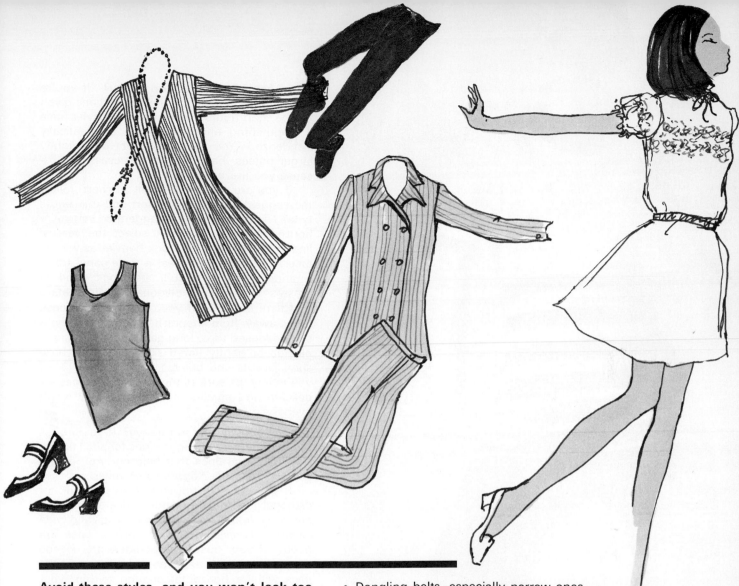

Avoid these styles, and you won't look too thin:

• Vertical lines or stripes that emphasize your slimness.

• Fitted styles that require more curves than you have to offer.

• V-necks, scoop necks, or off-the-shoulder styles.

• Severe styles or mannish outfits.

• Straight skirts, particularly plain sheaths or styles with a single center vertical.

• Overly large earrings or chunky jewelry if face is delicately boned.

• Long necklaces.

• Dangling belts, especially narrow ones.

• Sleeveless styles or shortie gloves if arms are extremely thin.

• Clinging fabrics, tight sweaters that offer no compensating fullness.

• Severe hair styles or angular hats. You want soft, feminine curving lines.

• Dark hosiery, especially in opaque styles.

• Chunky or ornate shoes that look too heavy for thin legs.

• Slinky, long-line knits that emphasize the slender figure.

• Long, scarves that are tied in a low V or that create vertical bisecting lines.

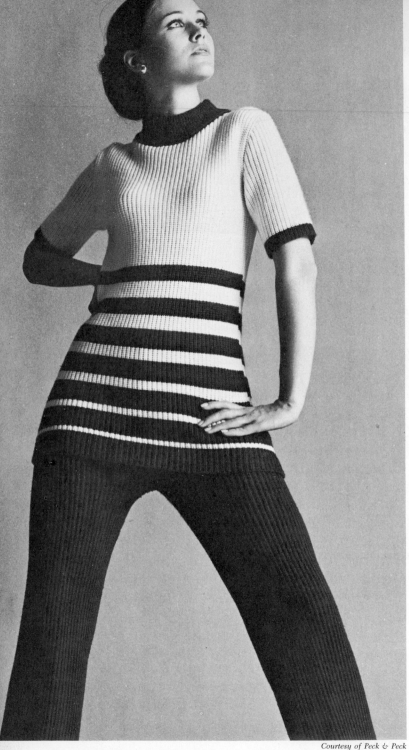

Courtesy of Peck & Peck

An outfit like this looks good on a tall girl, assuming she's not too hippy.

Short but too thin or too heavy? If you're short and heavy, follow the suggestions given for the short figure. Because these styles have a lengthening effect, they will automatically slenderize. You can, however, use slightly larger purses, hats, and other accessories because you are not so petite.

If you are too thin as well as short, follow the suggestions for both short and thin figure types. Instead of using exaggerated vertical or horizontal lines, however, select the vertical lines that will help you look heavier as well as taller—multivertical lines, a wide-panel front, a princess style. You'll also look good in dresses with yokes or diagonal seaming details that flare out toward your shoulders (Y lines). Steer away from mannish outfits and choose softer bloused tops, long gathered sleeves, and pleated or gently flared skirts. Slightly boxy short jackets and boleros are good. Because you're tiny, be sure all trims and accessories are delicate and small-scaled so that they won't overwhelm you.

Tall but too thin or too heavy? If you are tall but thin, follow the suggestions for a tall figure. The horizontal lines that help cut your height will also help your figure seem fuller.

If you are both tall and heavy-set, look for diagonal lines and off-center vertical styling with diverting details such as side closings and wide collars. Tunics with slim vertical lines are good. If your bust and shoulders are not too heavy, you can wear yokes and Y lines. These lines will be horizontal enough to trim your height but not enough to add apparent inches to your width.

✿ Notes on Necklines

A neckline should be chosen to flatter your face as well as your figure. If your face is not the "ideal" oval shape, the general rule is to avoid a neckline that repeats the shape of your face. A round face should avoid a round neckline, a square face should avoid a square neckline, and so on. Often a neckline that is not the most desirable shape can be changed to a flattering

156

line by the addition of jewelry, a scarf, or a collar. A high jewel neckline is not usually the best choice for a round face, but if it is teamed with a long rope necklace, the effect can be quite pleasing.

Round face. Instead of high necklines or round necklines, choose V-shapes and scoop styles. Pointed collars are better than rounded types. Narrow lapels are better than wide coachman styles.

Square face. A good-sized pin at the center of a collar will sometimes make the face appear more oval. Choose a V-shaped neckline or a round one. If you can't avoid a square neckline, round it out with the addition of a necklace or scarf.

Long face. Bateau or turtle necklines, peter pan collars, cuff collars, mandarin collars, and jewel necklines will all give desirable fullness. V- or U-shaped necklines will make a long face—and long neck—look longer. Such a neckline can often be filled in with a multistrand necklace. Long rope necklaces should be avoided because of their lengthening effect.

Long neck. Keep necklines high and look for stand-up collar styles, turtlenecks, and high neckline bows or ruffles. Scarves are excellent. Chokers and large, important-looking pins at the collar are flattering touches.

Bony shoulders. Steer clear of open, revealing necklines. Décolleté evening styles can be made more attractive if they are filled in with filmy stoles or bib necklaces.

Short neck. Most attractive are the deeper-cut U's and V's and the scoop necklines that allow the full length of the neck to show. Be sure that the neckline sits low in the back of the neck as well as in front. No high cascading ruffles, turtlenecks, or stiff cuff collars. Necklaces should always be fairly long.

❦ Camouflaging Figure Flaws

Narrow shoulders. Look for horizontal attraction at the shoulders—yokes, wide necklines, wide lapels, cap sleeves, puffed sleeves, wide collars, cape treatments, and short sleeves with big cuffs. Avoid halters, raglan sleeves, and sloping shoulder lines. Consider hats with brims to give more balanced proportions.

Wide shoulders. Select styles with vertical trim at the center front of the bodice and avoid all shoulder emphasis. Look for unmounted sleeves, raglan sleeves, sleeves without shoulder fullness, halter styles, V-necklines, narrow lapels. If shoulders happen to be padded, experiment with removing the padding.

Full bust. Play down a large bust by keeping the area from shoulder to waist as simple as

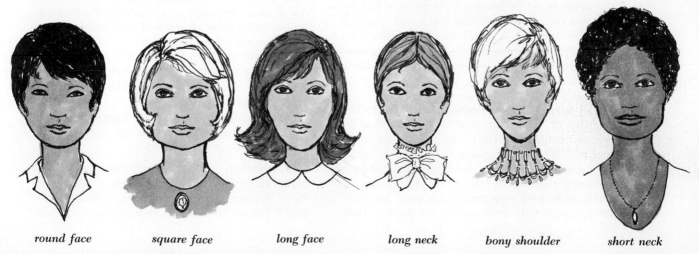

round face   *square face*   *long face*   *long neck*   *bony shoulder*   *short neck*

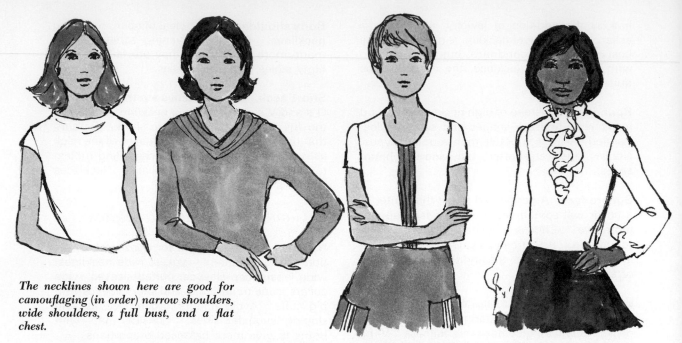

The necklines shown here are good for camouflaging (in order) narrow shoulders, wide shoulders, a full bust, and a flat chest.

possible and drawing attention to your face (interesting hairdos, hats) and to your skirt if hips are slim. You can do this by combining dark tops with light or patterned skirts and by choosing a dull-finish fabric for blouses and bodices. Pass up transparent fabrics or clinging materials (sweaters, jerseys, knits). Bodices should not be tight. Loose-fitting blouses, jerkins, and unbuttoned cardigans are all good. Look for vertical lines at the center front of the bodice and for V or scoop necklines. Please do not wear bows or flowers or large pins low on the bosom. Slightly flaring skirts with pockets or other details will flatter slim hips and at the same time help balance a top-heavy silhouette. Boxy jackets and A-line coats are best for a full-busted figure.

Small bust. Choose clothes that have bodice fullness of their own and avoid any that fit tightly through the bust. Look for yoke treatments, bib effects, pockets, full armholes, gathers, rows of ruffles, tucking, neckline bows, empire styles. Crisp fabrics will provide shape. Clinging fabrics only emphasize your problem. Select slips with gathers at the bust. Keep

accessory accents near your face or high on your shoulder. To help clothes gain a better line, consider a conservatively padded bra. After all, it is no more deceptive to provide a little more curve where Nature fell short than it is to girdle in bulges where figures are too generous.

High or low bust. These problems can often be camouflaged with accessories. A high bust will seem lower if you keep the accent high—wear a pin on your collar or high on your shoulder, a short necklace or a small scarf with ends flaring at the side. A girl with a low bust should keep accents lower and use accessories that will shorten the distance from bust to shoulder—a pin worn at mid-chest height, a longer necklace, a low ring scarf, or a large scarf tied with the ends dangling.

Girls with either of these figure problems should be sure that side bustline darts in bodices match their own contours.

Full stomach. Wear clothes that have some sort of fullness at the stomach area—skirts with front gathers, covering jackets, peplums, tunics. Rather than figure-revealing silhouettes, choose clothes that are slightly bloused above the waist and have easy skirts. Draw attention away from the waistline by using high accessory accents, lapels, and interesting necklines. Needless to say, a good girdle *is* helpful here.

Large hips. Aim for styles that have simple skirts and keep the accent high. Anything that broadens your shoulder line will make your hips seem in better proportion. Look for attractive blouses, interesting shoulder treatments, accents near your face. Try skirts that are darker than blouses and that have some flare. If you are tall enough, certain tunic and long-jacket styles can be flattering. Avoid tight slacks, bell-bottom and hipster styles. Wear long shirts, ponchos, tunics or other cover-ups with pants.

Short legs. Keep any horizontal lines high—jackets, sweaters, and overblouses should come no lower than the top of your hip bone. Be sure dress waistlines hit you at the proper spot. Separates may fit better than one-piece dresses. To make your legs appear longer, wear skirts fairly short and choose light or brightly colored hosiery. Avoid very high boots, long shorts, hipster styles, wide-bottom slacks.

Heavy legs. Choose eased skirts rather than straight skirts. Look for fabrics that have no shine. Slightly darker shades of hosiery will be most flattering. Try wearing skirts just an inch or so longer than current fashion, and stick to long shorts and to slacks that are not too tapered. Bathing suits with skirts are best.

Thin legs. Straight or slightly flared skirts are usually more attractive than billowing styles. Lighter shades of hosiery and textured or patterned styles give the illusion of fullness. Stick to shoes that are light in character.

Large feet. Keep shoes simple without too much ornamentation. Avoid chunky styles; look for graceful, curving heels. Horizontal details in styling will shorten a long foot. Vertical or diagonal stitching and trim will flatter a wide foot. In order to keep feet as inconspicuous as possible, stick to dark basic colors, choosing dull finishes such as calf or suede rather than patent leather.

---

1 *Examine your wardrobe, keeping in mind what you have learned about flattering lines for your figure. If any outfits possess undesirable lines, perhaps they can be altered in some way. If this is not practical, experiment with jewelry, separate collars, scarves, or other accessories to see if the unsuitable lines can be counteracted or hidden.*

2 *Go to a place that is frequented by smartly dressed women (an expensive store, a popular restaurant, a theater, and so on). Observe the women you see there and try to decide what makes them so attractive.*

3 *Study fashion advertisements and articles to see which versions of the new styles contain the lines you need.*

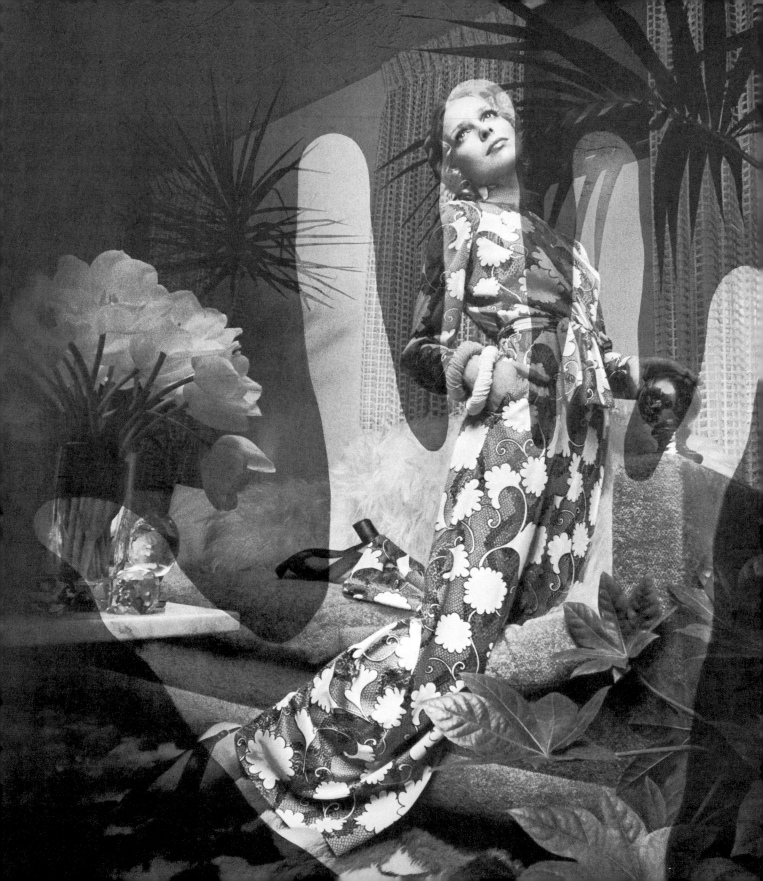

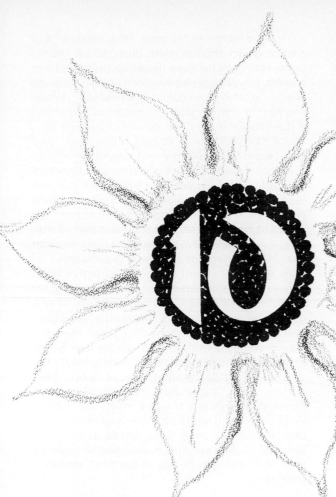

USE COLOR
WITH FLAIR

A flair for color results in a look of beautiful coordination that will do far more for your appearance than money by itself ever can. Chalk it up as the surest way to catch the eye of a man—and as foolproof allure that evokes compliments from all sides. Can such a flair be yours? Certainly! You've already learned to be an expert in using colors to create optical illusions that make your figure look more nearly perfect. Now you will learn how to combine colors and how to select the exact shades that will do the most for your beauty—for your eyes, for your skin, and for your hair. And you'll earn a bonus for your effort, too, because the ability to use color with flair is worth a goodly stack of dollars in the clothing budget. Although color in itself is a no-cost item, it can, when cleverly used, bestow a priceless look of chic on even an inexpensive outfit. The prerequisite for using color so dramatically is simply developing an expert eye for color. In other words, to put color to work for you, you must know it very well. The girl whose color schemes always win acclaim has learned to see each color for what it is—to distinguish all the various nuances of shading a particular hue can have. To her, blue is no longer just plain old blue. She carefully notes that it is a teal blue with tones of green or a periwinkle blue with tones of violet or a slate blue or a sky blue or a turquoise blue. When you have learned really to see color, you are able to select the precise shades that are most becoming to you, and you will also be able to combine and contrast these flattering colors with expert skill and artistry.

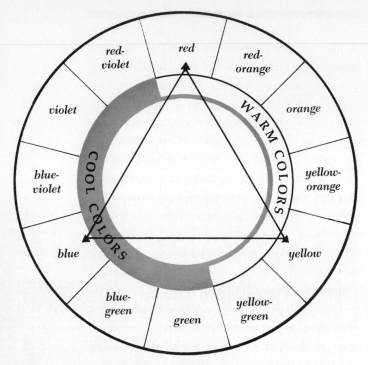

In this diagram the solid, straight lines point to the prime triad; the warm colors are toward the right, and the cool ones toward the left.

❦ Which Colors for You?

Your skin. Your skin and facial coloring are the most important considerations in choosing attractive wardrobe colors. The basic rule is to select colors that repeat the most desirable undertones of your skin and to avoid colors that repeat any undesirable undertones. For example, a girl with golden or olive coloring will usually look her best in shades that have a yellow cast to them (coral and orange-reds, yellow-greens, browns, greenish-blues).

Girls with pink-and-white complexions usually look best in shades that have a bit of red to them and in general are flattered by colors that have blue undertones rather than yellow (pink rather than orange, and blue-green rather than yellow-green).

If skin coloring is pale, the pastels and grayed-down shades (slate blue, forest green, dusty rose) will be more flattering than the vivid shades (royal blue, kelly green, red). Intense shades tend to drain color from the face. While this makes them a poor choice for sallow skins, it does make them quite desirable for girls with florid complexions. Beige, chartreuse, and mauve are other shades that can be unkind to a pale complexion. If skin is blemished or there are dark circles beneath the eyes or lines in the face, violet and purplish grays near the face should be avoided. These shades repeat the colors of natural lines and shadows and, therefore, emphasize them all the more. As you can see, healthy vibrant skin is a great asset. If your skin is clear and has no unattractive tints, almost any color can be worn successfully.

Brown, red-brown, and golden tan skins look good with intense colors, especially shades of red and yellow. Girls with lighter olive-tan complexions and auburn hair usually look better in yellow shades than in reds. Nearly black skin is flattered by softened shades of deep colors (copen blue, turquoise, champagne, rose). These subtle shades create a lovely soft effect. Vivid colors and white intensify and deepen the complexion and may seem harsh in contrast. Very dark colors are not recommended because they tend to subordinate rather than enhance dark skin.

Your eyes. The color of your eyes will usually be highlighted if you wear a shade that matches, or is slightly darker than, your eye coloring. If your eyes are quite pale, experiment with wearing a softer shade of your eye color near the face and a more intense shade farther away, so that your eyes will not be overpowered.

BLUE EYES (ALSO GRAY-BLUE, GREENISH-BLUE). Wear the color that matches your eyes, if possible, or one that accents the most desirable tones of your eye coloring. Since blue-green eyes tend to pick up green or blue in apparel, you can play up by your choice of clothing whichever tone is most flattering to you. Navy is often very flattering.

GREEN EYES. Wearing green, particularly dark shades, will deepen and dramatize green eyes. If they have a slightly bluish cast, this can be played up by wearing brown or blue-green colors. Grays are good for contrast, and reds, particularly yellow-reds, will emphasize your eyes.

BROWN EYES. Accent your eyes by wearing orange tones, perhaps those that pick up any golden glints in your eyes. Beige with brown touches should be flattering. Blue and blue-green will intensify eye coloring.

HAZEL EYES. Since most hazel eyes contain several colors, it is usually advisable to highlight the strongest color. Green, brown, blue, coral, and gold should all be flattering.

Your hair. To highlight your hair, you can choose complementary colors, those that fall opposite each other on a color wheel. These will intensify your hair color. Or you can select harmonizing shades. When using a harmonizing shade, however, you will want to avoid too vivid a hue, which might steal the show. Golden blonde locks, for instance, look lovely with pale yellow or soft gold, but team them up with vivid buttercup yellow, and they seem washed out. (In evaluating colors, remember that skin tone is more important than hair and should be considered first.)

BLONDE. Emphasize its beauty with blues, greens, and turquoise. Yellow in a paler shade is an excellent backdrop. Also good are navy, rust, browns, black. If your hair color is drab, wear grayed tones and pastels to brighten the hair by contrast.

BRUNETTE. If your hair has gold or red highlights, you can play them up by repeating this color in clothing. Blues, greens, reds, yellows should all be flattering, especially in the vivid shades for hair that is dark brown or black. If your hair color is a rather drab brown, do not use a richer brown close to the face; use it in a skirt or some other area at a distance from the hair.

REDHEAD. Greens should be wonderful for you—dark greens, light greens, blue-greens, yellow-greens, olives—also peach and yellow. Dark chocolate browns and black should be excellent for basics. Avoid blue-red tones.

PLATINUM BLONDE OR SILVER GRAY. Usually pastels and soft shades are most flattering. Rose, copen blue, turquoise, blue greens, and navy should all be lovely. If skin tone is not too pale, black and vivid colors can be quite dramatic. Avoid camel and yellowish browns.

Courtesy of Helena Rubinstein

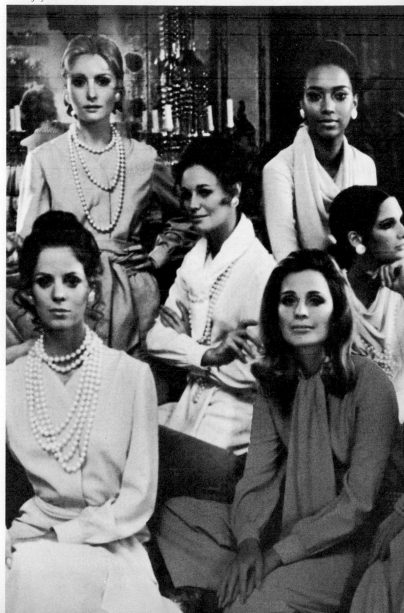

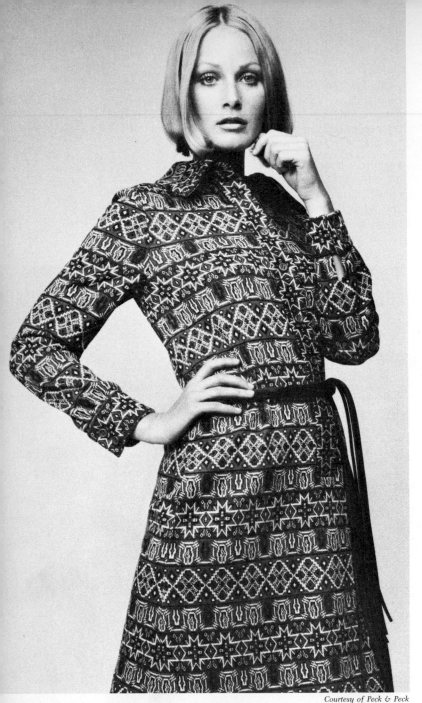

Courtesy of Peck & Peck

With a print dress make sure the colors are flattering and the pattern size is appropriate for your figure.

❦ Color and Your Personality

Color can have a strong psychological effect on us. Red and yellow are warm, cheerful colors. They are exciting, inspiring, and make us feel more energetic—happy colors to wear on a drab, rainy day. The blues, greens, and violets are restful colors. They are more calm, more cool-looking—good psychology for busy, hectic days. Black is considered dramatic, navy blue genteel and ladylike, purple regal, and so on. But the effect a color has on *you* is most important.

Above all, the colors you wear should feel *right.* They should make you happy, let you feel at ease, be an outer expression of your inner feelings. Bright red may disturb some more retiring girls because of its eye-attracting brilliance. Others find the much-touted "little black dress" far too drab to be the wardrobe mainstay they want. Perhaps you can't abide one of your recommended colors. Then skip it for now. Perhaps in time you will find an off-shade of it that will appeal to you.

When a favorite color isn't flattering, you needn't forsake it entirely. Save it for small accents—perhaps a scarf looped in your belt, a purse, or gloves—or use it for skirts so that a more flattering color can be near your face. The girl who loves colorful clothes but realizes bright shades make her look too heavy can compromise on the duller shades of her favorite colors—maroon instead of bright red, forest green instead of kelly green.

Don't be afraid to experiment with color. Possibly, now that you are more experienced with makeup, you will find that colors you had formerly ignored are quite flattering. In summer, when your skin tans and your hair brightens, you may be able to consider more brilliant shades. Widen your color horizon and you'll find a pot full of compliments at the end of your rainbow.

On the job. One day an attractive young girl was trying on a beautiful white coat from a clearance rack in a store. The coats were all reduced to the point where they were marvelous bargains. The white one was very becoming, and she seemed quite pleased with it. Suddenly she unbuttoned the coat hurriedly and put it back on the rack. "I don't know who I think I am to consider that coat," she declared emphatically to her friend. "It's certainly glamorous, but I'd need to send it to the cleaner's every week!" Cleaning bills can quickly erase such a bargain for the girl who commutes by train or bus or who works in the city. An impractical white coat or a light-colored non-washable garment can soon become a white elephant.

In business almost any tasteful color combination is acceptable. Loud plaids and shock shades are best avoided, but most employers no longer demand the dark dress as an on-the-job uniform. Just the same, it's a good idea to discover whether your boss has any color dislikes. Your colors shouldn't conflict with his personality either. You don't want to sashay into the office in your lovely new lavender dress only to find that lavender is his pet aversion. If he's irritated by a color you wear, chances are your day will be far less pleasant.

❦ How to Combine Colors

The trick in combining colors is to play one color against the other so that both will be enhanced. Put a bright kelly green with a brilliant tangerine and you have something fit only for a circus poster. Neither color stands out, the effect is loud and garish. Just change the shades slightly, however. Suppose you put pale green with tawny tan or use a soft shrimp pink with dark forest green—both colors look much better. Good taste is never loud. Combined colors should whisper compliments, never shout their rivalry.

Your colors will blend handsomely if you:

• Accent dark colors with a light or bright color.
• Accent light colors with a dark color.
• Accent bright colors with a neutral or dark color.

For instance, a dark outfit is dramatized and brightened when it is teamed with a brilliant

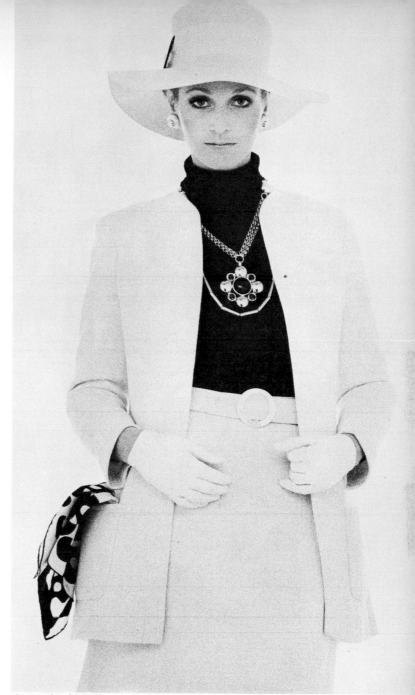

Courtesy of Lord & Taylor

Combining colors and knowing how to accent them is an art that will enable you to look your best.

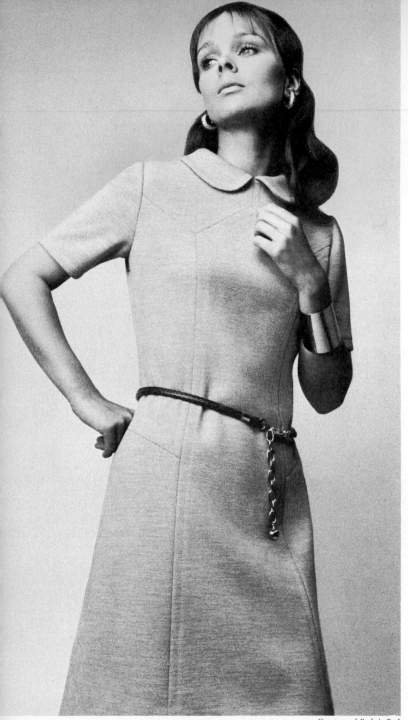

Courtesy of Peck & Peck

A contrasting color belt plus the glint of golden chain and jewelry are enough to accent this intricately seamed dress.

color (black dress, hot-pink hat). Pair black with navy and the effect is dismal. Black and brown are sometimes used together very effectively, but normally, basic dark colors (black, brown, and navy) should not be combined or used to accessorize each other. The girl who has brown shoes but not navy ones shouldn't consider buying a navy dress until she can afford suitable accessories.

Bright colors will look more vivid teamed with a dark color than with neutrals like beige or gray. A red blouse with a black skirt has intense brilliance. Switch to a light gray skirt and the red assumes a softer cast—an idea worth trying if you want to subdue a shade.

If two pastels, such as pale pink and blue, are put together, the effect is weak and rather candy-sweet. Teamed with a dark shade, each would come into its own.

Very striking results can be achieved by using just one color, particularly one of the neutrals. Many a top fashion personality has wowed the feminine population with an all-beige ensemble. Gray is also very sophisticated for a one-color-tone outfit, and sometimes blue can be handled effectively in this manner. With other colors a more dramatic effect can be achieved by using shades of the color varying from light to dark. The success of this look depends on a keen eye for color, because each shade must have the same undertones to avoid a clash.

The rules that have been given here are general rules. Follow them and your color success is assured. But occasionally they can be broken with stunning results. Every few years some fashion potentate seems to wax enthusiastic about pink with orange—a rule-breaker if ever there was one! Bright reds and blues are often teamed in summer wear, and bright turquoise with buttercup yellow accents and light blue with avocado are particularly attractive warm-weather combinations. An occasional variance of this sort can be handled successfully by the girl who is thoroughly grounded in fashion lore and who is experienced at judging just how appreciative her personal public will be.

166

❦ How Many? How Much?

How many colors should be used in a costume? Three at most, and two are sometimes better than three. A russet-brown suit with a yellow and orange scarf, orange hat, and brown accessories would be a smart combination using three colors. Suppose green shoes and a green blouse were added—the smartness of the color combination would be diluted. The result would be more of an autumn garden effect—lovely for gardens but too hodgepodge for fashion chic. Perhaps an even more attractive outfit could be created by using only two of the colors, such as russet and yellow.

In using three colors, the trick is to use one color in large doses, your second color in a moderate amount, and just an accent dash of the third color. As with the russet-orange-yellow combination just mentioned, one color (or shade of a color) must predominate. The dominant color (russet) is used for the large areas, the second color (orange) is kept to accessories (hat and scarf). Another use of the second color might have been an orange blouse and gloves with a russet hat brightened by orange and yellow trim. Your third color is usually a single smaller spot, such as a handsome pin or the trimming on a hat. Often it is merely blended in jewelry or in a print. Balance of this sort gives unity to a costume. If equal amounts of each color are used, there is no uniting color and the effect is choppy.

How many accents of your auxiliary color or colors should be used? Again, the fashion-wise number is three. Three places are usually sufficient for accents, two often better. A navy blue suit teamed with red hat, red earrings, red-and-white necklace, red belt, red purse, white gloves, and red shoes is at least three reds too many. The effect is blotchy. An all-navy costume sparked with red hat, red-and-white necklace, and white gloves would be far more attractive. Your auxiliary color should be used for accent and should not fight for first place. Color touches should emphasize your best features and not confuse your beholders with too many focal points.

167

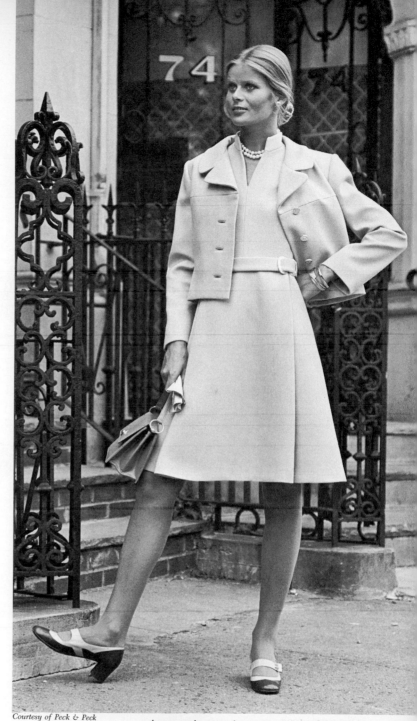

Courtesy of Peck & Peck

Accessories are important in achieving a complete "look." The color of your shoes and bag should match or complement your outfit, and your jewelry should harmonize with it.

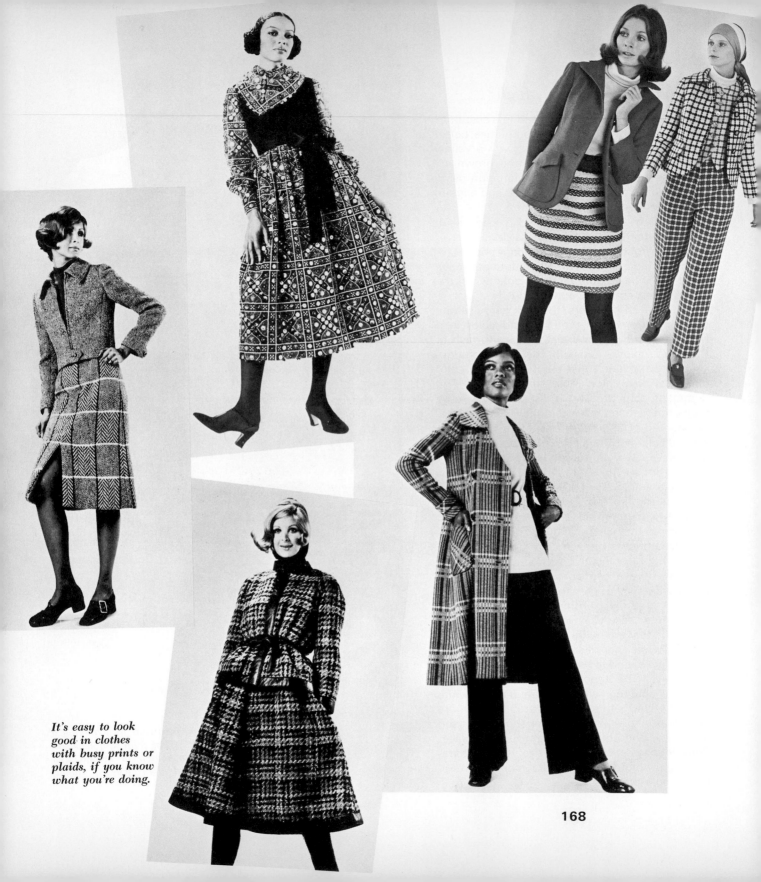

It's easy to look
good in clothes
with busy prints or
plaids, if you know
what you're doing.

168

Dramatic effects can be created by keeping an entire costume in one hue with the exception of a single use of a second color. In this case, the color accent should be important—a beautiful hat or a striking piece of jewelry or even elbow-length gloves. Too insignificant a spot of color is lost. A small blue pin may not be noticed on a dark dress. Show your good taste and color awareness by repeating this color in a second more prominent accessory (such as a blue hat or belt), so that both items will enhance each other.

When a costume is primarily a print or a plaid, a charming effect can be created by picking out the most becoming color of the print and keying accessories to this. Prints are, of course, combined only with solids. Stripes, plaids, polka dots, checks, tweeds, or other designs should *never* be used together. They create a busy and confused effect.

1 *Conduct a color clinic for yourself to see which colors and which color combinations will do most for your particular coloring. You've learned the colors that should be most flattering. Now you will want to test them to find the precise shades that are best. Check each color carefully to judge its effect on your skin tone, hair, and eyes.*

2 *Go over your own wardrobe to see if you have collected any really unflattering colors. If you have, eliminate them—perhaps by having a swap session with your friends (what's poison for you may be perfect for them).*

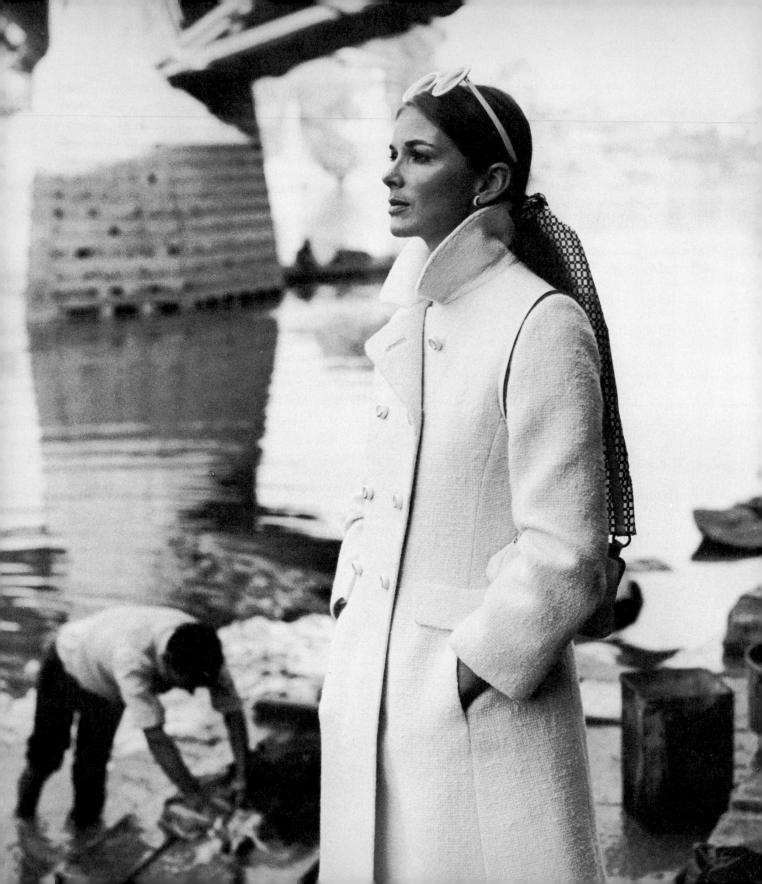

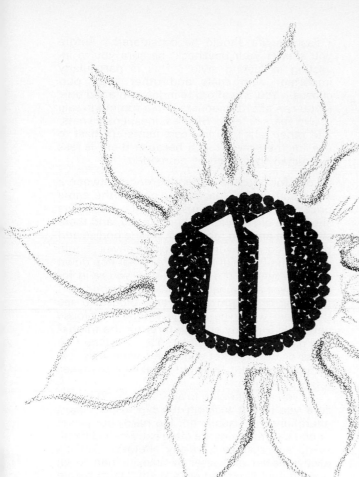

PLANNING
YOUR
WARDROBE

A well-coordinated, attractive wardrobe is a boon to any girl's charm. What's better for self-confidence than the assurance that you always have something marvelous to wear—something to give you a look of smartness and competence by day, something spectacular to make a substantial splash for evenings? You're ready for any change of plans, any big fun. And knowing you look your very best brings that priceless elation that allows you to forget clothes and to concentrate completely on being your most charming self.

Such a well-coordinated wardrobe is the result of clever planning and clearheaded shopping. The girl who plans her wardrobe well knows the wisdom of buying a few basic changeabout fashions that can lend themselves to many occasions and thereby save her enough money for the special splurges that make her appearance a standout. She shrewdly shops by color schemes, insists on good fit and practical fabrics. She knows where she should invest her money most heavily and where she can get by with unnoticeable skimping. She's always well dressed because she leans less on dollars and more on sense.

An important factor to consider in planning a wardrobe is the life expectancy of a fashion. Basic trends in styling, such as the skirt length, the shoulder line, the figure-fitted look versus the loose cut, come on us rather gradually and usually stay with us, with slight variations, from five to eight years. When the pendulum begins to swing in the opposite direction, fashion-wise women take notice. A new trend of this basic sort will be with us for some time, and wardrobe plans should be geared accordingly. These trends are factors that date a wardrobe—considerations you can't escape.

More changeable fashion features—the meanderings of the waistline, the shape of the sleeve, the flare of the skirt—have a shorter life-span, usually about three years. Pick up your cues when the fashion first shows its refreshing lines. Take a style to heart when it's past its prime, and you're stuck with the old dog that can't do new tricks for your wardrobe. This type of fashion is one that you can usually ignore if it isn't flattering. When the skirt length changes, yours must, too, but a three-year fashion usually isn't so pervasive that you can't find flattering exceptions.

The other type of fashion is the one-year fad. Here you tread lightly and invest as little as possible. This fad can be a color craze or it can be an extreme version of a three-year trend. Remember the Nehru jacket? Sometimes it's a jewelry fad, a hat style, a new scarf shape. These are the fashion touches that can make you look in-the-know. Smart girls buy less expensive versions and play them hard while they are stylish.

❦ *What Is a Good Buy?*

A good buy must meet several qualifications.

• It must do something for you. If it doesn't, pass it up—no matter how great a saving it offers. Almost every girl has had in her closet a wrong-type dress or a drab dress that she bought because she couldn't see past the marked-down price—a bargain, perhaps, but a drag on the ego every time she dutifully wore it.

• Any clothing item you purchase must also do something for your wardrobe. The most gorgeous sweater might as well belong to someone else if it goes with only one outfit and can be worn only on rare occasions. Ask yourself, "Will this blend with my color scheme? How many things will it go with? How often will I get to wear it? Will I get my money's worth out of it?"

• Fashion life should be considered. Before you shatter your paycheck, be sure you're investing in lasting style. This is particularly important with coats and other large purchases. You can afford to indulge in a fad only if you can afford to donate it to a rummage sale in two years or less. Blouses, inexpensive hats, and other relatively low-cost items are best to use for the timely touch because there is less loss when they become outmoded.

• Look for good fit. The difference between a so-so suit and a spectacular one at the same price may be merely a matter of fit. Shoulders should be big enough but not sloppy, and there should be enough room through the bodice and back for easy movement. Long sleeves should stop at the break of the wrist and not flop down over the hand. If a skirt is tight, you're in for lap creases and a baggy seat. It's a good idea to try on a straight skirt over a blouse to see that there won't be a ridge where the blouse ends. Is it roomy enough through the thighs? (No garter bumps, please.) The waistline of a dress or fitted jacket should hit your waist exactly all around. The right hemline also makes a big difference.

If you are planning to alter a garment, make sure you're not tackling too big a job. Skirt alterations are usually not too hard, but jacket or bodice alterations are often extremely difficult to do successfully. In any alteration job it's always easier and safer to take in than to let out. If you plan to let out a seam, check before you buy to see if it is wide enough. You'll want to be sure the seam isn't notched too deeply. Certain fabrics, such as satins, failles, moires, taffetas, and some cottons, hold stitch marks, and any let-out areas will show no matter how much you press them.

• Insist on good workmanship. Shoddy seams and unauthorized puckers can spoil the effect of the smartest style. Check to see that the seams are straight and that the sleeves and zipper are set in smoothly. Are the points of the collar even? Are the lapels cut correctly and reinforced? Is the waistband of a skirt stitched carefully and backed with a sturdier fabric to keep it from wrinkling? If its fabric is a loose weave, a slim skirt should be lined. Are the buttonholes finished properly? In buying a suit or coat, check also to see that there is enough

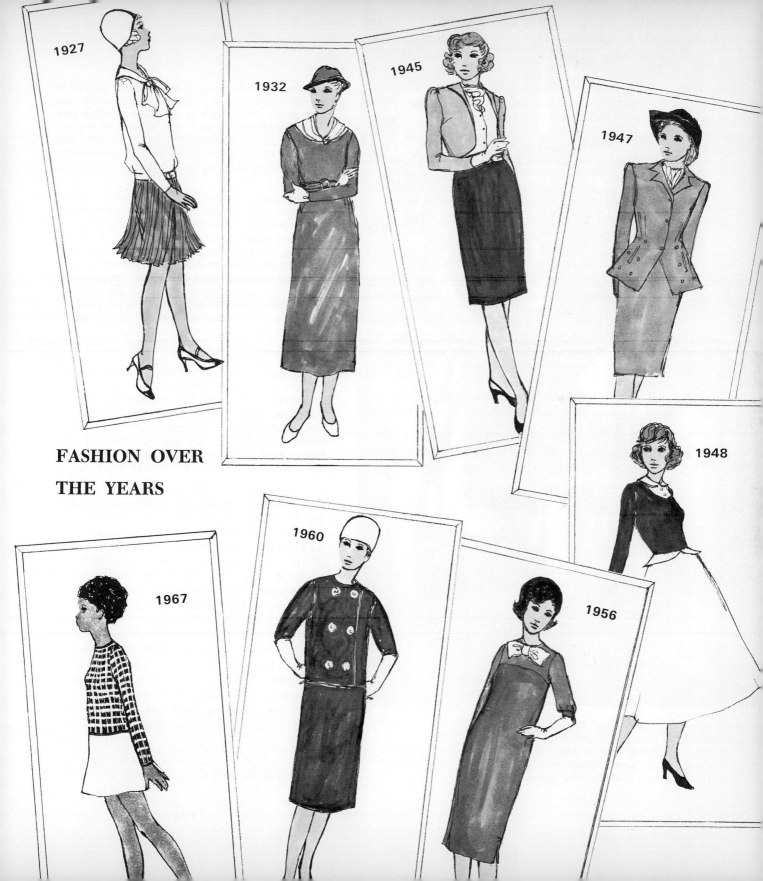

1927

1932

1945

1947

1948

**FASHION OVER
THE YEARS**

1967

1960

1956

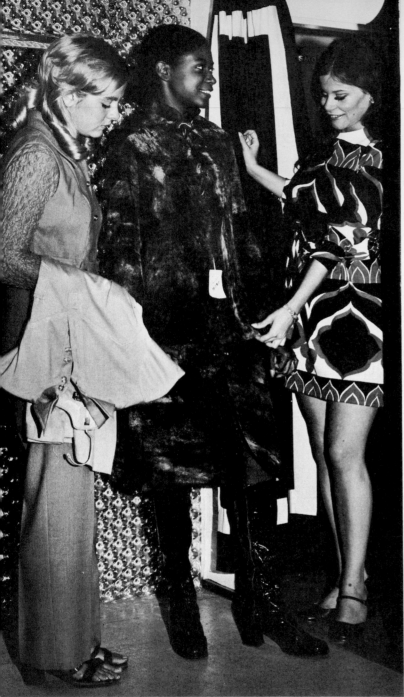

B. D. Unsworth

When buying clothes, there are so many things to consider, if you are to be sure you are getting a good buy. You may want to take some friends with you, so that you may consider their opinion.

fullness in the lining. Well-made garments usually have a pleat in the lining or extra fullness down the length of the back to allow leeway for easy movement and to prevent the lining from being strained. Check, too, that any stripes or linear patterns in the fabric are straight where they should be and match evenly at the seams.

• Good materials pay off. Put your money in materials that will be easy to care for and will hold up well. Look for labels that guarantee against fading, shrinking, wrinkling, spotting, sagging, and all the other undesirables. If a garment must be dry-cleaned, you should consider upkeep expenses as well as the purchase price. For good wear, look for flat weaves rather than nubby or fleecy fabrics and for tightly woven materials rather than loosely woven ones.

• Is it a good value? There are high-priced bargains and low-priced booby traps. The smart shopper learns to tell when a bargain really is a bargain. You don't need to spend a fortune on clothes, but the garment that is too cheap usually gives itself away. Some of the telltale signs of a cheap dress: poor fabric, harsh bright color, wavy seams, gimmicky trim. Sometimes it's wiser to splurge on one good dress than to buy two low-priced ones.

The girl who shops at sale time* gets the most value for her dollars. In many areas there are traditional big sale days. Election Day and Veterans Day are often special coat sale days, for instance. Look for early-in-the-season sales of manufacturers' samples if you want the newsiest selection. Look for end-of-season clearances for the really big savings. When you buy at the end of the season, you may not have a wide choice, but often you can pick up the better-quality clothes, which you could merely admire before, at marked-down prices you can afford. Look for classics of good material and cut at end-of-season clearances rather than for something that might become dated.

Where you shop often has a lot to do with the price tag on the merchandise. In most

° For a list of sale times, see p. 333.

cities there are the elegant stores and the bargain stores. It's fun to go to the prestige shops, and you can usually be sure of getting topflight merchandise, but if you don't mind walking on uncarpeted floors and trying clothes on in less glamorous fitting rooms, you can often find the same dress for several dollars less in a bargain house. You need a good eye for value (and a bit more stamina) to shop successfully in a bargain store. You must be able to sort out the real buys from what may actually *be* cheap, and you must inspect carefully for good workmanship, but the shrewd shopper can usually make some significant savings that warrant any extra effort involved.

• Will I get my money's worth out of it? Practicality should also raise its righteous little head when it comes to evaluating price tags. The girl on a budget must remember that a moderately priced nylon slip will do as good a job as an expensive one, but a cheap version that fits poorly is no bargain. She asks herself if she really needs to spend a great deal for a New Year's Eve dress. How often will she wear it? If her social life is filled with less formal affairs, she may settle on an inexpensive cocktail dress and save the rest of the treasury for clothing items that will get more frequent wear. Or perhaps the dress is so super-stupendous that it is worth twice its high price because of the wonderful things it does for her—and to him. Maybe her social calendar is dotted with many gala occasions when she can use the dress. Maybe this dress is the type she can vary so that it won't look the same each time. Or maybe it has a cover-up jacket that lets it do double duty for less formal occasions as well. Put your money where it will give you the *most* satisfaction if you want to be sure of getting your money's worth.

• Is a less expensive version worth considering? Certain accessories are so simple in design that they could be any price. In these items a medium- or even low-priced version may be as satisfactory as a high-priced version. This is often true in hats, patent-leather-type plastic belts and purses, and simple accessories such as scarves, gloves, and summer jewelry. In a year when everybody is wearing a beret or a pillbox or what-have-you, a simple velvet or

wool jersey version may be just as smart as an expensive felt. And white beads are white beads, whether they come from the five-and-ten or the fanciest specialty shop.

❦ Smart Shopping

In this chapter and the next you'll learn how to plan a wonderful wardrobe for yourself. After you've completed your plan, you'll probably find you'd like to make a few additions to

Often you can get bargains in a sale, but you must be careful. Sometimes you may think you are buying something at a reduced price when really it is merely inferior merchandise.

B. D. Unsworth

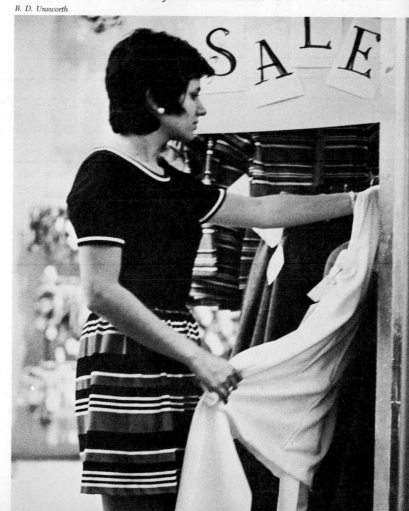

175

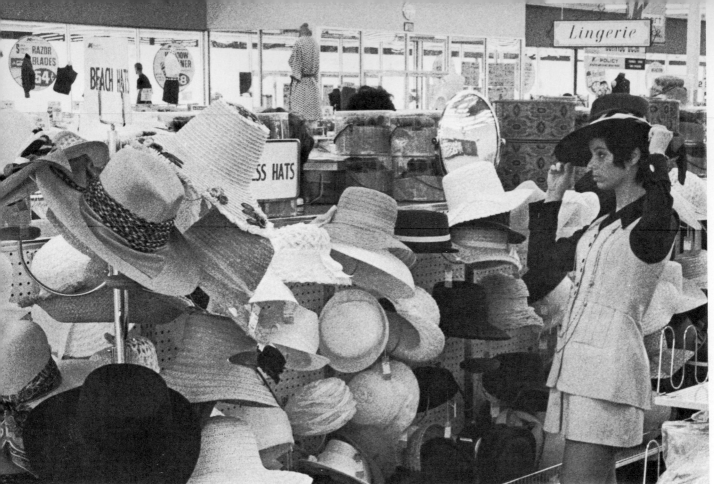

Courtesy of Merchandiser Publishing Co.

your present wardrobe. Smart shopping isn't easy. It involves stamina, clearheaded, unemotional reasoning, and a strong hold on all the nasty little mental meanderings that try to lure you into the purchase you'd later regret.

One of the best ways to fortify yourself is to start out with a priority list of the items that you want to buy, heading the list with essentials for daily wear. Thus you won't be tempted to splurge on a nice-to-have pair of date sandals when you badly need everyday shoes for school or business. You'll also have an idea of how many "must haves" are on your list and how you should allot your money.

In order to be a discriminating shopper, have a clear idea of what you want before you set foot in a store. Know the colors that will coordinate, the lines that will set off your figure, and the degree of casualness or dressiness that will

be suitable. Then you won't be tempted by a gorgeous color that goes with nothing you have or by a high-pressure salesgirl who coos that an unbecoming style is the newest fashion. If you know what you want, you'll have the sales resistance to hold off until you're sure the item is completely right for you—and your wardrobe.

When shopping for dresses, don't overlook the plain style that needs a pleasing shape inside to show off its good lines. Visualize it on you with your favorite necklace or a handsome belt or scarf. Gimmicky styles always clamor for attention but often are less satisfying and less versatile than the style that depends on superb lines for long-lasting appeal.

Allow yourself sufficient time to shop. Seldom is it wise to buy the first style that catches your fancy, unless you've done some careful window shopping beforehand. If you have any doubts, look further. Most stores will hold apparel for at least a few hours—time enough for you to check a few other stores to be sure you've selected the best buy. If a big date suddenly materializes at the last minute, don't rush out madly to buy a new dress. When you haven't enough time to shop calmly and carefully, it's usually better to postpone making any purchase. Desperation buying is seldom satisfactory. Couldn't you possibly get by with something pretty that's already in your closet? Or in an emergency perhaps you could borrow the right accessory to give a new look to something you already have? It's better to do without than to be stuck with a not-quite-right outfit that will seem all the more disappointing when you later spot a perfect outfit that you can no longer afford.

❦ Take Stock

The first step in formulating a wardrobe plan for yourself is to see just what you have to work with. Go through your closet and bureau and make a list of every speck of clothing you own. As you come to each garment, examine it carefully to see how much life is left in it—how soon it will need to be replaced. And as you read through the following sections, note any items you need to buy to provide yourself with a well-balanced, well-coordinated wardrobe.

❦ Be a Successful Color Schemer

Any girl, unless she can afford as extensive a wardrobe as her heart desires, is wise to develop a color plan. A color-planned wardrobe far outstretches a hodgepodge of solo items and assures a cleverly coordinated look at all times.

A wardrobe color scheme should begin with the choice of a basic color (usually black, brown, or navy). A girl on a limited budget can do splendidly with even one basic color. This becomes her choice for shoes, purse, and everyday gloves, and the rest of her clothing

177

selections are keyed to go with them. Quite possibly her coat will be in the basic color, also. Girls who work in the city or who travel on trains and buses a great deal find that dark or bright colors are most practical for outer wear because dirt and soot show up so readily on light colors.

Of the basic colors, black is most popular. It is the easiest to use if you are limited to one basic color, because it allows the greatest variety. There seem to be more prints with black

Courtesy of Peck & Peck

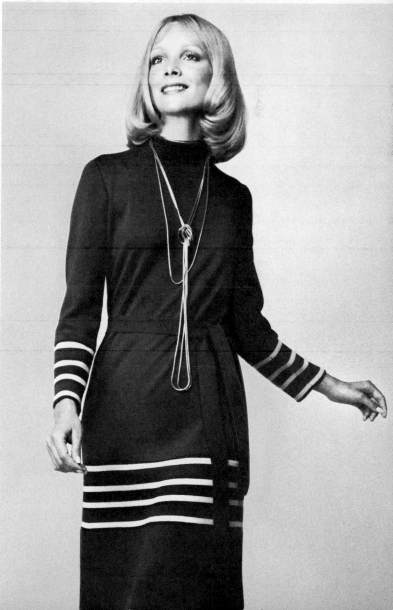

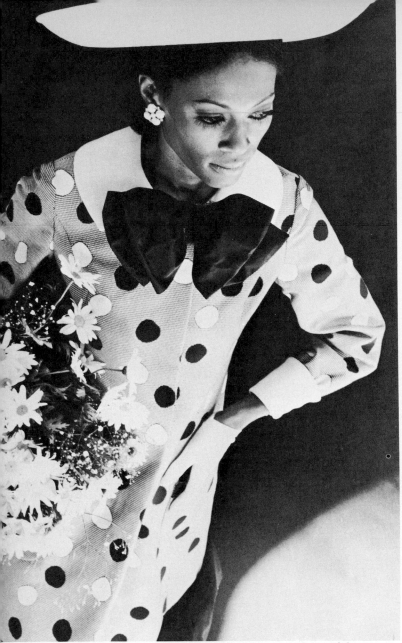

used only for accessories such as shoes and handbags that are not near the face.

Navy is a softer background color than black. It is generally very flattering for all but dark skins and mixes well to make some lovely color combinations.

Brown, too, lends itself to marvelous color harmony and is generally flattering. Rusty browns and beiges are excellent basic colors for dark skins. Brown is a bit more difficult to work with because fewer ready-made outfits are patterned or trimmed in brown. The prints and plaids that are available are usually quite interesting, however, and many combinations, such as the black and brown prints, can be very sophisticated. Brown tends to be slightly more sporty than the other basic colors (mink coats to the contrary). If brown is selected for the basic color, a rust or beige coat that could also be teamed with accessories other than brown would be more adaptable than a dark brown coat.

Once you have selected your basic color, you can build on this, choosing clothing and accessories that are interrelated. Each clothing purchase you decide on should be in a color that is not only flattering to you but is keyed to the other items in your wardrobe. Because a coat must blend with everything in your wardrobe, you can save yourself much trouble by choosing it in a neutral color or your basic color.

In making your plan, you'll want to correlate your winter wardrobe with your summer wardrobe. During the in-between days of spring and fall, you'll be mixing winter coat with spring hat or spring jacket with winter dress, and all should blend attractively.

❦ Building on Basics

The wardrobe that stretches furthest and always looks best is one that has a backbone of a few ever-dependable basics. A basic is a simple fashion with superb lines that can be dressed up or down to suit a variety of occasions. It's not in the show-off category that immediately reminds everyone that this is the same dress you

in the design and more dresses trimmed with black buttons and belts than there are in either navy or brown. Black is usually very flattering to girls with vivid coloring, dark brunettes, and redheads. It may tend to be a bit severe for young girls or those with paler coloring and does nothing for those with dark brown or almost black complexions. In these cases it should be

WITH BLACK AS THE BASIC COLOR

Color accents—blue, gold
Shoes and purse—black

FALL-WINTER

Coat—charcoal gray
Hats—black, blue
Suit—slate blue
Dressy dress—black
Tailored dresses and skirts—royal blue, gold,
   green and blue print, blue and purple tweed

SPRING-SUMMER

Coat—dark royal blue
Hat—natural straw
Dressy dress—gold
Tailored dresses—light blue, pale green, rose

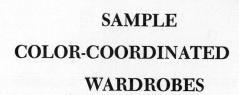

SAMPLE
COLOR-COORDINATED
WARDROBES

WITH NAVY AS THE BASIC COLOR

Color accents—red, yellow
Shoes and purse—navy

FALL-WINTER

Coat—bright navy
Hats—navy, red
Suit—dark navy
Dressy dress—blue
Tailored dresses and skirts—gold, bright
   green, red and navy pincheck

SPRING-SUMMER

Coat—light gray
Hat—white straw
Dressy dress—light blue
Tailored dresses—navy, violet, aqua

WITH BROWN AS THE BASIC COLOR

Color accents—yellow, rust
Shoes and purse—brown

FALL-WINTER

Coat—rust
Hats—rust, brown
Suit—brown and rust check
Dressy dress—green
Tailored dresses and skirts—light blue,
   gold, brown print, brown

SPRING-SUMMER

Coat—gold
Hat—yellow straw
Dressy dress—royal blue
Tailored dress—dark green, tangerine, pale
   yellow

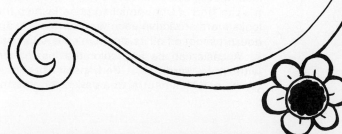

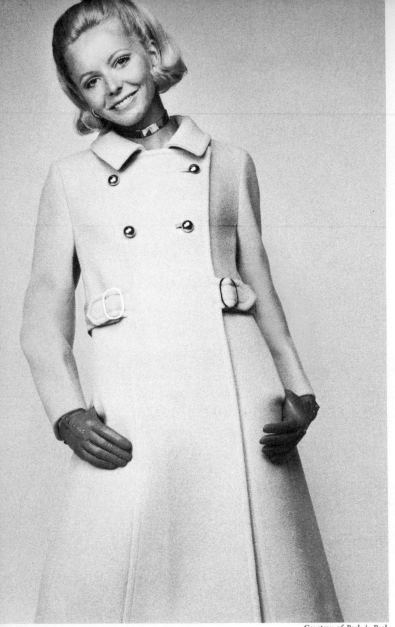

Courtesy of Peck & Peck

This coat may be worn in the daytime as well as to evening events.

even a red. (Red, because of its brightness, has a look-at-me quality that usually makes it a less versatile choice.)

A basic coat. In cool weather many people see you only with your coat on. They must judge you by the coat you wear rather than by the lovely dress it covers. Your coat makes the first impression. It is an important investment and should be the best you can afford in style and quality.

To be more flexible, your coat should be so basic that it can look as right with a cocktail dress as with a sweater and slacks. It should have no dressy trims, such as fur or velvet, and should be in a solid color rather than a tweed or plaid that dubs it as strictly sporty. Contrasting color in buttons, collar, and the like will make it less adaptable. A dark or neutral color is likely to be easiest to coordinate, but if your wardrobe consists mainly of dark colors, a bright coat can be a snappy contrast.

If your coat is to take a lot of hard commuting, a smooth, tightly woven fabric, such as wool broadcloth or flannel, will be most serviceable. Cashmere, high-pile fleeces, and nubby or loosely woven fabrics succumb too quickly to hard wear. (Chinchilla cloth, despite its nubby texture, is such a hard-finished fabric that it gives excellent wear.) You might also consider one of the imitation fur coats in a simple style.

Before making a choice, you will be wise to consider your height and the clothes that you will wear with your coat. Girls who live in the city need more highly styled coats than those who live in the country.

SHORT COATS AND JACKETS. Jackets, car coats, and shortie coats are popular for casual wear, but they are difficult to pair attractively with dresses. A flared or boxy jacket looks good only with a slim skirt. *Never* wear one with a full skirt. A much better silhouette is created if the full skirt is combined with a Spencer or a battle jacket or a close-fitting bolero, or some other waist-length style. These are the only styles that look good with both full and sheath skirts.

wore Tuesday, nor need it have the kind of plain look that gives it a why-bother ordinariness. It's the kind of ungimmicked good fashion that looks more attractive each way you wear it and doesn't shoot off all its steam in one quick pouf.

A basic can be any color that harmonizes with your wardrobe. Perhaps it is blue or green, maybe a neutral or a dark color, possibly

180

Some girls, especially if they are city dwellers, find that a bulky-knit cardigan sweater is a more satisfactory—and generally more basic—jacket choice.

Short girls look best in the shorter length jackets that hover near the waistline. Tall girls can cut their height if they wear longer jackets and three-quarter length coats.

A basic dress. A basic dress is the dearly beloved mainstay of a well-planned wardrobe. It can go from desk to date with equal aplomb, and even if the date turns out to be two-on-the-aisle at the theater instead of top bleacher seats at a night ballgame, you'll be well dressed. It plays up perfection of line rather than gadgetry and seems stunning each way you wear it. To allow you the greatest fashion mobility, it should have no contrasting trim that is not easily detachable. The neckline should be simple so that you can bedeck it with jewels for festive occasions and alter it with scarves for daytime wear. In spring add a crisp white collar for a fresh, timely look. The dress can be in any flattering color that coordinates with your wardrobe.

To avoid pattern conflicts, your dress had better be solid in color if your coat is not. Wool and wool blends are the most versatile fabrics for cold weather. Silks, failles, crepes, nylons, and the miracle-fiber jerseys are good for milder days, with cottons, rayons, and polyesters among the summer favorites.

Some girls are such masters of changeabout tricks that they multiply a few basic dresses to amazing proportions. A clever receptionist in an advertising agency is famous for her quick-change devices. She once knit sleeves and a turtleneck dicky for last year's sheath. She made big puffy sleeves to snap into a summer sleeveless dress. Her wool jumper is worn to work with a blouse but goes to dinner later with pearls replacing the blouse. She has also made a filmy overskirt that she adds to simply styled dresses for festive affairs.

A basic date dress. Here's where you want drama—whether your personal prescription

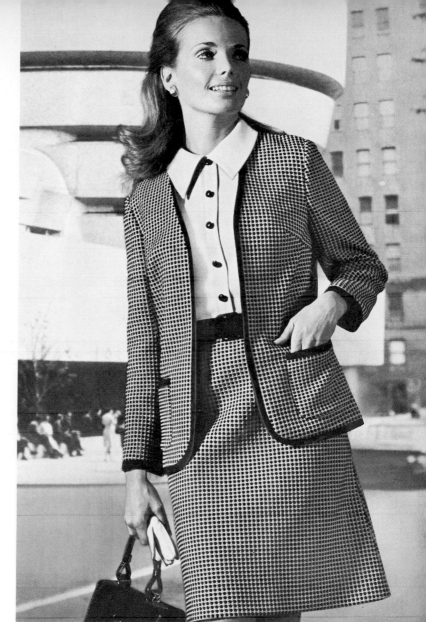

Courtesy of Peck & Peck

Although this suit is simply styled, the checked pattern limits its versatility.

calls for grand entrance effects, subtle sophistication, or beguiling femininity. To do the trick, look for a beautiful color in a simple style or, just the reverse, a glamorous cut in a dark color. The most usable style is a beautifully cut dress in a fabric that spans seasons easily (no velvet or organdy, for instance). A fairly formal dress with a jacket, as mentioned before, will

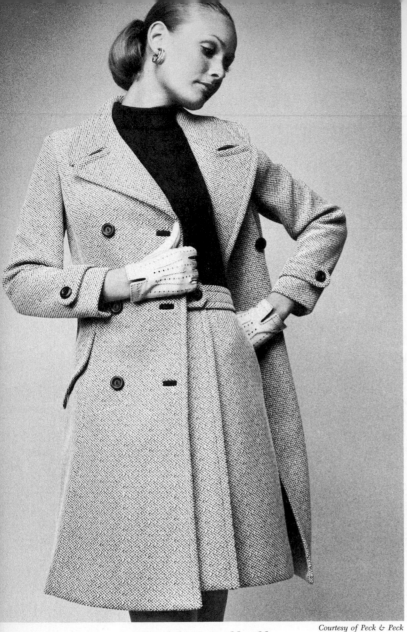

*A coordinated coat and skirt ensemble add
up to high-caliber fashion.*

fitted suit with the slim skirt. This style weathers the whims of fashion, while pleats and flared skirts come and go. Look for good lines and good fit. The most adaptable suit is one in an all-season solid color, or perhaps in a muted tweed. Two-tone effects and contrasting trim limit its flexibility. The neckline should look good with a variety of blouses and should also be attractive without a blouse. To allow freedom in accessorizing, there should be no large jeweled buttons, no fur collar (unless detachable), or other restricting decorative trims.

Your nonbasics. No wardrobe needs to consist entirely of basics (although many of the best ones do). Every now and then you find a dress that looks so perfect you wouldn't dream of changing it, or a blouse that makes such a beautiful ensemble when worn with one suit that you don't mind if it doesn't go with any other skirt in the closet. But, being a woman, you probably will want change—and only a wardrobe with a good supply of basics allows this flexibility. A dress with fussy details or ''cute'' trim is eye-catching at first but may soon become boring because it allows no change and remains the same forever and ever and ever. Scan the photos of the women who are rated best-dressed. Nine times out of ten these women, despite their wealth, are wearing basics—superb simplicity at its best.

A basic wardrobe, then, presents a good takeoff point for any flights of fancy. After you have acquired the essentials, you can go for the extras. And basic styles save you money because they can be transformed so easily that you need fewer clothes. Once you've acquired your minimum quota of good basics, you'll have saved enough to indulge in some of the other nonbasics you might not otherwise have been able to afford.

allow your date dress to double for many occasions.

A basic suit. A suit provides a look of efficiency and style that makes it rate high with business girls. Suits are available in so many forms that they can fill a large number of social requirements as well. The most basic style is the softly

🌸 *Multiplication with Separates*

By mixing and matching separate blouses, skirts, and jackets, many business girls provide themselves with a wardrobe that, even if small, allows a great deal of variety. As with short coats, care must be taken to create a well-balanced silhouette. Full skirts and dirndls require tucked-in or waist-hugging tops. Bulky or boxy tops are good with slim skirts or those with low controlled fullness or pleats.

The most successful combinations are generally a detailed blouse with a simple skirt, or a plain blouse with a more decorative skirt. Both items should be neither too plain nor too fussy. The best effects are achieved when only one element seeks the spotlight.

In teaming separates, take care that the same degree of formality prevails. No one would wear sneakers with an evening dress, yet we occasionally see a very dressy blouse with a sporty skirt or high heels with pants. Such pairing up is completely incongruous.

A print top with a plain skirt creates a smart twosome, but the styling, color, and texture must all be carefully cued to one another. It is best to avoid fabrics that are difficult to coordinate, such as gabardines, slub textures, or bold weaves.

❦ Pants

Pants play an important part in the wardrobe of many girls. They are comfortable and practical, and the right style on the right girl can be very attractive. From well-tailored ski pants to gracefully flowing wide-legged ensembles for evening wear, pants are available in a variety of styles and fabrics.

Fashionable women wear well-tailored pant suits for city wear, as well as in the country, although some city restaurants and other staid institutions still will not admit women in pants. Practical as they are, they are not allowed in every office. A pant suit with a matching skirt is a versatile choice for a career girl who feels she cannot afford to invest in a pant suit for leisure wear only.

In selecting flattering pants, let your figure be your main consideration. The wide-legged ones have a shortening effect—the wider the flare the more height is required to offset them.

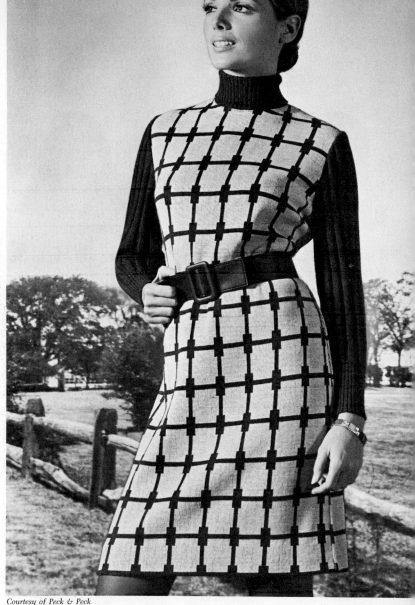

Courtesy of Peck & Peck

No wardrobe need consist entirely of basics. It should have some drama also.

They also look good only on slim-hipped figures. The short or stocky girl will be more attractive in a straight-legged or tapered style. Wide-legged pants won't look right unless they are the proper length. Although you can get by in tapered pants that are a little short, wide-legged varieties must be long enough to touch the instep and the back of the heel.

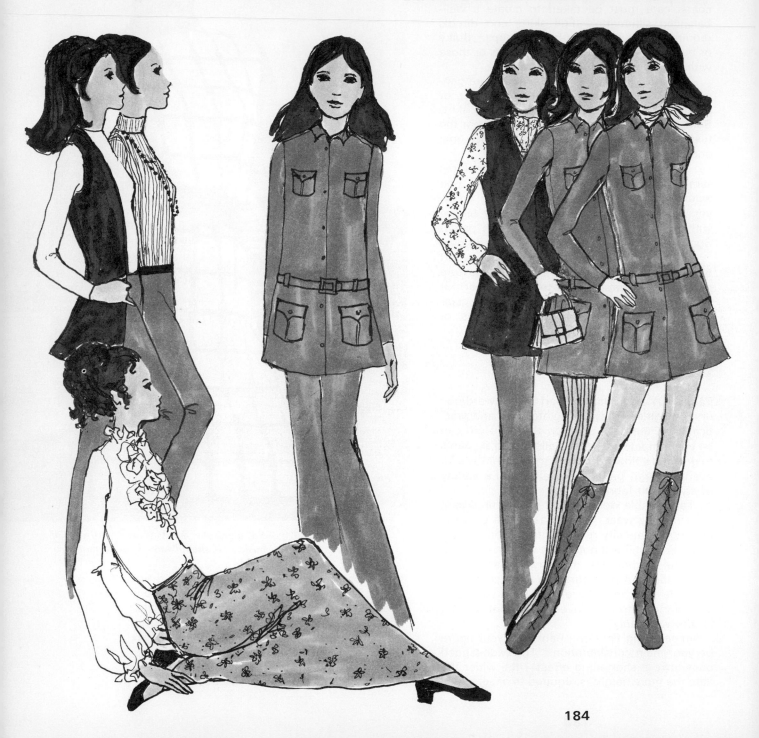

WITH SEPARATES

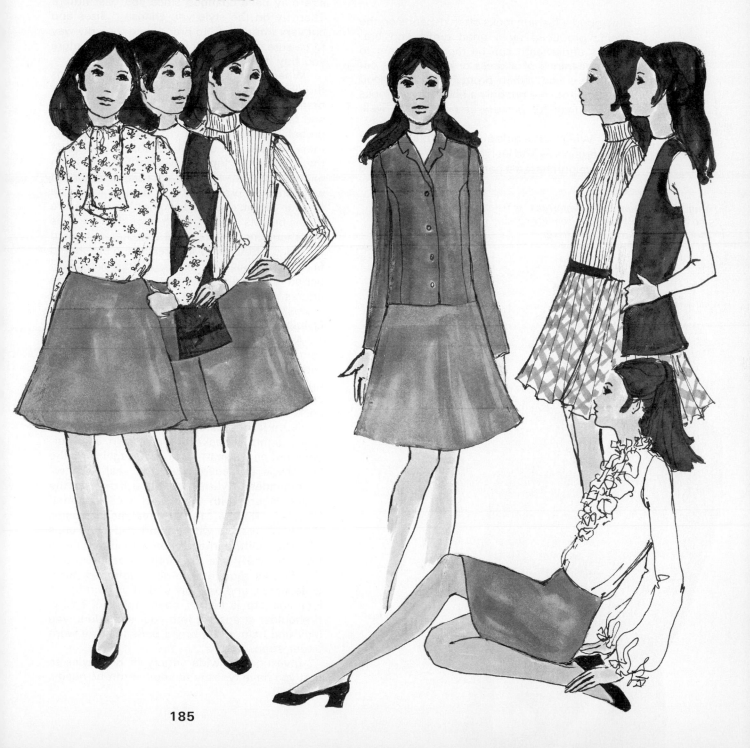

❦ Foundation for Good Fashion

How good a fashion looks often depends on the effects produced by a good girdle and bra. What's underneath can be more important to the appearance of a dress or suit than its cut or fabric. And, when properly fitted, a good bra and girdle are not only a boon to good looks but do much for posture and morale as well.

Bras. When some girls purchase a bra, they ask for a certain size and let it go at that. But unless you have purchased a particular style and brand

Your foundations are important when you wear a knit dress or something else that is particularly form-fitting.

Courtesy of Peck & Peck

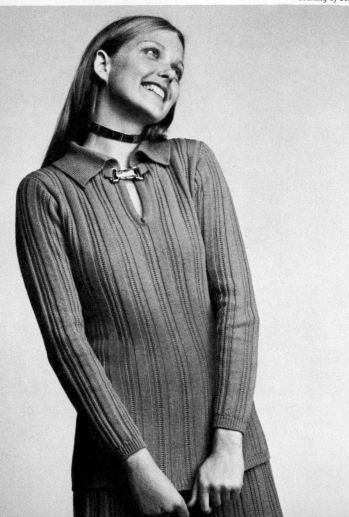

recently, it is best to be measured, because your size may have changed since your last fitting. Then try on the style you choose. Sizes and cut vary from brand to brand, and the only way to be sure of a good fit is to try on a bra before you buy it.

When you try on a bra, put your arms through the straps and lean forward so that your breasts slip into the cups. Then straighten up and fasten the band. The shoulder straps will probably need adjusting. If a bra fits correctly, there will be firm uplift from the underside of the cup and the top side will not put any strain on the breasts. This is especially important with strapless bras. Wires or boning should be fitted to the rib cage and shouldn't put pressure on the breasts. Your breasts should fill the cups but should not be crowded together or toward the sides. Between your breasts the bra should fit right against your chest. Bras with elasticized undercups are good for between-size figures. If you're quite small, you may want to consider a padded bra to help your dresses fit better.

A bra that fits well should give you a lovely contour, and it should be comfortable. It shouldn't interfere with deep breathing or ride up when you lift your arms, and it should not cause bulges under the arms or across the back. You should be able to run your finger easily under the band of the bra; otherwise, it is too tight. Check your profile in a mirror. Then put on a sweater and check again. Is the bra shape attractive? Do any seams show?

A bandeau style is probably sufficient for the young figure with high and well-separated breasts. Mature, more developed bosoms should have a bra with a band under the cups for extra uplift, perhaps even a style that fits to the waistline if the diaphragm needs control. Full figures require built-up, reinforced cups, wide straps, and possibly underbust wiring. A long-line bra is best if your midriff is fleshy. If shoulder straps dig into your shoulders, you may find help in the broad pads that are worn under straps.

Investigate a wide variety of bra styles so that you have types to fit your wardrobe needs.

186

There are bras with wide-apart straps for scoop necklines, halter bras for halter necklines, strapless bras, brasalettes for princess-line out fits, low-underarm bras for sleeveless dresses, backless bras, and bras with more rounded cups for wear under sweaters.

Girdles. Whether a girl struggles into a size 40 dress or slithers into a size 8, she needs a girdle for a smooth look. Even the slimmest models wear girdles because they realize that even their lean figures need the light controlling touch that refines curves and presents an attractively molded silhouette.

The type of girdle you choose depends on your figure. Your girdle *size* is based on your waist measurement, but if you require anything more elaborate than a simple two-way stretch, you will need to know which style and length is best. Garments with no-stretch or vertical-stretch panels must be fitted carefully. The *style* you need is determined by the fullness of your hips and the length that best suits your frame. The difference between hip and waist measurements is about 8 to 10 inches for the average figure. Full-hipped figures may measure 11 or more inches larger and require a girdle that is designed for full hips. Slimmer figures (with less than an 8-inch difference between waist and hips) can wear a straight-hip style. Proper length can make the difference between a sleek line and border bulges. The measurement is taken at the side, from the waist to the thigh, and is sized as follows: 14 inches or less—short; 15 to 16 inches—medium; 17 inches or more—long. If your stockings feel strained, the difficulty may be either that your girdle is too short or that your hosiery is not long enough.

For accurate and comfortable fit, always consult an experienced corsetiere. She knows the special features of each brand and style and which one will do most for your figure. Tell her whether you intend to use the garment for sports or for business and dress wear. A lightweight girdle is excellent for sportswear but may not give you the firm control you want for other clothes.

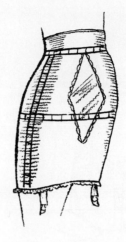

A slim, willowy figure needs the least amount of control and can usually get by with a simple all-elastic, pull-on style. A fuller figure will need panels that give more control. There are girdles with special front panels for tummy control, with nonstretch side panels for hip bulges, and with strong back panels for derrière smoothing. Heavy thighs require a longer length girdle with firm side panels or an extra long-legged panty. (If thighs are very full, however, you will probably find a regular girdle more comfortable than a panty style. Panty legs that fit too tight can sometimes cause unpleasant circulatory difficulties, especially if your work requires you to sit a lot.) High-rising styles control spare tires at the midriff. For heavier figures the corsetiere may suggest an all-in-one (a corselet) to give a smoother, more defined line. Light-control, all-in-one body stockings are favored by slender girls to provide a slinky smooth, uninterrupted line under knits and figure-revealing outfits. All-in-ones are sized for figures in which the bust and hips are in proportion. If yours vary from the norm, consider a long-line bra to team with a high-top girdle.

Before making any final decision, try on the girdle and fasten your hose properly—do the front and side garters while seated, the back garters while standing. Then try a sitting test. Does the girdle dig at the waist, produce a spare tire, or strain on stockings? If so, it doesn't fit

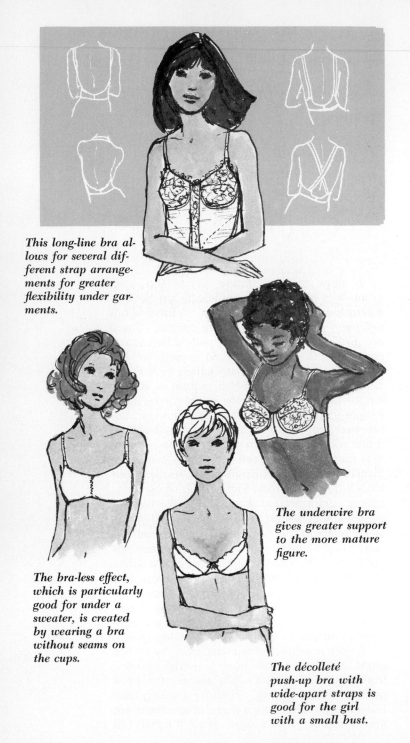

This long-line bra allows for several different strap arrangements for greater flexibility under garments.

The bra-less effect, which is particularly good for under a sweater, is created by wearing a bra without seams on the cups.

The underwire bra gives greater support to the more mature figure.

The décolleté push-up bra with wide-apart straps is good for the girl with a small bust.

properly. Try the bend-over test also. Does the girdle ride up or poke your middle? It shouldn't. Here are some other points to check. The garment must either be rejected or altered if it does not pass with a perfect score.

• Does it fit snugly at the waist without gapping or squeezing? You should be able to fit three fingers under the girdle front, four if it's boned. Too large a waist can be corrected by taking a dart at the waistline.

• Does it prevent a spare tire? If a girdle is too tight or is not built up high enough, an unpleasant bulge around the waist is sometimes the result.

• Are boned sections comfortable? There should be a finger-width space under the boning at every point where the body bends.

• Can you walk forward and backward and move comfortably without constriction or without the garment riding up?

• Does the crotch ride up or do the legs cut into your thighs? If so, you need a longer length or a style with longer legs.

An all-in-one should be checked to see that the bust cups fit comfortably. If there is any downward pull over the bust, the corselet is probably short. Are the shoulder straps comfortable? Too much strain on straps can rub your shoulders raw. An all-in-one foundation should fit properly so that no roll is caused at the top edges, particularly across the back. Check to see that it fits smoothly through the waist and hips and is long enough to allow you to sit comfortably.

Do you know how to put on a girdle? Often more damage is done by the strain and struggle of getting into a girdle than by weeks of wear. The simplest and safest method is to pull the girdle partway up over your hips and then grasp the lower edges and flip the girdle inside out as you pull the entire garment up above your waist. (A bit of swivel at this stage makes the job easier.) Then smooth the waist section into position and, grasping the bottom edges of the girdle, slide them down again (right side out) over your hips. By pulling the girdle down from above your waist, you are working with Nature instead of against her, and your flesh is smoothed into proper position, not all squeezed up to overflow in a roll at the top.

Be sure that your girdle is centered on your figure—that the center panel is really in the center. With so many of the lightweight elastic pull-ons, it's easy to don the girdle off-center. Unless it's on correctly, you'll be uncomfortable and won't get maximum support. If your garment has a zipper, don't try to close the zipper before you've fastened all the hooks beneath it. Fasten from the bottom up—never from the top down.

Panty girdles can't be put on in this flip-the-bottom-up manner, obviously. Instead, first fold the garment in half, top to bottom. Step in and smooth the folded girdle up over your hips to the right position. Then roll the top up to your waist. This makes the tugging much easier.

Some girls mistakenly believe that the longer their foundations go without washing, the longer they will last. On the contrary, dirt, oils, and perspiration cause elastic to deteriorate and discolor. Suntan lotion, for instance, is especially destructive; it's a good idea to wash off all traces from your legs before putting on your girdle. In laundering your garment, gentleness is the rule. The villains are hot water, harsh soaps, irons, radiators, and rough handling. Do be sure zippers are zipped. Soak in mild lukewarm suds for about seven minutes, rinse thoroughly, and roll in a towel so that excess moisture is absorbed. To dry your girdle, close the garters over a hanger and hang it away from heat or direct sunlight. Fabric sections can be ironed, although this may not be necessary. Never iron the nylon or elastic. If you want to use a washing machine, put your girdle in a cheesecloth or nylon bag for protection and be sure the water is not too hot.

The average girl needs at least two girdles—one to wear, one to wash—with another, perhaps, for sports. Alternating foundations helps them last longer, for it gives the elastic time to rest and regain its shape between wearings.

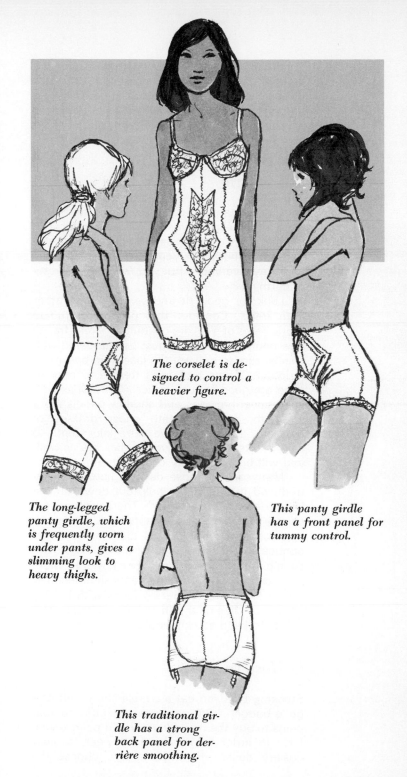

The corselet is designed to control a heavier figure.

The long-legged panty-girdle, which is frequently worn under pants, gives a slimming look to heavy thighs.

This panty girdle has a front panel for tummy control.

This traditional girdle has a strong back panel for derrière smoothing.

When you take off a girdle, inspect it for rips or loose garters. It's disconcerting to anyone's poise to have a garter pop at an inopportune moment. Small rips should be repaired before another wearing. Try to let your girdle air for a while before putting it away.

❦ Lingerie

Your slips, panties, pajamas, robes, and such need not be expensive, but for the sake of your morale, they should be attractive and neat. Perhaps nobody but your family sees them— and they love you—but you *feel* best in pretty underthings.

Look for good fit and serviceability rather than frills. Consider that pleated or ruffled fabric hems of slips are opaque, whereas fragile lace hems are not and must be laundered with special care to prevent the lace from becoming ragged. Taffeta or fabrics treated to prevent cling are good for use under knits. Slips with lined cover-bra tops and shadow panels are a must for wear beneath sheer dresses or blouses. Dark slips give extra inky depth to dark outfits and if you wear a dark bra as well, you will be completely coordinated.

Many dual-purpose designs have been introduced in lingerie to help cut down on the layers of clothing you wear. There are bra slips, culotte slips, petti pants, panty hose, and garter belts or light-control briefs attached to nylon panties or half slips, to name a few. There are even panty girdles with attached hosiery. More practical, however, are the panty slimmers that attach to separate long stockings with hidden garters or clips or that have special elastic leg-bands to keep stockings aloft.

❦ Hosiery

Stocking bills can eat a sizable chunk out of a girl's budget. *Pfft* goes a run and *pfft* go your plans to buy the new blouse you'd been saving for! In order to get the most wear for your hosiery dollar, it's important to choose the proper weight and style for each occasion and to obtain the type and size that fits best.

Many women consistently wear dress-sheer hose for all occasions. This is pretty fragile stuff, not intended for the hard abuse of career or classes. Hosiery manufacturers advise "daytime" or business" sheers for greater daytime longevity. Better wear can usually be obtained from mesh or textured stockings. When these are snagged, a hole may develop-but they usually will not run. A tiny hole in a hidden spot can be dabbed with colorless nail polish and forgotten, whereas in regular stockings it would mean a run.

Many hosiery troubles arise from poor fit. Your stocking should be long enough so that when it is on the foot it can be pulled out about a half inch at the toe, heel, or instep. A stocking that fits too snugly may cause a burning sensation on the sole of the foot, and it is prone to runs that start from the toe.

Correct length and proportion also affect comfort and wear. If stockings are too short, there is uncomfortable strain, and breaks at the knee soon develop. If stockings are too long, they will wrinkle and wear excessively at unreinforced points. Even though two women may be the same height, one may have fuller legs and will require a longer stocking than the other, whose legs are slim. Several manufacturers offer proportioned nylons so that very slender and very heavy legs can have a smooth, comfortable fit. Stretch hosiery, because of its elasticity, and mesh hose, with its flexible knit, also help solve this problem.

Whenever you purchase stockings, always get three or more pairs alike. This allows you to wear them in rotation and to match up any leftovers when one in a pair gets a run.

Panty hose or hiplets are a must with short skirts. The latter give you the long, unbroken leg line of panty hose with the advantage of combining leftovers when one stocking sprouts a run.

Non-skintone hosiery—colored stockings and tights with interesting weaves or shiny finishes—is often quite effective with short skirts. These look best on girls with long, slen-

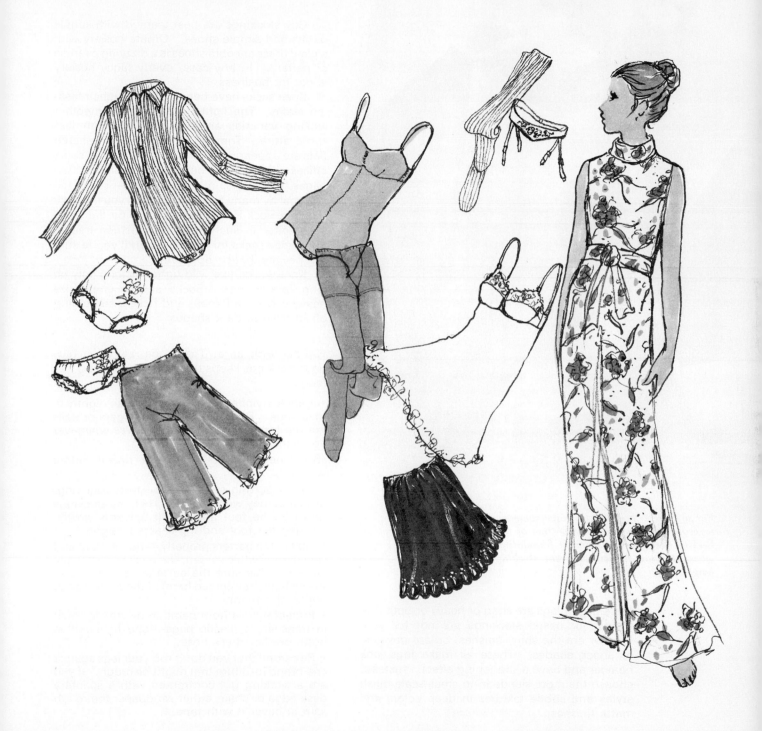

191

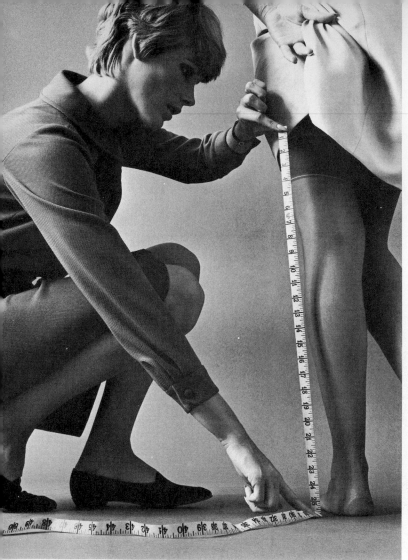

Courtesy of E. I. DuPont de Nemours & Company

For a correct stocking fit, have someone measure your leg from the bottom of the heel to the garter. Different foundation garments may require different stocking lengths.

der legs. If legs are short or heavy or both, the whitish or pastel stockings are not for you. Neither are the shiny finishes, ornate designs, or shock shades. These all make legs look heavier and have a shortening effect. Instead, choose the more slenderizing small-scale mesh styles and subtle textures in deep colors and matte finishes.

Gay stockings are best teamed with simple outfits and simple shoes. Ornate hosiery with a plaid dress or cobra shoes is a dizzying overuse of pattern. In any case, overly fancy hosiery is not for business.

Knee socks have been expanding their fashion realm. The lighter weaves and smoother looking varieties are being shown with less rustic attire. Trim socks paired with tailored flats are appearing on city streets, even in some offices. Since most bosses don't read fashion pages, such styles may well be considered too informal by many firms. Although you may like the knee-sock look, it's unwise to be the office style setter in such debatable fashion trends. Save knee socks for weekends until you're sure the powers-that-be approve.

Knee socks, like wild tights, belong only on long, pretty legs. Socks always emphasize heavy calves and knees and have a shortening effect even in dark shades.

Handle with care. The tender care you give your stockings keeps them pretty and snag-free longer.

• Handle nylons with caution. Wash nightly in mild suds. Don't rub. If your fingers or nails are the least bit rough, wear gloves whenever you handle stockings.

•Brand-new nylons should be rinsed before wearing.

• When putting stockings on, turn your rings in so that they won't catch. Then roll stockings down to the foot and unroll upwards slowly, keeping the foot and leg seams straight.

• Fasten the garters properly—do the front and side garters while seated, the back garters while standing. Be sure the garters are fastened in the welt (top reinforced hem) of the stocking but not on the seam.

• Protect nylons from damage by storing them in transparent plastic bags—one for daytime hose, one for dress hose.

• Be careful that you don't rub your legs against chairs and furniture that might be rough. If you are a working girl confronted with a splintery desk edge or chair, either sandpaper the rough spot or cover it with tape.

✾ Shoes

Many attractive shoe styles are available in a variety of heel heights. Good-looking low heels are quite appropriate for office wear and are especially good for the girl who must be on her feet much of the day. Choose the trimly tailored styles with a slight heel. Loafers and similar casual flats are not considered businesslike. High heels are appropriate for all but very informal occasions. They make feet look smaller and calves and ankles look prettier.

The most versatile shoe is a simple medium-heel opera pump. Fashion trends come and go, but this unadorned closed design is always in style and always appropriate for every costume. Calf or kid are best for every day wear because they can be repolished to gleaming beauty, whereas suede or buckskin may become water-scarred if caught in the rain. Some of the glossy patents hold up well also. Sandals and similar fancy cutout shoes and gold or silver leathers should be reserved for dressy occasions. They are not appropriate for business.

Keeping your shoes in good condition is very important for good grooming. Scuffed shoes, run-down heels or tips, and smudgy suede can spoil a smart appearance. For emergency cleanups try facial tissue to restore a shine or paper towels to brush suede. A soft eraser removes marks on buck.

Fit first. Good fit is essential to comfort. No matter how attractive a shoe, don't buy it unless it feels right. In the shoe store make a point to walk off the thick carpet to a spot where you can give your shoes the hard-floor test. Be sure there is no pressure and that there is wiggle room through the toes but a snug fit at the heel. The ball of your foot should come exactly at the widest part of the sole, and your instep should be well supported. If your foot rides forward, the salesman can put in a metatarsal pad or a foam rubber sole cushion, which often helps a low-arched foot.

For surest fitting, it is best not to buy shoes early in the morning. As the day progresses and we walk around more, our feet swell. This is particularly true in warm weather. What may seem a perfect fit at ten may be causing you agony by six. Never, never buy cheap shoes for daily wear. Shoes that are poorly made give out fast and result in aching feet, a short temper, and an anguished expression that is detrimental to any girl's charm. Foot specialists advise that we have at least two pairs of daytime shoes so that we can alternate them. This adds to foot comfort by giving your feet a change and

193

B. D. Unsworth

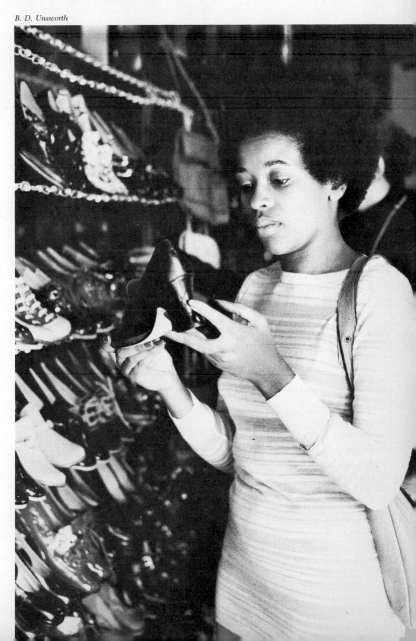

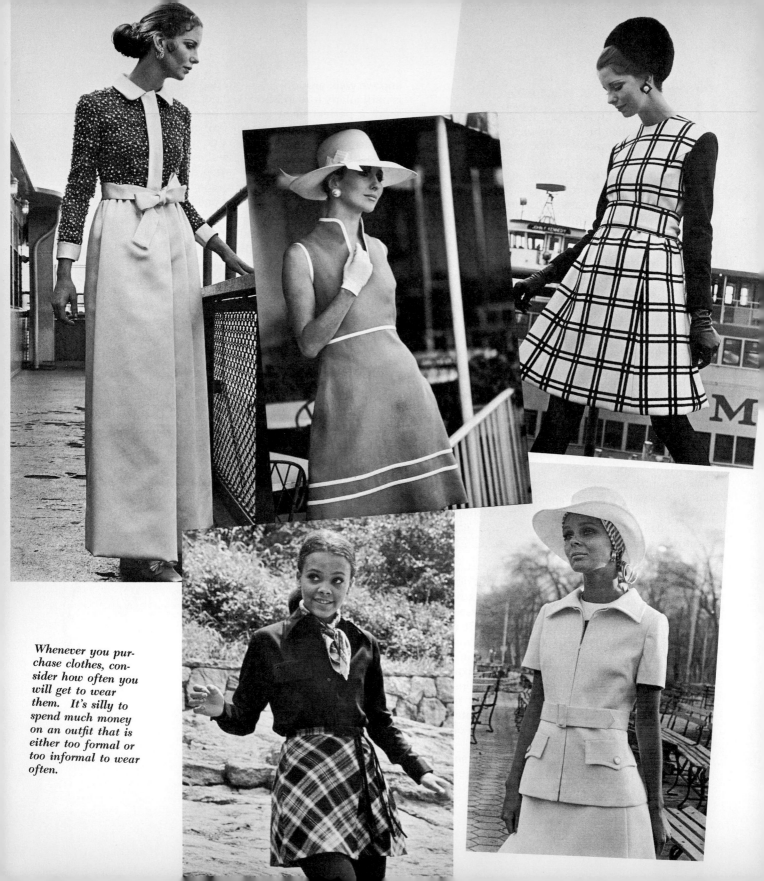

Whenever you purchase clothes, consider how often you will get to wear them. It's silly to spend much money on an outfit that is either too formal or too informal to wear often.

adds to shoe life by giving the leather a chance to rest and to air out.

❧ *Boots*

Boots look marvelously dashing, and they're eminently practical for foul weather. If you want to wear them in wet or snowy weather, however, be sure they are marked *waterproof.* Leather and some synthetics are merely water-repellent, which isn't enough for slush or puddles. When selecting boots, don't choose too heavy a lining if you intend to wear them in moderate weather or while commuting by bus or train. Heavy linings are great for snow but can be too hot for comfort any other time. Lighter linings can always be insulated by wearing extra socks in your boots on frigid days.

While some of the most attractive boots come in leather, good ones are quite expensive and poor-quality ones are not recommended. To maintain their smart appearance, you must treat leather boots frequently with saddle soap and polish, just as you do leather shoes, and you should guard them from rain and salt, which may stain. As with shoes, the tips and heels of your boots should be kept in good repair.

Black or brown boots in a classic style with a comfortably low walking heel are most versatile. Long, slender legs can wear the swashbuckling knee-high or higher styles, but short or heavy legs look best in a boot that just covers the curve of the calf. Before you buy any of the mid-calf or higher styles, try climbing a few stairs with them on to make sure they don't cut or bind you when you bend your knee.

Boots, of course, should not be worn in the office. If you carry your shoes, use a pretty shoe tote or perhaps an interesting flowered case or shopping bag that can also hold your newspaper and other extras. Girls with large-sized shoes should be sure that a shoe tote is large enough before they buy it. Some are not generously sized.

1 *Try to become acquainted with the characteristics of good-quality clothes. Examine the clothes in the windows or on display in better stores. See what factors you can observe that warrant the expensive price. The girl who is familiar with the look of quality will be a better shopper even though she buys in a lower-priced department. She will be able to appreciate a true bargain and to recognize shoddy merchandise.*

2 *Work out your own color-coordinated wardrobe plan based on the clothing you have on hand. Note any new items that may be required for proper balance and coordination.*

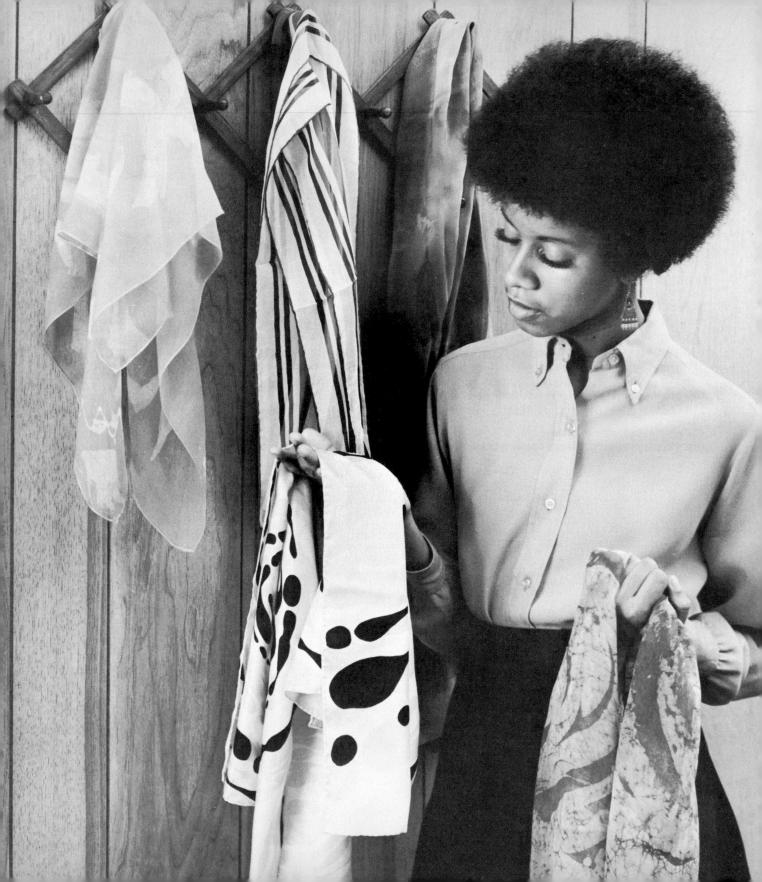

12

ACCESSORIES MAKE THE DIFFERENCE

The accessories you select and the way you wear them reveal your personality—particularly your cleverness and your good fashion sense. Some girls can give a high-fashion look to the simplest outfit by the way they use accessories. The difference between one girl's shirtdress and another's may hinge on a marvelous belt. Perhaps a handsome bag sets off the whole effect. Or maybe it's the scarf tucked in at the neckline or her unusual color combination. Smart accessories are a wise investment. They aren't limited to one costume but can be used to spark several different outfits, paying their way in compliments for years to come. In using your accessories, keep in mind that the total effect must be one of perfect harmony—accessories and dress must agree with each other in degree of formality. They must also blend into a happy oneness. Too many eye-catchers splinter attention.

The more elaborate the outfit, the simpler the accessories—and vice versa. A detailed or frilly dress requires only the simplest accessories. A plain dress can use more lively accents. Finally, use dramatic accessories to play up your best features. A girl with big hips cleverly avoids tricky purses, saving her fireworks for hats and face-flattering jewelry.

Back in January, 1849, a famous Parisian couturier pronounced in *Godey's Lady's Book* that no lady should appear in a street costume that was comprised of more than fourteen eye-arresting elements. This Rule of Fourteen has been used by fashion experts ever since.

Accordingly, you should be able to count no more than fourteen items that are visible

COSTUME SCORECARD

dress, one piece (one color)   1
—plus 1 for each additional color
suit or two-piece dress (one color)   2
—plus 1 for each additional color
blouse   1
hat, plain   1
hat trimming   1 for each color
hat, flowered or feathered   2 or 3
hose   1
—with clock or design   2
shoes, plain   1
—high style or decorated   2
purse, small   1
—large   2–3
gloves   1
coat   1
buttons, self-fabric, simple matching   0
—other   1 for each
belts, self-fabric   0
—leather, plastic, etc.   1
scarf   1
necklace   1 or 2
earrings, small   1
—large   2 or 3
pin   1
bracelet   1
ring with stone   1
wristwatch   1
glasses, plain   1
—with trim   2

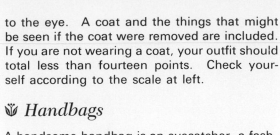

to the eye. A coat and the things that might be seen if the coat were removed are included. If you are not wearing a coat, your outfit should total less than fourteen points. Check yourself according to the scale at left.

🌷 Handbags

A handsome handbag is an eyecatcher, a fashion accessory as well as a necessity. The most basic type of bag is, of course, a one-tone leather bag in your basic color. In summer a tailored white, patent leather or neutral plastic bag, or a casual basket is a pleasant change to blend with any color scheme. Prints, stripes, and multicolor effects are fun but are often difficult to coordinate unless you have several solid-color outfits in shades that will match.

Quality is an important factor in the life of a handbag. Fairly inexpensive leathers are available, but a better-quality leather is a wiser choice. Cheap leathers scrape off and scratch too easily. If your budget is limited, a good-quality leather-look plastic or fabric bag will give better wear. Check the frame—is it sturdy? Does the catch close tightly?

A daytime bag should be large enough to hold all your totables without bulging and yet be in proportion to your size. Larger bags may get the fashion nod, but small girls are wise to keep to ones of fairly moderate size. A bag that can look quite smart on a tall girl will seem like a suitcase when hauled by a short person.

In addition to your basic bag, you will probably need a small one for dressy evening occasions. Faille, satin, silk and other dressy fabrics in a dark color are most versatile, but a gay little clutch in a hot pink, tangerine, bright blue, or other vivid color adds zip to a dark outfit, especially when teamed with one other accent in the same shade. Needless to say, since our gala occasions are not too frequent, the major investment should be in a daytime bag rather than in a dressy one.

Gay tote bags are fun and offer an easy way to carry newspapers, shoes, purchases, even lunch. If you carry a separate handbag, be sure your tote bag blends with it. Your tote bag should, of course, always be coordinated attractively with your outfit and your other accessories.

If you have any figure flaw, don't call attention to it by carrying your bag at that spot. For instance, a girl with a large bust shouldn't tuck her bag under her arm, a girl with a large waist won't choose a shoulder-strap bag, and a girl with a hippy figure looks more so if she dangles her bag at the side.

Here's a tip for carrying strap or handle styles. When you put your hand through the strap, go from the outside toward your body—don't aim out away from your body. When you aim in and then keep your arm against your waist, your bag can be held securely and won't bob back and forth as you walk. Ever had your hat knocked askew by somebody's bag when you were seated in a bus? If you carry your purse properly, you'll never be guilty of causing such mishaps.

❦ Gloves

Every girl needs a pair of simple, not-too-tailored, not-too-dressy gloves in her basic color and about three pairs of white ones. But for fashionable fun you may want a couple of extra pairs in gay accent colors. A black outfit with a daisy-trimmed white hat takes on extra sparkle when yellow gloves are added to pick up the yellow of the daisy centers. Beige or gray can be spiced with turquoise or rust, and so on.

Fabric gloves are now made in such attractive and smooth-fitting styles that they go everywhere, and they are often better choices for budget watchers than leather gloves. If you buy leather ones, look for the washable label. Otherwise, they must be dry-cleaned—a sure way to limit their circulation. Most leathers are dressy, but pigskin and similar textured skins are reserved for tailored wear. Insewn seams also are more dressy than outsewn styles and are more flattering for large hands. Broad hands look best in styles with vertical designs. Be sure you purchase the correct size. Too tight a glove will constrict your fingers uncomfortably and will actually make your hands feel much colder in the winter.

Many girls do not know how to decide on the length of glove that is most suitable for the sleeve they are wearing. You will have little trouble choosing the proper glove if you remember these guides.

• Outer wear (such as coats and suits)—your glove should meet the end of your sleeve.
• Short sleeves or sleeveless dress—a shorty glove is preferred.
• Three-quarter-length sleeve, informal dress—a shorty glove.
• Three-quarter-length sleeve, sophisticated dress—a glove that meets the sleeve.
• Formal evening wear—an over-the-elbow-length or shorty glove.
• Formal daytime wear—a shorty glove. (Over-the-elbow length is only for nighttime.)

Incidentally, in regard to glove etiquette, it's perfectly permissible to shake hands with your gloves on. It's considered poor taste (and rather precarious) to smoke, eat, or drink while wearing gloves. If you are wearing long gloves at a formal affair, you can unbutton them to the wrist so that you can slip your hands out; then tuck the fingers back into the wrist to keep them out of your way. At a public banquet or a dinner in a friend's home, you would remove them completely.

❦ Scarf Tricks

Whenever a dark dress looks too dark or a basic seems too basic, it's time to dig out a scarf and twist up something special. A girl with a long, slender neck will look marvelous with a gay ascot tucked inside her collar or twined around her throat. Watch the fashion magazines and the scarf counters at department stores for new ways to wear scarfs. Instead of letting the ends dangle, experiment with new tricks yourself. Try looping the ends into a bow or making a pouf by tucking each end back through the tied section and pulling out a little puff of the material.

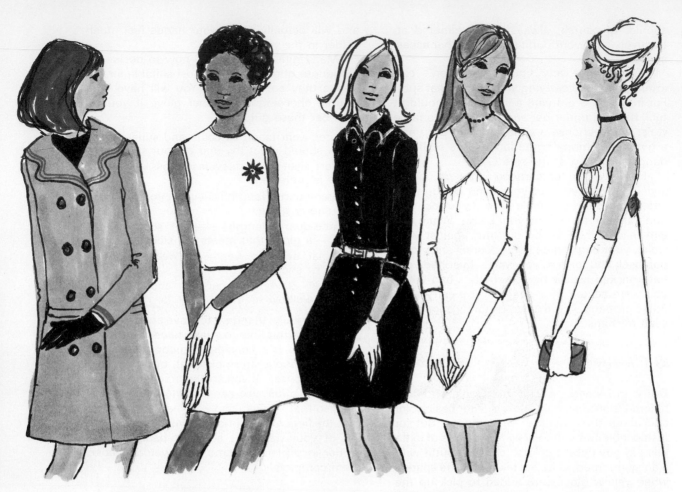

Neckline scarfs should be anchored in some way so that they don't twist out of place. A scarf that goes inside a collar will stay put when the ends are tucked under your bra straps. If you are wearing a dress or jacket that buttons in front, you can tuck the scarf ends in at the collar and let them peek out between the buttons. A necklace is also good for holding a scarf in place. A small scarf can be twined in and out of pearls. A larger one can be slipped under a two- or three-strand necklace or a long chain. Hold a ring scarf in place by pinning it to the shoulder seams of your dress—perhaps using one decorative pin and one hidden safety pin.

One ingenious scarf addict snipped enough fabric from the hem of a dark dress to make a loop about an inch and a half long and an inch wide. This she sewed vertically just below the center of the jewel neckline of the dress. This loop is an excellent spot to adorn with a pin, and it provides attractive anchorage when she wears a scarf. She loops scarf ends back and forth through this loop to make a variety of attractive bows, poufs, and ties and uses a pin atop the loop to keep them from slipping.

This loop trick can be tried by girls with shorter necks, too. To give a lengthening V-line, the loop should be sewn (or pinned so that it would be detachable) a little lower on the chest.

A girl with a really short neck will look too bundled up in a neckline scarf. She should save scarf accents for other areas—perhaps looping one around her waist as a cummerbund (if she is tiny), pinning it in a skirt pocket to let the ends flare out as a colorful note, or fastening it to a belt.

❦ *Jewelry*

Well-chosen jewelry is like the bow on the gaily wrapped birthday present. Many a dress looks unfinished until the proper piece of jewelry is added.

So many attractive designs are available that inexpensive pieces can look many times their value. If your budget is small, choose one metal color for all your jewelry—either gold or silver—and stick to it. The two are not to be mixed in one costume. Gold has the advantage of being generally more dressy, but inexpensive gold-plated jewelry is more subject to discoloration. (A light coating of colorless nail polish can be used to help prevent tarnish.) Sterling silver jewelry often gives you quality at moderate prices. Although silver will tarnish, it can easily be cleaned with a silver polishing cloth and will always keep its beauty.

Many girls couldn't get along without a pearl necklace and earrings. Pearls are always in good taste, and their soft glowing luster is flattering to every complexion.

Costume jewelry with stones or fake pearls should be chosen with care. Very inexpensive pieces give themselves away by large glassy stones and poorly finished settings. In the low-priced group, it is usually advisable to stick to small stones, with your best buy being pearls. When you buy a pin or earrings with rhinestones or colored stones, you usually get much better value and more realistic appearance if you pay more. Rhinestone jewelry is, of course, strictly nighttime glitter.

As with all your accessories, proportion is again important here. Chunky jewelry overpowers the small-boned face and weighs down the diminutive figure. Tiny pieces look inappropriately doll-like on a tall or full figure.

Necklaces. Remember the effect of a necklace line on facial contours? A quick review:

• The thin face and long neck profit by the illusion of width created by a choker length.
• Multistrand necklaces are excellent for filling in a bony neckline.
• If you aim to slenderize your face, choose a length that comes below the base of the throat. Long ropes also have a slimming effect, the only exception being with the bosomy figure. A rope swinging in space below a large bust merely emphasizes its size.
• Even the shape of the bead can affect your appearance. The larger the bead and the rounder it is, the more it gives an illusion of width. Round or oval beads soften angular features. Irregularly shaped beads are recommended for full faces. Small features need delicate beads; chunky jewelry is overpowering.

Earrings. Your earrings should match or blend with your necklace or pin. They need not be matching in design, but they should have the same general feeling—plain tailored style worn with heraldic emblem on a chain, more decora-

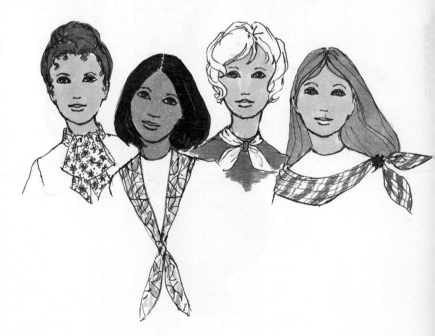

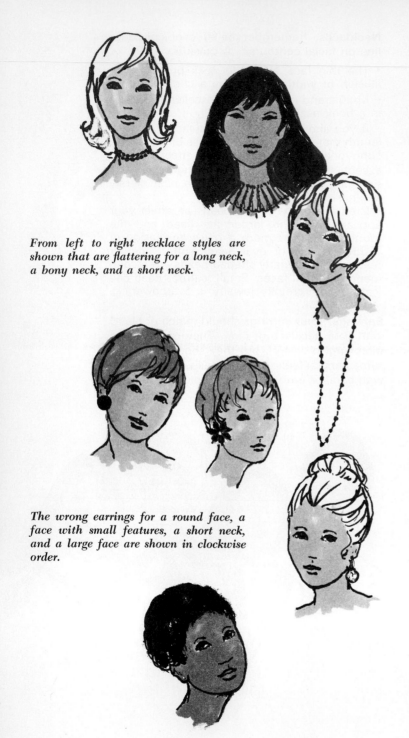

From left to right necklace styles are shown that are flattering for a long neck, a bony neck, and a short neck.

The wrong earrings for a round face, a face with small features, a short neck, and a large face are shown in clockwise order.

tive design with a dressier stone-studded pin, for example. As with all jewelry, they should fit the mood of your dress.

The most generally flattering earring is the upslanting wing shape that follows the curve of the ear. If earlobes are large, a bigger earring is preferred. Girls with small lobes need dainty styles and should look for screw-backs or magnetic-type backs if they have trouble keeping earrings on.

If a clip-type earring seems too tight, don't resign yourself to letting it just sit in your jewelry box. Many styles can be adjusted by bending down the arm that joins the clip to the back so that the clip won't snap so tightly. Your jeweler can probably fix it for you very easily, but if you try it yourself, use small pliers (or tweezers) and bend the arm just *slightly.* Strong-arm methods can do damage.

The earring style you choose should also balance the lines of your face. As you have probably figured out by this time, there should be no round earrings for round faces, no bulky styles for small features, no dangle designs for short necks. Drop earrings are the most difficult to wear. Although they lengthen a face, long or bulky drops can swallow up any but a long, swanlike throat.

Small girls and girls with delicate features should be careful to choose only drop styles that are delicate or light in character. On the other hand, tiny drops for pierced ears do nothing for a large or chubby face. Better balance is achieved with flat buttons or hoop styles.

Thinking about having your ears pierced? With so many marvelous pierced-look styles available, this hardly seems necessary any more. Before you take action, be sure you want those permanent holes in your ears. When the fad passes, as it did in grandma's day, the holes remain and all those with pricked ears are permanently—and conspicuously—dated as members of a bygone era. Remember, too, you must keep wearing pierced-ear earrings, no matter how tired you become of them, or the holes close up. If you do decide to have your ears pierced, be smart and have them done by a doctor. Too many cases of serious infection have resulted from do-it-yourself attempts or hasty jobs in jewelry stores.

Pins. Perhaps a pin is *the* most versatile bit of jewelry. Show your fashion flair by imaginative placement of pins. Instead of always wearing a pin on your lapel or collar, show it off on a hip pocket, let it adorn your hat, cuff, or belt, or loop it through a chain to make a pendant. When you want to make a simple pin more dramatic, you can back it up with a cockade of ribbon or display it badge-fashion atop striped grosgrain.

In choosing a place for your pin, remember that it is an attention-getting accent. Use it to direct all eyes to your best features. Wear it on your best side, or near a tiny waistline, for example. To create width for your face, perch a pin high on your shoulder. To give length, center it, preferably two or three inches below the base of your neck. If your bust is large, don't plunk a pin at the base of a low V-neckline.

Some large pins are too heavy for jerseys and other soft fabrics. You can often keep a pin from pulling by fastening it through your slip or strap as well as through the blouse.

Bracelets. These are excellent for long, thin arms—the best being slim styles, charm bracelets, and more delicate links. A heavy arm with a short hand needs a wider type of bracelet, one that gives the effect of being solid without creating too much bulk, such as larger link bracelets and those with openwork designs.

During office hours avoid wearing jangly bracelets. Your watch on one wrist and one wide or two or three narrow bracelets on the other are maximum. Never wear a bracelet with your watch.

Gems on display. It's easy to fall in love with jewelry. Occasionally a female with a kindergarten sense of fashion tries to display too much glitter at once. Incorrect adornment would be a three-strand necklace with matching earrings, a shoulder pin, a watch, bracelets, rings. Ornate or jeweled buttons and metal or jeweled

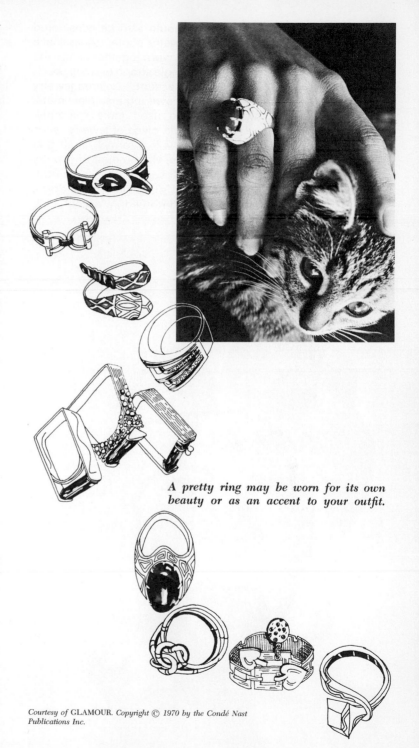

A pretty ring may be worn for its own beauty or as an accent to your outfit.

trim on eyeglasses should also be considered when tallying your jewelry quota. A necklace and pin are usually not worn together unless the necklace is merely a single strand of small pearls and is not an obvious accent. Colored jewelry tends to be more overpowering than plain metal pieces and should be used more sparingly. Sometimes just a single piece of jewelry, such as dramatic earrings with a formal, is all that is required. Of course, the amount of jewelry you should wear will vary with each outfit. Jewelry can be out of place on a busy dress, but simple dresses often need an accent.

Courtesy of Tampax Inc.

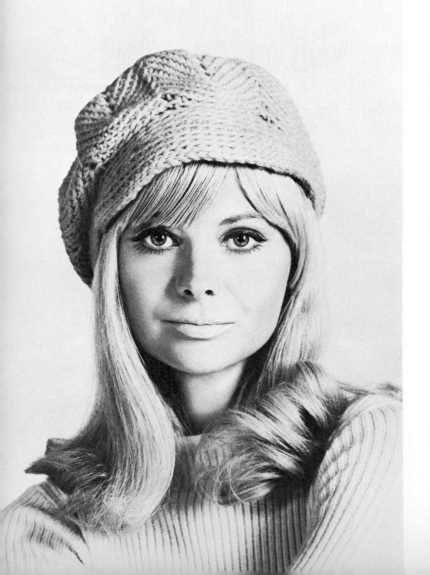

☙ *Hats*

A hat can be fun. A hat can be pretty. Few accessories can add the drama that a striking hat can impart. And few can do as much for your face and figure as the right hat.

Hats are required wear for formal teas, and either a hat or pretty veil should be worn in church and at weddings and funerals. Other than that, hats have been relegated to the ear-warmer or sunshade category—you can take them or leave them. But hats can provide so much flattery and are such great mood makers that they shouldn't be ignored.

Hat lines. A hat that does something for you complements your face and figure—those old camouflage techniques again. As with hairdos, the lines of your hat should not repeat undesirable body or facial flaws but rather should have lines that counteract any flaws. For balance your hat should be at least as wide as your face or hairdo but never wider than your shoulders.

Round shapes such as bretons, cloches, or round-crowned styles are good for square or diamond faces but not for round faces. Berets, angular styles, or hats with one-side-up-one-side-down brims flatter round-, pear-, or heart-shaped faces. If your face is long, choose low-crowned styles and turned-down brims rather than toques or other high-crowned styles.

Particularly helpful for a prominent nose is a hat with a brim that extends beyond the nose to balance it. Long noses need brims that slant upward and outward. Pug noses need narrow, down-slanting brims.

A receding chin can be built up with hat lines that are shallow at sides and curve up off the face. Play down a protruding chin with brims that reveal most of the forehead in front but are wide enough in back to balance the chin in profile.

Your hat wardrobe. Your basic hat should be fairly simple—neither too dressy nor too tailored to go with most of your outfits. Some girls produce stunning effects with a simple hat by making several snap-on hatbands or other detachable trims in colors that coordinate attractively with their wardrobes. Often a basic style can be made to double for dressy occasions by the addition of a simple small rhinestone or pearl pin. A spring hat (which, incidentally, takes on special attraction if worn very early in the season) should be a gay fillip. If it is to serve for summer, too, you might look for a style that depends on line and color for its appeal. The posy-covered bonnets that catch the eye at Easter may seem tired and too much in July.

How to buy a hat. If you are shopping for a hat that is not a standard color, try to wear the outfit it must blend with or have a bit of the fabric along to guide you. In many cities health department regulations forbid the return of hats, so you will want to be certain any new chapeau is a good match before you buy it.

When trying on a new hat in a store, note how the salesgirl adjusts it. She knows what the latest fashion quirks are and how each design is intended to be worn. But don't stop there. You know your face and the lines that will flatter it. Sometimes, if a hat doesn't look right, just a bit more tilt here or a twist there is all that is needed. Be sure the hat you choose is the correct head size. If it is too small, it may not sit down as far as intended or may be snug enough to become uncomfortable after you have been wearing it for a while.

Before you decide on a hat, check it from all angles. How does it look in profile? The big floppy-brimmed hat that looks quite dashing from the front may seem to smother a small face from a profile view. A drooping brim can also create a no-neck look. Some of your neck should be visible in back below the hat brim. As you know, the sides of your face differ. Your best side can be emphasized by a design that concentrates trim on that side.

If you wear glasses, keep them on while hat shopping. Some styles that look right alone may crowd the face when glasses are added.

How is the full-length view? Never buy a hat until you can see yourself while standing.

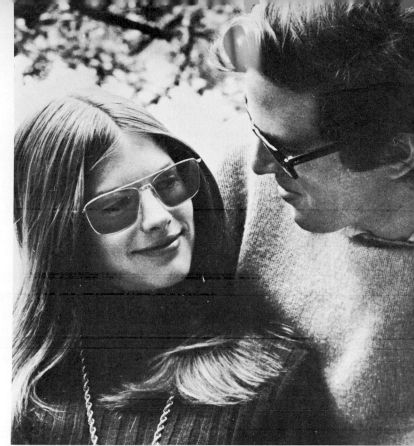

Fashionable glasses add a striking note of drama to your appearance.

The correct hat must be in proper proportion to balance your figure. A short girl in a wide-brimmed hat resembles a walking umbrella, but she will seem taller in a hat that is the same color as her outfit and is small in size but has uplifted lines. An upflung feather, stand-up flower, or bow can give an illusion of height without overpowering bulk. Tall girls can cut their height with hats of contrasting color and with good-sized brims. If shoulders are thin or sloping, avoid droopy brims; upturned brims provide better lines. Upslanting brims are also good for hippy figures.

🌷 Glamour with Glasses

Today eyeglasses are so attractive and come in such a variety of shapes (to flatter all faces) that they have become a charming beauty accessory instead of a beauty hazard. No longer need a

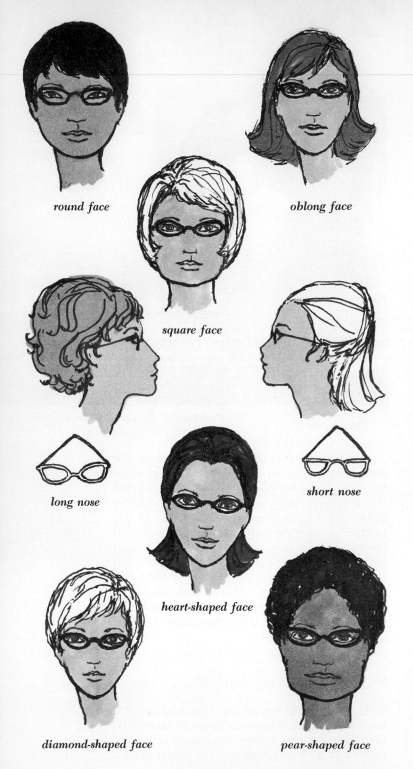

round face

oblong face

square face

long nose

short nose

heart-shaped face

diamond-shaped face

pear-shaped face

girl take off her glasses when the man of her life draws nigh. The right glasses enhance her good looks—and who isn't prettier when she doesn't squint, and more graceful when she can see clearly where she's going? If you wear glasses, make the frames a definite accessory and you won't be tempted to keep whipping them off.

If you depend on glasses, it makes good sense to carry an extra pair with you so that you won't be lost if the pair you're wearing breaks or is mislaid. This is especially important if you drive a car. When you select a second frame, choose a different style so that you can have one pair for everyday and one for dress. Since your glasses are so much a part of your costume and your general appearance, it is not extravagant to build up a wardrobe of frames that suit you and the life you lead. One of the most practical extensions of your glasses wardrobe is a pair of prescription sunglasses. They are useful all year and can be a glamorous fashion accessory. When you choose sunglasses, be sure that they are big enough to prevent glare from entering around the sides.

Choosing the frames. Whether you are choosing sunglasses or reading glasses or all-the-time glasses, be sure that the frames complement your features. The frame color should blend with your skin and hair, and the size of the frames must be compatible with the size of your face. If they are overpowering, they give you a beetle-like appearance. Lenses, however, should be large enough to show off the whole eye, including the lashes at the outer corners. The bow (sidepiece) should fit close to your head so that it can be partially covered by hair without disturbing the line of your coiffure. If you have only one pair of glasses, choose a simple frame that does not have too much decoration. Not only is this type best for office wear, but it is also less likely to conflict with jewelry and other accessories. Colored frames must, of course, be coordinated with the outfit you wear.

Fads come and go in eyeglass styles. Often a new craze such as the oversize round lenses is more striking than flattering. If you are buy-

206

ing prescription glasses, be very careful about investing a lot of money in a fad style. Your first consideration should be, "Are they flattering?"—not just, "Are they new?" The shape of the frame should be governed by the shape of your face.

OVAL FACE. No problems here; almost any shape will be flattering.

ROUND FACE. Counteract the roundness with frames that have sharp angles or squared-off bottoms, and ones that sweep up at the sides.

SQUARE FACE. Avoid frames with squared-off lines. Choose a style that has a gently curving upsweep.

OBLONG FACE. Give width by choosing glasses that extend beyond the broadest part of your face. They should be softly curved without too much upslant.

HEART-SHAPED FACE. Choose oval lines at top and bottom. Avoid harlequin styles.

DIAMOND-SHAPED FACE. Select a style that adds breadth to your forehead. Frames should be wider at the top than at the bottom and should have a definite upsweep.

PEAR-SHAPED FACE. A frame with a heavier top piece that slants slightly upward is flattering. The bottom should be oval and should not be as wide as the top.

LONG OR SHORT NOSE. A long nose can be visually shortened by wearing frames with a low bridge. A short nose seems longer if you choose a frame with a high bridge.

---

1 *Pay particular attention to the way fashionable women use accessories. See how many attractive new ideas you can find.*

2 *Experiment with your own accessory collection. Don a basic dress and conduct a mirror study session. Can you find four different places to put a pin? What different styles of necklaces could be worn? How could you dress your outfit up or down with belts? What scarf ideas would be flattering? Have you any separate collars or ties you could add? Don't overlook the possibilities of pairing up a matching jacket or knit cardigan to create an ensemble.*

3 *How successful a wardrobe planner are you? Based on your clothing inventory and your list of needed items, make yourself a three-year purchase plan that will provide a balanced, well-coordinated wardrobe. Note which items should be purchased each year for the next three years.*

Consider that the life expectancy for each coat, suit, dress, blouse, or skirt is three years. Shoes, hats, handbags, and other accessories can usually be counted on for about one year's wear. Plan to purchase a winter coat every three years, and apportion your expenses so that a suit or other major expense comes in an alternate year.

Part Four

Your Sound Effects

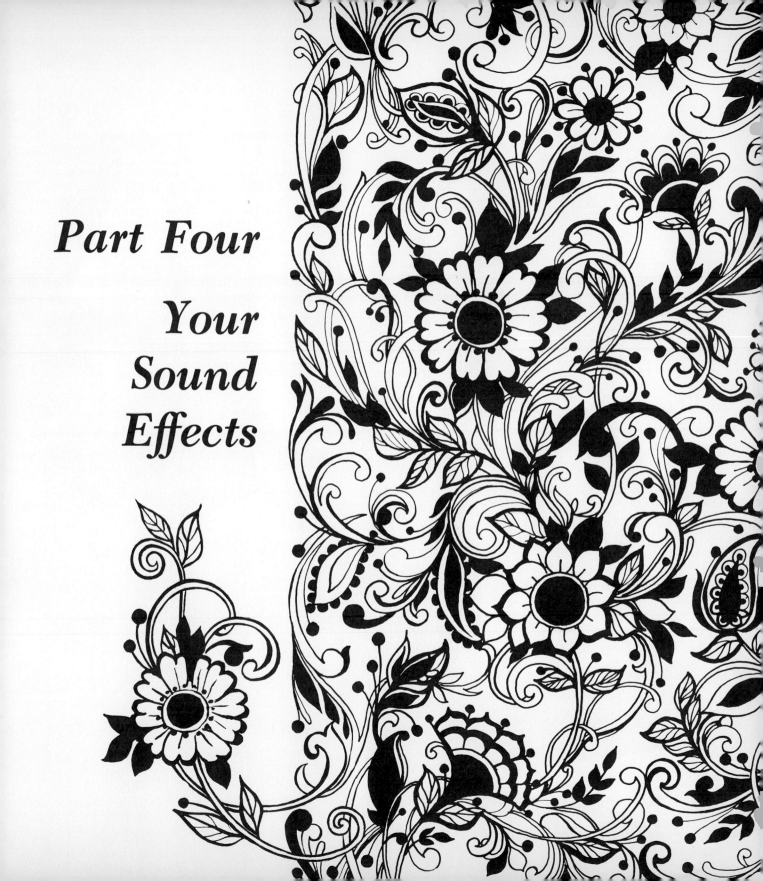

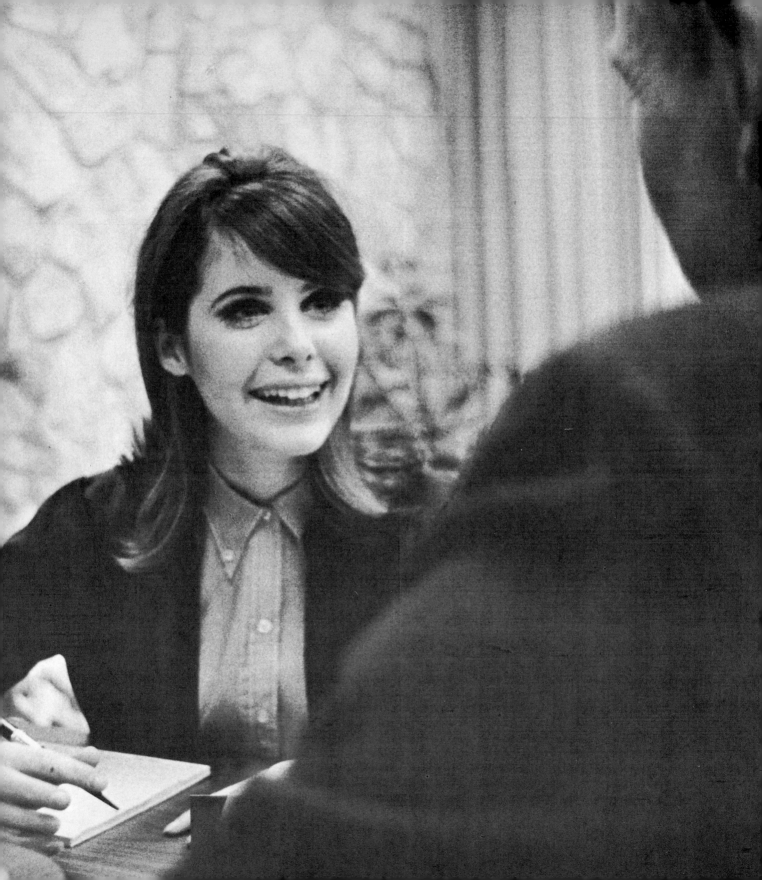

YOUR VOICE SPEAKS FOR YOU

A warm and pleasing speaking voice is an asset almost anyone can have—and a good voice is truly a great asset for charm. Acquiring one is not difficult. The only requirements are learning how best to tune up your voice and then putting good habits to work to drive out any bad ones. By concentrating on achieving a melodious, happy voice, you can make yourself a lovelier person. Almost any voice can be improved. There's probably no other area of charm that is so neglected, yet offers such rich rewards.

Voice is the result of the vibration of the vocal cords in your larynx, or Adam's apple. The force that provides the vibration is air expelled from the lungs. This is why good breathing habits—something few of us have—are so important to good speech. The sound produced by your vibrating vocal cords would sound rather flat if it weren't for your built-in resonators. Musical instruments all have resonators of some kind. The throat, the mouth, and the nasal and sinus cavities are—forgive the connotation—the holes in your head that serve as resonators to give your voice full tone and quality.

The first and most important step toward good speech is proper breathing. Unfortunately, few people breathe correctly except when they are asleep. Correct breathing begins with the diaphragm, the web of muscles that controls breathing. (To locate your diaphragm, place your hand just above your stomach, right between your lower ribs. Then cough slightly, moving your hand until you feel the spot where the diaphragm pulls in when you cough.) Make these muscles do the work of breathing. They should push your abdomen down and out to allow room for the lungs to expand as they take in air. Then, to expel the air, the diaphragm pushes up and the abdomen is pulled in. This is called *diaphragmatic breathing.* To feel diaphragmatic breathing in action, lie flat on your back for a few minutes and let your mind wander to any subject except breathing. Then note the way you breathe—this is the natural and correct way.

Women, especially, tend to be upper-chest breathers. Breathing from the upper chest

As opera singers know, proper breathing is essential for good voice control, whether they are singing or speaking.

Courtesy of Fred Fehl, New York City Opera

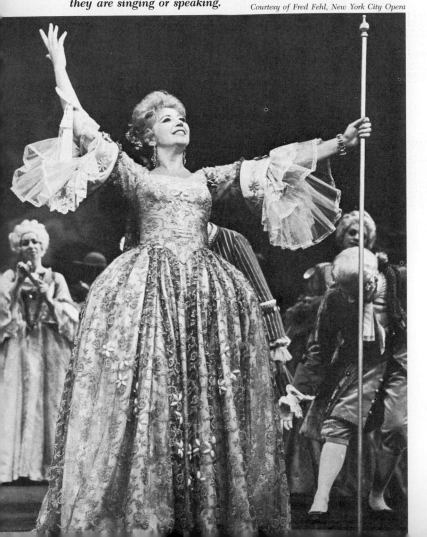

cannot produce the steady flow of air needed to control the strength and steadiness of tone and resonance. It also causes tensions that interfere with good voice control.

To establish good voice control, you do not need to inhale great gulps of air. Neither should your chest rise and fall with each breath. Your diaphragm should do all the noticeable work. Help it along by lifting your chest high (which is, of course, part of good posture).

Try this exercise to develop good diaphragmatic breathing habits and to increase the airstream that will produce good, clear speech. Sit tall and breathe slowly from the diaphragm. Check your posture—chest up, hips against the back of your chair. Get comfortable, not rigid. Try to remain completely relaxed. Inhale slowly and deeply from your diaphragm. Hold your breath a few seconds; then count aloud slowly and evenly as you exhale. Continue to count as long as possible. If you can only get to fifteen, you should practice frequently until you can do better, perhaps twice as well.

Good breathing habits make a world of difference in both health and speech. Practice diaphragmatic breathing every time you think of it during the day. If you find yourself forgetting, provide little reminders for yourself. Leave yourself notes or wear a certain piece of jewelry as a reminder. If possible, get good, fresh air in the process and your energy and spirits will improve, too. Soon deep, diaphragmatic breathing will be a welcome new habit.

❦ The Mellow Tones

Your resonance chambers give your voice its full, rich quality. If they are not functioning properly, as when you have a cold, your voice becomes flat or distorted. But resonance is also under your control—at least partially. If, for instance, your mouth is not open wide enough for the vowel sound *oh,* you lose resonance and the resulting sound is dull and flat.

You also have control of the soft palat at the rear of your mouth—you use this for the nasal sounds *m, n,* and *ng.* Too much nasal resonance produces a twang; too much throat resonance, a guttural sound. Helped by the lips and tongue, your mouth becomes a resonating chamber of infinite variety. So many possibilities exist that no two human voices are exactly alike. You will want to do all you can to improve your resonance so that you develop your voice potential and get all the mellow, rich tones possible.

Try humming to help improve resonance. Can you feel the vibration in your nose? You should be able to. Also practice saying the nasal sounds *m, n, ng.* Add a vowel to them and make up words such as *pong, bong, dong, kong,* holding the sound long enough to hear full resonance. Using the same consonants, vary the vowel sound to include the other vowels; for example, *pang, peng, ping, pong, pung.* Keep practicing until you can get rich resonance with all the possible combinations.

Too much resonance will produce harsh, nasal tones. Avoid this by being sure the throat is open wide, not constricted and tense. A good exercise to eliminate nasal harshness is to practice the type of exaggerated singing that imitates the open tones of an opera singer. Of course, this is strictly for your private moments, but let yourself go and have fun—all in the cause of a charming voice.

❦ *Listening In on You*

The best way to find out how you sound to others is to tape or record your voice. Does your school have a tape recorder for this purpose, or can you borrow one? If you work in an office, perhaps you can use your boss's dictating machine. When recording your voice, be sure to converse normally—forget about the recording and let your natural, unconscious voice speak. Only after listening carefully to the recording several times should you begin analyzing your voice.

If you are unable to record your voice mechanically—or even if you are able to—listen to your voice the next time you are in a lively

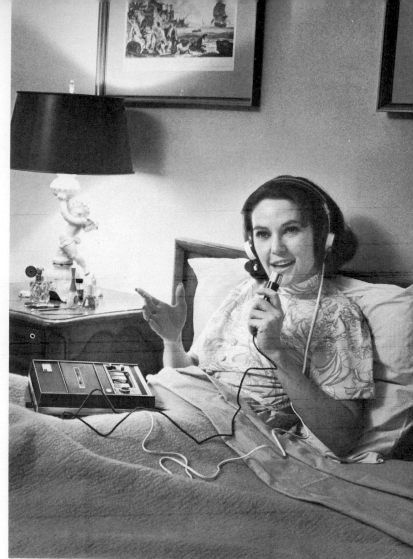

Courtesy of the Linguaphone Institute

Many people tape their voices because listening to one's own voice is the best way to improve pronunciation and speaking techniques.

conversation. Listen critically not only to your own speech but to the way others speak. Sometimes you can spot flaws in others and then realize you do the same thing. Listening to the way words are spoken will make you aware of both good and poor speech habits.

Voice qualities. Whether you listen to yourself or others, the following are the qualities—and flaws—to listen for.

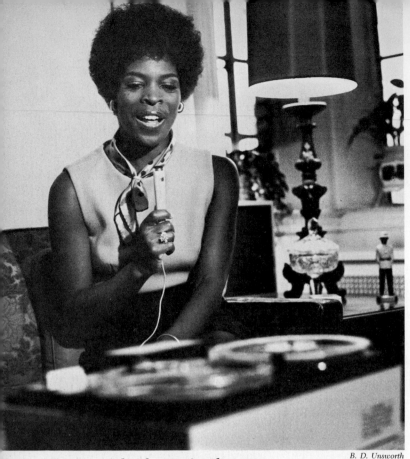

For Roxy Roker, here taping the poems of Langston Hughes, voice training has been the key to opportunities in music, acting, and television production.

PITCH. This means the position of your voice on the musical scale—how high or how low it is. Your voice operates within a certain range. You raise or lower pitch to suit your mood or to emphasize meaning. If you feel light and gay, you will use a higher pitch. When you are serious or sad, you lower the pitch of your voice.

Listen to whether your voice sounds warm and mellow. If it is pitched too high, it may sound shrill or squeaky; too low, and it becomes unfeminine. Your ideal speaking pitch should be about one-fourth of the way up from your lowest possible note. You can find your vocal range—your highest and lowest possible notes—on the piano. About a quarter of the way up from your lowest note is the point where your pitch should center. If in doubt, it is usually best to *lower* the pitch of your voice.

When you speak softly and tenderly, your voice naturally has a lower pitch. Just be sure you don't make it so low that it becomes unfeminine.

ENUNCIATION. Do you speak clearly? Or are you a mumbler and an ending-dropper? If people have to ask you to repeat what you say, faulty enunciation is apt to be the cause.

Do you say "acrost" for "across," "libery" for "library," or "gonna" when you mean "going to"? Poor enunciation is unattractive, and it is easily misunderstood. If you have this fault, you can correct it by speaking slowly and carefully. Make a real effort to avoid running words together, and try to pronounce every sound in a word that should be pronounced.

Saying tongue twisters is also good practice for making speech more distinct. Announcers and others who must enunciate clearly find them an excellent exercise. Try "A big black bug bit a big black bear." You probably know many more. Here are a few others you can try.

• Theophilus Thistle, the thistle sifter, sifted a sieve of unsifted thistles.
If Theophilus Thistle, the thistle sifter, sifted a sieve of unsifted thistles,
Where is the sieve of unsifted thistles Theophilus Thistle, the thistle sifter, sifted?
• Bring Bruce some brown bread.
• The old scold sold the school a coal scuttle.
• She stood on the steps inexplicably mimicking his hiccupping and amicably welcoming him in.
• Amidst the mists and coldest frosts
With barest wrists and stoutest boasts
He thrusts his fists against the posts
And still insists he sees the ghosts.
• The sixth sheik's sixth sheep's sick.

EMPHASIS. Do you give proper or sufficient emphasis to words? Individual words or groups of words within a sentence take on different meanings according to the emphasis they receive. Try saying the sentence "Give me my book" four times, each time emphasizing a different word. Did you get four different meanings?

Correct emphasis gives richer meaning to speech, but care should be taken not to use too much emphasis, because this slips into exaggeration and loses its effectiveness.

INFLECTION. Inflection—or change in pitch—gives life to your voice. We use a rising inflection to signify a question or an incomplete thought. A positive assertion is generally accompanied by a falling inflection—a signal indicating completeness or finality. Most of us could use more varied inflection in our speech to liven it up. Nothing is more boring than a lifeless monotone. On the other hand, overuse of inflection will, of course, produce an unpleasant effect.

RATE. How fast do you speak? Speech that is too rapid tends to become shrill, and the meaning is apt to be lost or garbled. Speech that is too slow bores us. About 150 words a minute is a good normal rate for ordinary conversation.

Although you have a customary rate of speech, you vary it to suit your mood or purpose. If you are tired and morose or contemplative, you naturally slow down. With friends at an exciting basketball game, you speak much faster. In intimate get-togethers, your rapid conversation can be easily understood, but if you address a large audience or use an electronic voice reproducer such as a telephone or public address system, you must speak slowly in order to be understood.

Variety adds spice to your speech, and changes of pace in speaking can effectively stimulate your audience, large or small. Try consciously to pace your words to the mood you are trying to express.

PROJECTION. Do you have to cup your hands and shout to make your voice project? A good actor can make a whisper be heard far back in the balcony seats. The secret is combining

Be the bright, lively charmer, who uses a variety of facial expressions and gestures to enhance her words but happily avoids going to extremes.

B. D. Unsworth

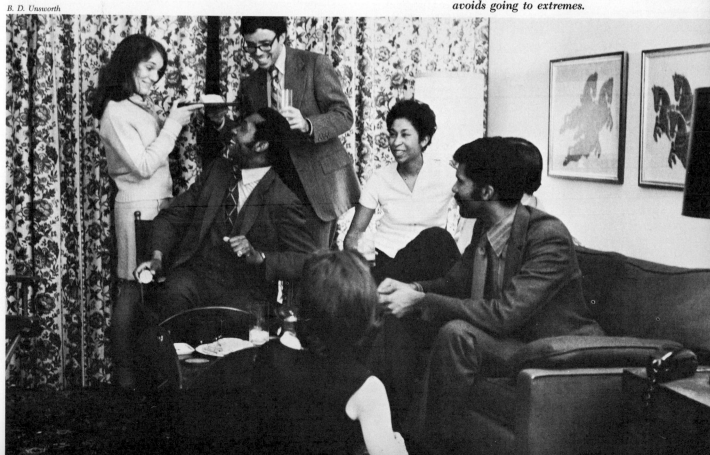

proper pitch, rate, and enunciation. But most important is diaphragmatic breathing. Clear, unmuffled tones must come from the diaphragm.

VOLUME. No doubt you have wished for the ability to adjust someone's volume control—either up or down. Loud voices are irritating and grate on the nerves. The too-soft voice is wildly frustrating. Neither does anything for charm. Try at all times to keep your volume at an appropriate setting. The woman at the next table who talks too loudly is probably completely unaware of how she sounds. Charm requires consideration and control at all times.

Your voice personality. As you listen to your voice, be on the alert for any traits you dislike.

Does it sound whiny, singsongy, timidly apologetic, harsh, brusque, belligerent, depressed, indifferent? Does it have some other undesirable quality? Would you be attracted to that voice? Most voice flaws are easy to correct, and when we detect any in ourselves, we should make every effort to abolish them as soon as possible. If you have any serious voice flaws, by all means consult a speech therapist. You will find it well worth the time, effort, and money.

❦ Perfect Pronunciation, Please

Often we are completely unaware that we are speaking English poorly. Take the work *English* itself. Is it pronounced *English* or *Inglish?* A look at your dictionary will show that the second pronunciation is correct.

Different situations require different amounts of vocal volume. Make sure your voice is neither too loud nor too soft for your surroundings.

B. D. Unsworth

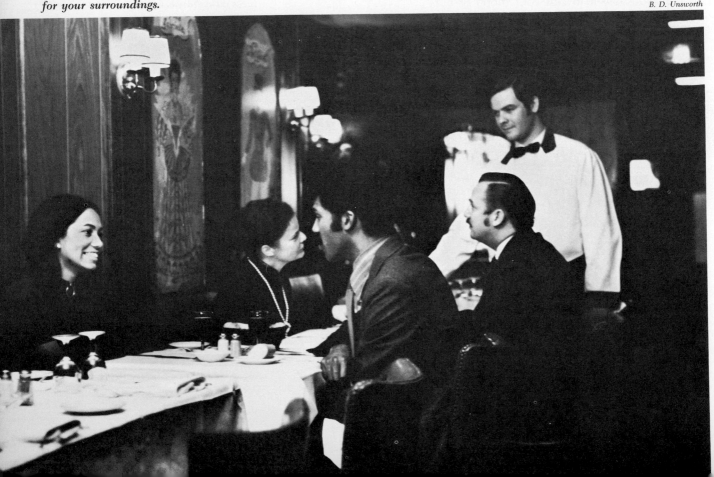

Perfect pronunciation is required for good speech. Whenever you have any uncertainty about pronunciation, save yourself possible embarrassment by avoiding the word for the moment and looking it up at the first opportunity you get. In the dictionary correct pronunciation is shown between slanted lines after the word. The key to pronunciation is usually found along the bottom of the page and also in the front of the book.

🌷 Accents

Have you ever admired the lilt a French- or English-born girl gives to her English speech? If so, you've probably also tried to imitate the sound and discovered that even if you could do it perfectly, the accent still isn't *you.*

Too often Americans don't realize the charm and color of their own native accents. Instead of considering yours a handicap, why not make it an asset? Listen to outstanding speakers, preferably women, whose accents are similar to yours. Do these speakers exaggerate some sounds, soften others, perhaps weed out a few? Try imitating them, but keep in mind that they have adapted the accent to express their personalities, not yours. Since your accent is natural to you, you'll soon distinguish the nuances of sound that best express your moods and personality.

But making the most of your accent is only part of the job. In business, particularly if you work for a large corporation, you will often speak personally or by telephone with people whose natural accents are quite different from yours and whose ears are not attuned to the way you speak. These conversations will be frustrating indeed unless both you and they can control how much accent is used. Such control is a business skill, and like other business skills, it may well be a job requirement.

To learn accent control, try to imitate national radio and television announcers. Because they must be understood by Americans of all accents, their speech is a model of "accentless" English, or Standard American. You'll

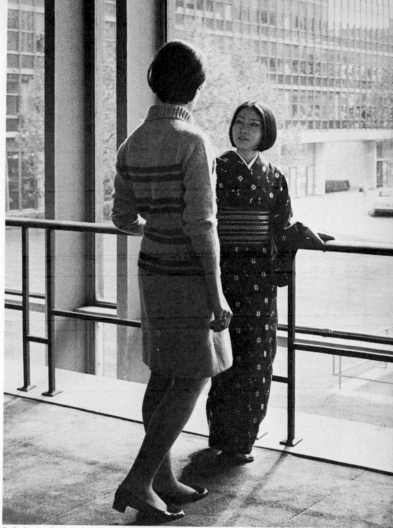

B. D. Unsworth

Guides at the UN have studied hard to control their accents because they have to be easily understood by people from so many different regions and places.

learn the new speech more quickly and thoroughly if you abandon your natural accent entirely for a time. Later, when you have mastered your control, you'll be able to switch to your natural charming accent just as easily as you switch from business clothes to at-home attire.

If your accent is quite different from Standard American, the chore of learning the new sound may require all your persistence. But keep in mind that this skill is an asset in social meetings as well as in business. In our highly

217

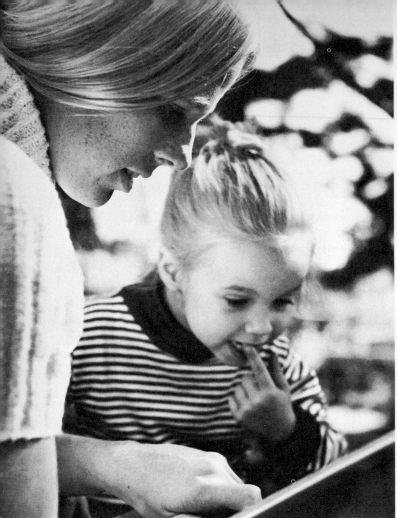

Reading aloud can be useful in that you get used to hearing yourself use good grammar and talk in complete sentences.

B. D. Unsworth

mobile society, you are sure to meet many people who speak with different accents, but with your new skill you'll converse with them easily and confidently.

❦ Know Your Grammar

Poor grammar is certainly a blot on anyone's charm. The person who slips into "he don't," "I don't want none," and similar bad constructions not only gives a poor impression of her intelligence but also crosses herself out from competition for interesting meet-the-public jobs or for any other work that involves letter writing

or telephoning. Anyone who is shaky in grammar should take a good course in Standard English or study a book until she is sure of the rules.

Listening closely and being guided by those you know use English properly will also be helpful. Grammatical errors can be corrected easily if you are aware of the problem and concentrate on improvement.

Good practice for tuning your ear to proper grammar as well as to a rich choice of words is reading good literature aloud. (Read to a child, to an elderly person, or to someone who is ill, and you get double benefit from your practice.) As you read, try to notice the construction of the sentences and the clear, logical order used to express an idea. Association with the best in both the written and spoken word can do a great deal to help develop the good speech that is essential to charm. And it can aid pronunciation and enunciation, too.

❦ Follow the Leaders

One of the best ways to develop correct and vibrant speech is to study the experts and follow their examples. Listen carefully to the top television and radio announcers. Of course, they use good grammar, they speak distinctly, and their tones are pleasant, friendly, and well controlled. But notice also how expressive their voices become through appropriate change of pitch, mastery of the dramatic pause, and clever change of pace to heighten a mood. Effective speakers give thought not only to what they say but to *how* they say it.

❦ Let Your Best Voice Speak

Your voice is so important that it should always sound its best and never betray unwanted emotions. Next time you are upset, try these hints to keep your voice level while you struggle to smooth out your emotions. If you are irritated, take a deep breath before you speak. This helps relax your vocal apparatus—as well as your nerves. Another good suggestion is to yawn—a big, wide yawn—and your voice will come out sounding more like the natural self you want it to express. Or you might try humming (softly to yourself if you are in an office or any place where you might disturb others, but as loudly as possible if you are alone).

Humming improves your voice and provides immediate release for tense feelings.

Next to appearance, voice is the most important factor in creating a good impression and deserves much conscious thought. Like facial expressions, voices reflect inner harmony or discord. Let your voice represent your best self.

1 *Hold practice sessions in which you speak as loudly as possible. Start talking in normal tones. Gradually increase your volume until you are speaking in full, loud, robust tones. Breathe deeply and watch your pitch so that your voice does not become shrill. Practice against the noise of a vacuum cleaner or dishwasher, and you will be spurred to even greater vocal accomplishments.*

2 *Make a conscious effort for the next two days to listen to your speech. If you discover any flaws, start an immediate campaign to correct them.*

3 *Concentrate right now on breathing from your diaphragm. Breathe deeply and slowly for at least two or three minutes. Then find someone to talk to—or talk aloud to yourself. As you speak, make a determined effort to continue to breathe properly.*

4 *Listen to the speech of those around you and to your own talk. See how often you notice slips in enunciation, pronunciation, or grammar.*

5 *Read aloud, either to yourself or others, using your best enunciation and expression. Practice good breath control, pausing for breath (if possible) only where the punctuation indicates a period, comma, or other pause. As you speak, listen to the words. Note the various constructions used by the author and how skillfully the words flow together.*

6 *In all your reading—aloud or silent—note any words whose pronunciation you aren't sure of and look them up.*

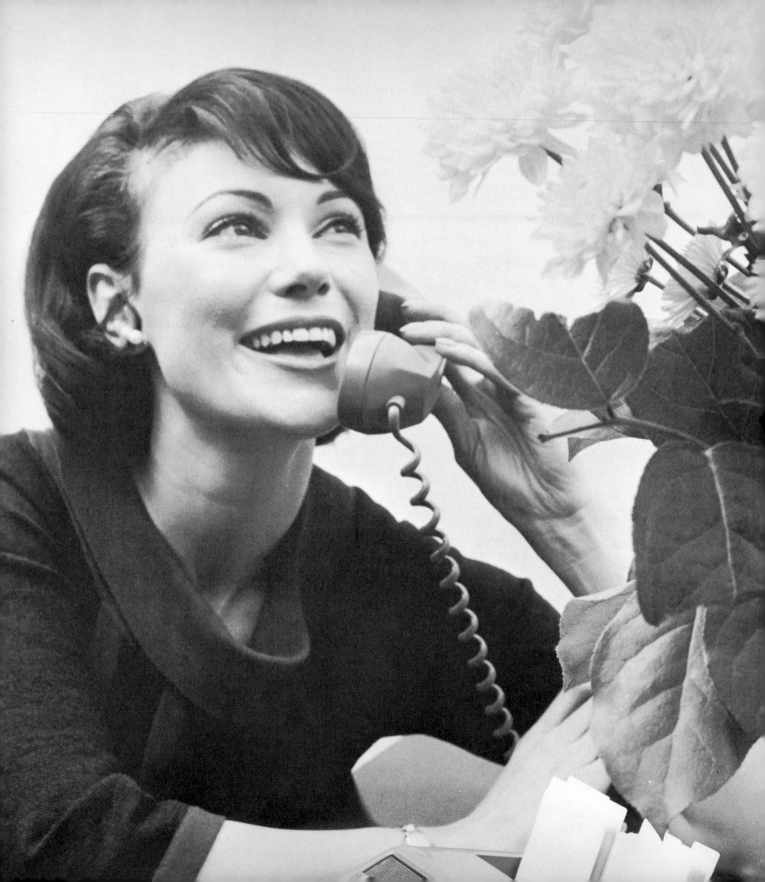

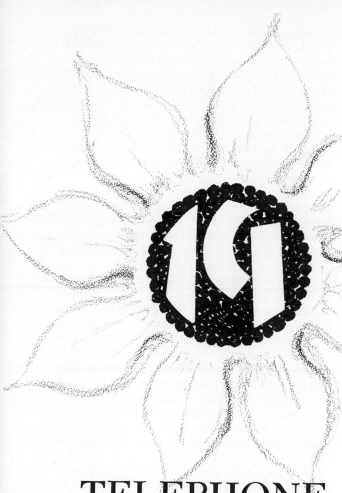

TELEPHONE TACT AND TACTICS

A definite premium is put on a business girl's voice quality. As far as a telephone caller is concerned, when you pick up the receiver, you *are* the company. He can't see the efficient staff, the modern equipment, or even your stylish dress—everything depends on your voice. The telephone has become so important in the business world that a pleasant voice, good speech habits, and correct telephone etiquette are essentials for good office performance.

Although your listener can't see your expressions or gestures, you can put a smile in your voice. How? Simply by smiling when you speak. Prove it to yourself. Smile and try to sound unpleasant—pretty hard to do, isn't it? A smile was considered so important to telephone technique by one large department store that a mirror was put in front of each girl in the telephone order department. When she saw her expression sagging, she knew her voice was not at its best and was reminded to brighten her countenance so that her voice would again smile a welcome to customers.

Being pleasant is usually easy the first time you pick up the phone in the morning. But it's that ninety-ninth call just one minute before quitting time that determines your caliber. The words you use may be the same, but even "May I help you?" can sound like "What on earth do you have to bother me about!" Just the tone of your voice is most important. A pleasant voice has been known to take the wind out of the sails of an irate customer and to diminish many a potential problem. An irritated voice will just make problems greater.

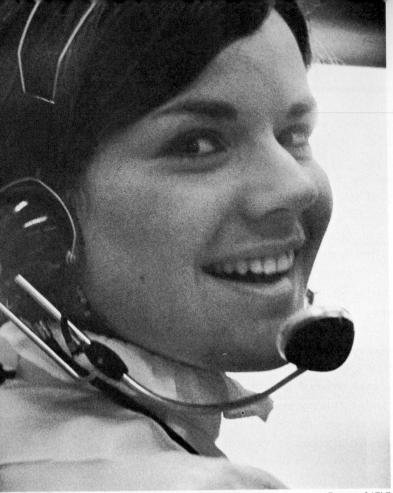

A switchboard operator has to answer the telephone hundreds of times a day and sound pleasant to everyone. Her cheerful greeting often makes her callers more pleasant.

❦ Handling the Boss's Calls

Whether you are a secretary or another kind of worker in the department, you should be skilled at taking calls for an executive. Few chores elicit more praises or complaints from employers than the way their telephone calls are handled. To put yourself in the praiseworthy category, begin by finding out how your boss wants you to answer his phone and how much screening he wants you to do. Then answer his phone promptly and properly.

You might say, "Mr. Perkins' office," or perhaps "Mr. Perkins' office, Miss Wilson speaking." Some secretaries feel it helps establish the caller's confidence in their ability if they identify themselves when they answer the phone. If you are as capable and as helpful as you should be, the caller will be able to rely on you for help in the future, and you will be able to save your boss many precious minutes. A plain "Hello," no matter how dulcet the tones, is useless in business. It gives no clue as to whether the caller has reached the right office or person.

Some executives like to answer their own phones when they are free to do so, and others like to have all calls put through to them for the sake of goodwill, but most bosses like to have their calls screened. This job will require all the tact and charm you can muster.

Start by asking your boss for a list of the people he will always want to speak with no matter how busy he is. Others he may wish to have referred to an assistant. You should soon catch on to the types of calls he takes and the ones he wants to avoid. Just make sure you extend the same courtesy to both the least and the most important persons who call. Even if you know your boss doesn't want to speak to someone, don't let the caller know it. You can make a friend for your company and still protect your boss if you handle the situation tactfully.

Ask your boss what he wants you to do if you have doubts about whether he will want to take the call or if the caller does not give his name without being asked. This is a delicate situation. You won't want to bother your boss needlessly, but nothing enrages a caller more than to know that the person he wants to talk with is there and chooses not to speak with him. And he will have a pretty good idea that this is the case if you get his name, sign off to check on whether your boss is in, and then come back with a negative reply. Of course you know whether or not your boss is there—at least you should. And the caller is fully aware of this.

You and your boss might decide to make it a rule to say automatically that he is not in, at a meeting, or away from his desk if you doubt that he will want to take the call. This will assure the caller that your boss is not in for anyone, and you can then proceed to find out who he is and what are his reasons for calling. When you find out the nature of his business, perhaps you can handle the matter yourself or can refer the call to one of your boss's subordinates who will be able to take care of it. Just make sure that you handle the situation in a way that makes the caller think you are trying to be helpful to him rather than protective of your boss. Few things are as annoying as the officious secretary jealously and gleefully guarding the portals to the Great One's presence. If you decide that your boss probably will want to talk, you can always spot him "just coming in" or you can check with him and return the call in a few minutes.

A word to the wise: Always get a caller's name right! If he mumbles or if you are uncertain, don't be afraid to ask him to spell his name. Then spell it back to him and pronounce it, saying, "Is that correct?" If the name is not familiar and the caller doesn't offer any other identification, you can add, "Thank you, Mr. Soandso. And what is the name of your organization, please?" No matter how bombastic a caller may seem, you want to have the right information to relay to your boss. You'd feel pretty foolish if Mr. Perkins answered the phone expecting to talk to Mr. Brandt, a top customer, only to find it to be Mr. Grant, a persistent and unwelcome salesman.

Once you know a caller's name, use it when you address him. Nothing is sweeter to his ears at this point than his own name and the knowledge that he has made sufficient impression to be recognized as an individual.

A good rule for your boss's phone calls: *Reveal as little as possible about your employer.* You must be careful to give no clue as to whether or not he is in until you know he wants to take the call. If your boss is out of town, you must still be discreet. Play safe and merely tell callers that Mr. Perkins isn't in. Such an innocent remark as "Mr. Perkins is in Detroit on a business trip" might be a solid gold tip for a rival company.

If your employer is busy on another line when a call comes in, ask the caller if he wishes to hold on or if he would rather leave a message. If he decides to hold on, check back with him frequently. This assures him that you haven't forgotten him and left for lunch (which has happened!). It also gives him an opportunity to give you a message or to ask you to return the call should the wait be too long. You will also want to be alert to see that your boss takes the call as soon as he is free.

You'll win friends for yourself and your boss if you maintain a natural and sympathetic attitude. Some girls annoy callers by their officious manner and artificial or stuffy phraseology. The caller is made to feel that so unworthy a one as he is indeed fortunate to be put through to Mr. Big-Big. This is extremely poor public relations. Let your charming manner make even the lowliest caller feel that he is being treated with special consideration.

❧ Taking a Message

What's complicated about taking a phone message? Not much, yet an amazing number of mangled messages agitate the blood pressure of bosses every day. Probably one of the most important points to remember is to *write down the message,* preferably on a telephone message pad. If your office doesn't provide a specially designed message pad, keep a separate pad—perhaps one with colored paper—beside your phone. Never trust a phone message to a stray scrap of paper or to the back of an old envelope. Too many harrowing tales have been told about the message that got away—usually because it was thrown by mistake into somebody's wastebasket.

Particularly disturbing can be too brief a note, such as "Call Mr. Harris" when the boss can recall no Mr. Harris. "Who's he with? What's his phone number? What does he want?" are disturbing questions that quickly switch any boss's mind from thoughts of how much you deserve a raise. Make sure you always include the following information.

- The name of the caller.
- His firm (or other identifying information).
- His phone number (in case your boss should need to call back).
- A brief report of what the caller wanted, anything you might have done to help him, and anything that might still need to be done.
- The date and time of the call—so your boss won't need to worry about when the call came if he should mistakenly shuffle your message in with other papers.
- Your name or initials—so he can check with you if he has any questions.

Write legibly when taking a telephone message so that your boss won't have to spend time deciphering it later.

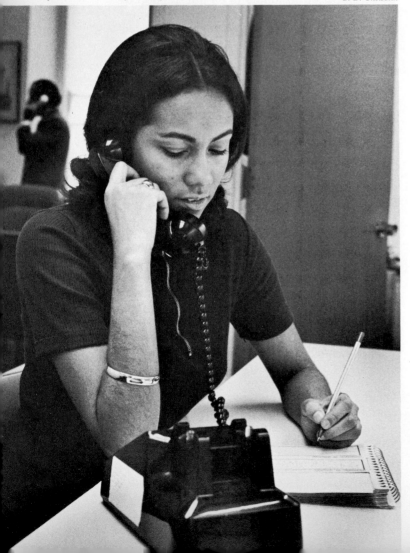

B. D. Unsworth

♉ *Pleasing Your Party*

Your telephone will win friends for you and your company if you observe the following suggestions.

- If your job requires that you answer telephone calls yourself rather than relay them to your boss, always identify yourself when you pick up the receiver by saying, ''Advertising Department, Miss Smith.'' Even though a good many of the calls you receive may be of the informal, interoffice variety, you will still want to begin with a businesslike identification. Just when Susie Smith is expecting Laura Mae in the filing department to call right back and answers with a breezy ''Hi!'' it is sure to be her boss's boss.
- Make a special effort to speak distinctly. Background noises and other interferences may make it difficult for you to be heard. Hold the mouthpiece so that it is about half an inch away from your lips. Many people are hard to understand because they don't hold the mouthpiece close enough.
- Be sure that you explain as fully and as carefully as possible. When everything depends on your voice, misunderstandings can easily arise and an innocent remark can take on quite a different meaning from the one intended.
- Be helpful. Take the extra moment it may require to give the caller complete information or assistance. It is wiser to spend a few minutes keeping a customer than months regaining him. If the caller is upset, don't argue with him. Attempt to soothe his ruffled feathers, and calmly express regret for any misunderstanding in a manner that allows him and your firm to save face as much as possible.
- Whenever more than a few moments will be required to get the information the caller requests, offer to phone back. If he decides to hold on, use your hold button if you have one. Otherwise you must be particularly careful of what you say while the receiver is lying on your desk. Idle chatter often comes in loud and clear. When you return to the phone, be sure to say, ''Thank you for waiting.''
- If you must transfer a call, be as tactful as possible and explain to the caller the reason for doing so. Calls to big corporations sometimes bounce from one department to another like

224

tennis balls, especially if the problem doesn't fit neatly in any one person's particular domain. "Pass it to somebody else" is the all-too-prevalent psychology. After the caller has explained his story even a couple of times, he doesn't relish hearing the familiar "Hold on, please—I'll transfer you." Try to ascertain first whether the department you are transferring him to can actually help him. If necessary, offer to check further and call him back.

• Keep alert. The antics of the office clown or other nearby distractions may be far more interesting than the caller's problem. Courtesy demands that you be attentive and listen carefully—even though you think you know what the person is about to say. Considerable confusion—and irritation—can be caused when someone wrongly anticipates what will be said.

• Include a happy ending. "Thank you for calling; goodbye," closes a conversation with a feeling of friendship. The person who ends with an abrupt "Okay" or who merely lets his voice fall and then hangs up often leaves the caller talking to himself, much to his embarrassment and resentment. He may think twice before calling again.

• Before you make a call about an involved matter, make a few notes of what you want to say. This helps you get complete information and avoids delays, omissions, or embarrassing call-backs.

• When you are placing a call for someone else, find out first what you should do if the person called is not there. Should you leave a message? call back? This way you won't have to keep the person who answered the phone waiting while you find out the answer. And, unless your boss instructs you otherwise, try to get him on the phone *before,* or at least at the same time as, the person he is calling. Since he placed the call, it's only courtesy not to keep the other person waiting.

---

1 *Whenever you make a telephone call, practice putting a smile in your voice. Notice how much more cooperative the person on the other end of the line becomes.*

2 *Check your telephone technique. Do you make a special effort to talk clearly and distinctly on the phone? Do you hold the mouthpiece close enough? Do you explain carefully and completely, so that others understand you fully?*

3 *Whenever someone is rude to you on the telephone because of something that is not your fault (perhaps he is annoyed at your boss, your firm, or his own inability to get the information he wants), keep in mind that you personally are not the real target of his anger. Remind yourself that he is mad at something else—not you—and endeavor to train yourself to overlook such rudeness so that you can maintain your composure and can reply calmly and courteously.*

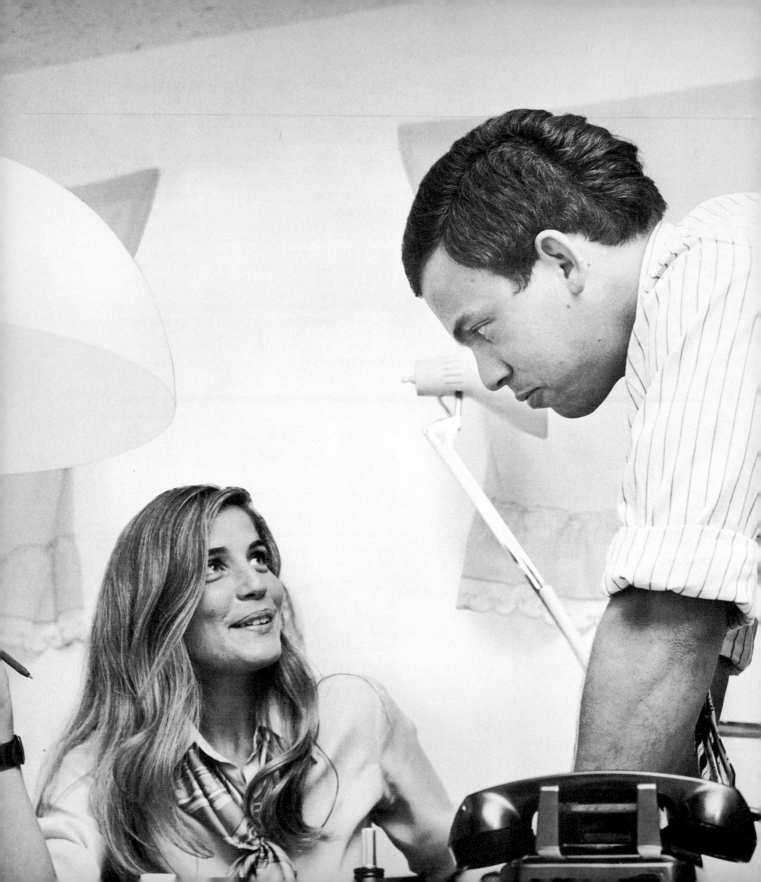

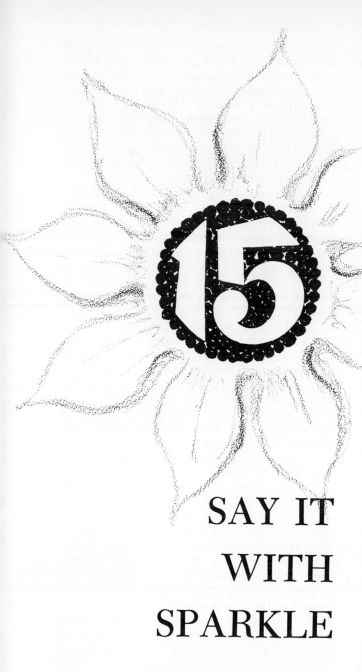

SAY IT WITH SPARKLE

Just about everyone learns to speak well enough to make himself understood, but a surprising number never learn to be the interesting talkers they could be. They plod along using the same dull, worn-out words in the same dull way. When they meet someone whose speech is a brilliant, fast-paced flow of sparkling phrases, they attribute it to a special gift that somehow wasn't in their genes.

Anyone can learn to develop more vivid speech. Just stir up your imagination and mix with a wide variety of words. Sound easy? It is! The reason most of us go on using the same old humdrum expressions is that we're lazy, we don't bother to seek out new words, and we stay in the same old rut using the same old familiar phrases.

Some girls collect stuffed animals; Some collect diamonds. Far more negotiable in charm benefits are collections of good words. Be on the lookout for catchy words, colorful words, expressive words, and new words whose meaning you aren't sure of. As you listen to people or to radio or television programs, notice the words that are used. When you hear a good one, give it an extra check in your brain and try to fix it in your vocabulary by using it in several different conversations. When you have used a new word three times, it is yours, the saying goes.

The words you select needn't be unusual six-syllable jawbreakers nor foreign phrases. Actually, these may merely cause raised eyebrows because they tend to sound affected. But don't be afraid of using a precise, colorful word just because it's a little different or because no one else in your crowd uses it. Your speech should sound like you—but the liveliest, most interesting you.

Good speech, like poor speech, is extremely infectious. When you listen to a stimulating speaker, you will find all sorts of colorful phrases popping into your own thoughts. Read a good writer and you are likely to catch a case of good-word-itis without even trying. In fact, many writers warm up by reading something clever that will start their own thoughts perking. Humorous writers such as James

Listen to the lyrics of songs. Often words are used in strange ways to create new and meaningful images. You can do the same thing in your conversation.

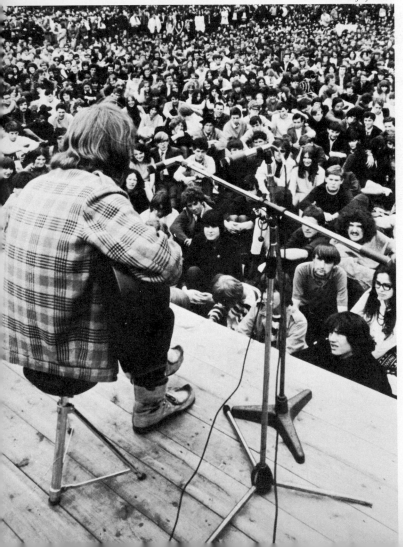

Thurber and Cornelia Otis Skinner are good stimulants, and there are many best-selling authors and newspaper columnists whose styles are marvelously incisive and expressive. Reading poetry, whether it be Ogden Nash's or Shakespeare's, is a particularly good way to enrich your vocabulary. Poetry, which deals largely with feelings and descriptions, is restricted by rhyme and meter, so that only the richest words can be used.

In all your reading, notice how the author expresses himself, how he uses words, how he evokes feeling or emotion, how he gets an idea across. Read slowly so that you can get the full appreciation of the style and language. Jot down the words that seem particularly good so that you can practice using them. They needn't be new words or extravagant words. Most of them will probably be simple expressions that are quite familiar to you but that somehow are not part of your active vocabulary. Many times our talk seems trite, not because we don't know the meanings of a wide variety of words but merely because they don't occur to us at the proper time. We can "say it with sparkle" only when the sparkling phrases are on the tips of our tongues. A little awareness and a little practice will put them there.

When you come across a new word that you don't know the meaning of, take a moment to look it up. There is still no substitute for consulting the dictionary. Particularly note prefixes and suffixes, and learn how they affect meanings. You may meet the same word root in many forms and will have a clue to its meaning from your knowledge of prefixes and suffixes. While you are looking up a new word, check its pronunciation so that you can say it properly as well as use it properly.

Word collecting can be extremely satisfying. Develop a love for words, and you won't settle for the rags and bones of talk. You'll soon know the pleasure of having on hand the exact word to express your precise shade of meaning. Words will come easily. Your speech will be vivid and lively. Often the difference between a meager vocabulary and an excellent one is only a few hundred words. With so

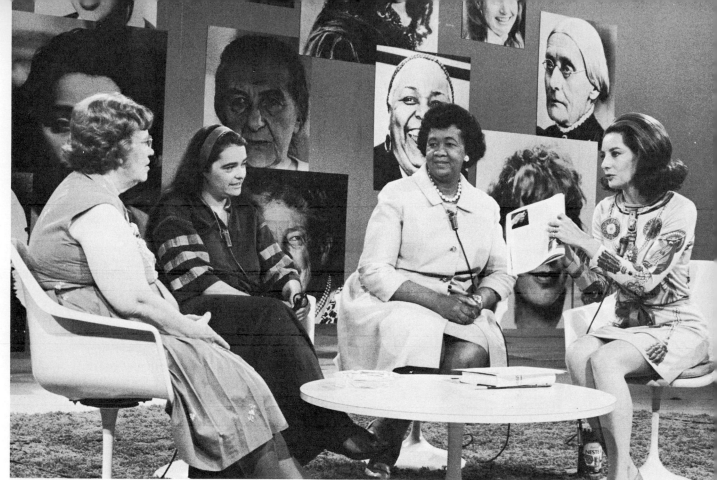

Courtesy of NBC

Listening to television discussion shows is one way to get new ideas and learn new words. On this program Margaret Mead, Kate Millett, Dorothy Height, and Barbara Walters discussed the status of women in today's society.

many words available from all sources, any vocabulary can be flourishing in a very short time.

❦ Open for Impressions

Sparkling speech depends on emotions as well as words. Often a speaker develops a sense of kinship in his listeners because he makes them share his feelings as well as his thoughts. Alert yourself to the details of life surging around you. Be aware of how you and others react to what is going on. A story about your trials and tribulations on a lunch-hour shopping jaunt comes alive when you include such details as the suffocating perfume of the customer

ahead of you, the interminable time the salesgirl took to sharpen her pencil, or how, in order to get the right-size box, you had to go back to some dusty, dingy corner of the store to a man who looked as though he dealt only with customers whose accounts were long overdue. While too much detail can hamper a story, a few choice impressions—told briefly—help your listeners share your emotions with you.

An awareness of the surrounding sights, sounds, and smells, hopes and joys, fears and frustrations lets you live life fully and helps you express it better to others. Picturesque words are required to portray these feelings, and you will find your own imagination kindled by the circumstances.

❦ Stretching Your Imagination

Your imagination quickly responds to exercise. The more you use it, the more flexible it becomes. Put it to work often, and it will provide you with the apt and lively words you want.

Good exercise is gained when you practice describing what you see. Some people look at nothing but the advertising posters every time they ride in a bus or subway. Instead, examine the people and scenes around you. Describe them to yourself in a few brief terms, such as *a laborer, stocky and ruddy; a poodle, frisky and fun-loving; a day, brilliant with sunshine.* This sort of quick labeling improves your power with words. Make your descriptions so succinct that they paint the scene in a few bold strokes. Appearance, motion, setting, and emotion should be noted. By such enforced brevity you will also learn to highlight the important points quickly and will protect yourself from the effusiveness that is a bad habit of tiresome talkers.

❦ Weed Out the Humdrum

Any vocabulary improvement program should begin with a check to see if there are certain phrases that you habitually use over and over again. Probably you know the girl who describes everything as ''terrific'' or ''cute'' or who throws ''you know'' into every other sentence. Even the most divine expression when used by the most divine people is not the least bit divine when it is overdone! Other people make pets of such words as ''really'' or ''very,'' which are usually just as well omitted, or they tag on meaningless endings like ''yet'' and ''already.''

Tiresome, too, are those who cram their talk with hackneyed clichés. There's the character who will tell you you look like a doll, are as good as gold, hit the nail on the head when you said it was easy as falling off a log to look cool as a cucumber, etc., etc. Most of these clichés were probably considered pretty clever way back when they were first said. Since then they have been mouthed so often that they have lost their luster. When you stop to think, it's actually quite easy to come up with better and more stimulating language. If, in a pinch, you can't find anything better, try speaking in a simple straightforward manner rather than repeating the same old ho-hum expression. Saying just plain ''You look so cool'' sounds much better than piping ''You look cool as a cucumber.''

Word games are an easy way to increase your vocabulary and have fun at the same time.

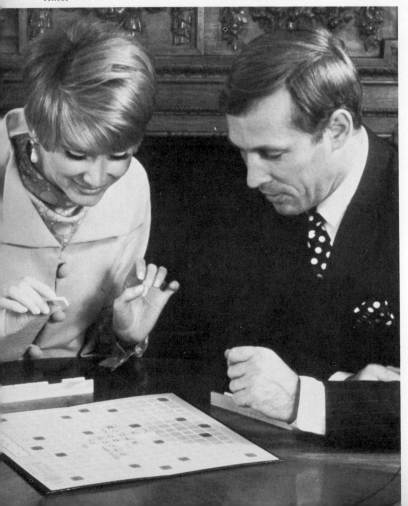

❧ Slanguage

There's a certain type of slang that shows you are "in." It's the latest colorful phrase that capsules an idea—the slang used by smart and sophisticated people. You'll hear your boss use a bit of it; you may even have noticed your teachers using some. The important point is that *they use only a bit.* Slang is like garlic: a little adds savor, but too much—no, thanks!

The type of slang used is also extremely important. The juvenile slang that sounds so smart around school is likely to be frowned on in the adult world. The wisest course for any business girl is to feel her way cautiously and to stick to the language she knows is genuinely acceptable until she is sure of what is right. You can never go wrong in the office if you restrict your use of slang words, and you may find that using "regular" words gives your speech much more punch.

❧ Learn It—Bury It

So far in this section on voice improvement, you've been advised to watch your pitch, your volume, your breathing, your grammar, your enunciation and pronunciation, and your choice of words. These all require your attention, but thoughts of them should be stashed away in your subconscious during conversation. When you are talking to someone, you don't want to be so conscious of how you are expressing yourself that your speech sounds studied or artificial. If you are overcareful, your speech is robbed of its spontaneity, which is in essence the warmth and charm of conversation. If you learn to love words and if you practice using them correctly, they will come readily when you need them. Direct, simple talk is far more desirable than stilted speech, no matter how splendid the words and how elegant the diction may be.

---

1 *Select a good book to read. Choose one that has a lively writing style and read it analytically for style and word choice as well as for meaning and enjoyment.*

2 *Read a little poetry every day for a week. Let it be humorous or light verse one day, more serious poetry the next. Look for the beautiful image-creating words and the lovely sounds formed by various word combinations.*

3 *Examine your speech carefully for an entire day to see if you overwork any words or expressions.*

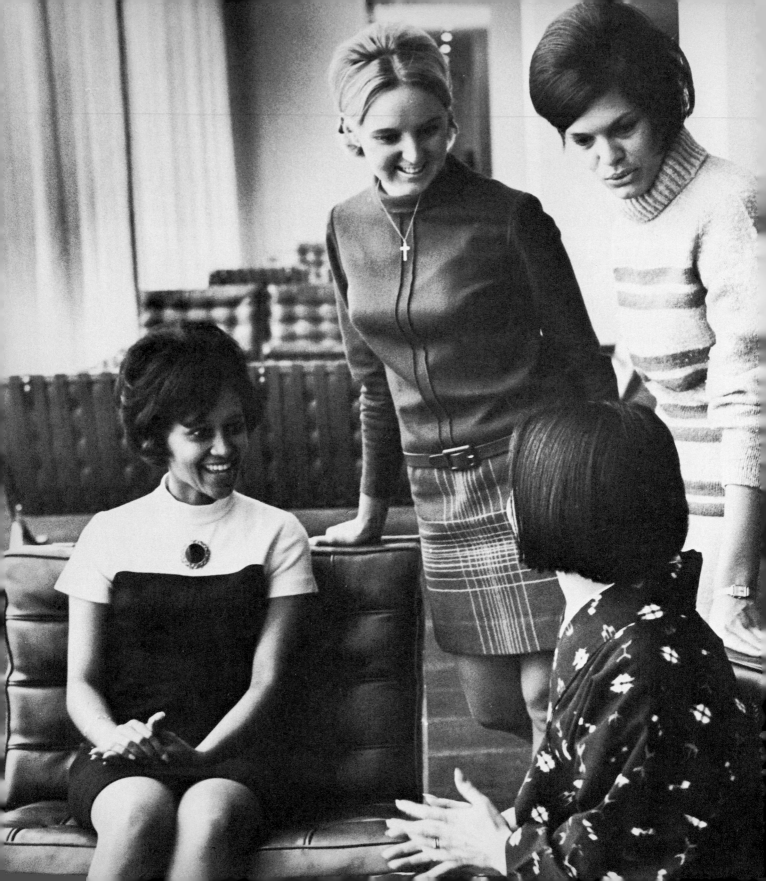

TALENTED TALK

The girl who is easy to talk to is always popular. Her friendly manner attracts and delights. Her conversation relaxes her listeners and inspires them, bringing out their best. As a result, friends flock to her and respond to her as to catchy, lilting music.

The secret of many a girl's charm is that she is literally easy to talk to. *She makes it fun for others to talk to her.* She is a good listener; she has the ability to suggest interesting conversational subjects and to inspire others to contribute their best. And she willingly lets others have the stage and do their share of the talking. She is always ready to contribute to the conversation, but she never monopolizes it. When necessary, she can add the proper remarks that keep the ball rolling and can guide conversation to lively topics. She has a storehouse of interesting anecdotes and observations that enable her to contribute something interesting and vital.

The reason she is so easy to talk to is that she is sincerely interested in other people. She is considered excellent company because she cares about what *you* would like to talk about, what would make *you* happy. And she allows the other person to say his share without extraneous interruptions or stories of her own that sidetrack the conversation. Her own talk is often of an impersonal nature that draws others in and encourages them to share their feelings and experiences.

The benefits of such an approach are many. It provides the surest cure for any charm-stifling self-consciousness because it forces you to get your mind off yourself. When you set for your-

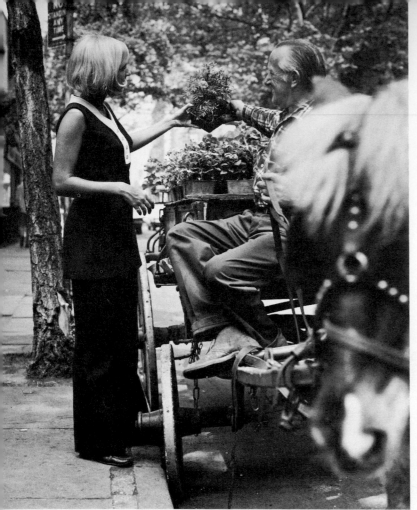

Your life can become so much more interesting if you engage the people you meet during the course of the day in conversation.

B. D. Unsworth

self the goal of making *others* happy, you must become so completely involved with *you*-thoughts that there is no opportunity for *me*-thoughts and for haunting self-appraisal. And as your guest warms and responds to your charm, you cannot help gaining confidence and expressing the best of yourself.

Another benefit is that through encouraging good conversation and playing the straight man more often than the star, you can learn many things. After all, you already know the anecdotes and experiences that you can relate. Give the other person the opportunity to talk, and you will glean many new stories and ideas.

❦ Grand Opening

The opening remarks that start off a conversation can dispel any awkwardness or strangeness if they lead quickly to a pleasant discussion. But what shall the topic be? Find the solution by asking yourself what the other person has been doing that he would like to talk about. Perhaps he's just returned from vacation, has an interesting job, is a bug on photography or sports. What was he doing when you last spoke to him?

A compliment is always a gracious beginning. Is there something you can admire about a person's appearance, about his recent accomplishments or activities, or about his home if you are a guest? Needless to say, sincerity is essential. It gives warmth and feeling to compliments and also protects you from any tendency to overdo.

Another technique is to ask someone for imformation or advice. Anyone who is even a small authority on some subject is usually delighted to share his knowledge. There's always the girl who can tell you about the newest books, the artist who can suggest the proper paints for some project you might be undertaking, the bargain specialist, the girl who sews or knits well. Almost everybody has some field they've investigated a bit more than the average person—and how it does their hearts good to have a chance to expond to an interested listener! When you can direct the conversation to a person's favorite topic or specialty, you can be sure the conversation will have plenty of momentum for quite a while.

But suppose you are confronted with the problem of making conversation with a complete stranger, someone whose interests and activities are unknown? A compliment is a good beginning, or perhaps a favorable comment about your surroundings. When you are in someone's home, a remark such as ''Lynn has such a wonderful record collection'' can give you many convenient handles for conversation. You can talk about Lynn and her musical interests, new records, favorite musicians or singers, the best places to buy records, lyrics of certain songs, and so on. The good conversationalist can usually find several directions a subject can be turned to strike a responsive feeling.

Choosing openers. Here are some specific subjects that usually help break the ice.

THE WEATHER. Don't be afraid to talk about the weather. The cavemen probably discussed it, and long after we're gone, it will still be a topic of interest and concern. Very often it can serve as a convenient wedge to lead into other subjects.

FOOD. The way to a man's heart may be through his stomach, but talk about food usually interests both sexes. Good restaurants, favorite foods, foreign dishes, memories connected with different foods, recipes, new products on the market, food advertising—all are good for spirited talk.

ANIMALS (PERHAPS PETS) OR CHILDREN. If discussing a younger brother or sister, please include only the kindly comments, however.

A RECENT NEWS ITEM. If something such as the political situation or the status of world affairs seems too heavy for the occasion, you might well find a lighter feature of more interest. Perhaps you might discuss a personality in the headlines or some recent occurrence, such as an act of heroism or a scientific development.

LOCAL HISTORY. An outsider might be interested to know that during the Revolution a local parson once tore up the hymnals and used the paper as wadding for the muskets used to hold off the redcoats. Or perhaps some famous person once lived in your area or an interesting event took place in the vicinity.

SOMETHING OF COMMON EXPERIENCE. A feeling of kinship can be aroused when we share sentiments about a common experience. It might be merely the problems of commuting, but more fascinating topics are travel and the places you both have visited. Strange supernatural occurrences (ghosts, telepathy, palm readings come true) and fears are also engrossing. Per-

haps you have some friends in common from your schools, churches, or neighborhoods, but remember not to make any unkind remarks.

Stick to the impersonal. The best subjects—and the safest ones—are impersonal topics. Unless you have lived an extraordinarily rich and full life, talk about yourself usually is bound to be rather unexciting. And perhaps you've noticed that even the people who have led the most interesting lives often avoid overemphasis on the personal, preferring to tell about things and places they have seen rather than about their own accomplishments. Occasionally we come across the individual who can't seem to get away from ''I.'' No matter how vast the topic, at the first opportunity she will narrow it down to some trivia in her own experience. While there are many occasions when our own feelings and reactions are pertinent, often a story would be more interesting if unencumbered by ''I'' references.

Conversation is the activity that, more than any other, will show just how charming you are. Pay attention, look interested, and, most important, have something to say.

B. D. Unsworth

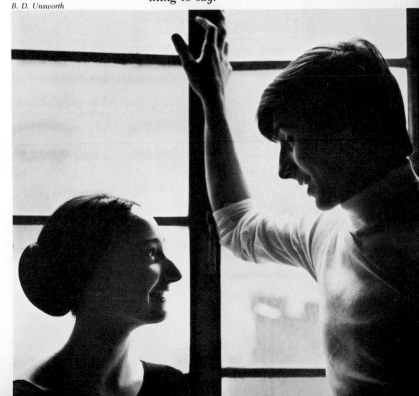

235

❦ Expanding Your Repertoire

The more things you know and the more things you are interested in, the more versatile you will be as a conversationalist. The person with a broad background can easily find common ground for conversation with others, for she has a rich and varied supply of material to draw on. A broad background doesn't require a European tour and a Phi Beta Kappa key. It can be acquired by listening closely to what is said and by observing and absorbing what is going on in the world. Conversational ability comes easily to the person who reads a good newspaper daily, listens to some informative TV and radio programs, reads good books, keeps up on new movies and plays, and is alert to what's going on around her.

Fascinating material can be gleaned from many sources if you are on the lookout for it. Some people can get more interesting material from a short bus ride than others gather from a coast-to-coast trip. Next time you walk down a busy street, see if you can't observe at least five little human dramas. With a bit of practice you will probably find even more.

Salespeople are sometimes a gold mine of information. If, for instance, you encourage a perfume salesgirl to talk, she might be able to tell you stories about ambergris (a substance secreted by whales and used in perfumes), its rarity, and the fabulous price it commands. You might be surprised at how much interesting information you can gain from service people such as dry cleaners and repairmen. Rich sources are all around us.

Ideas for conversation often elude us because of our woefully weak memories, but you *can* remember anecdotes if you really try. As soon as you have a quiet moment, think about what you've seen or learned during the day. Perhaps you can tell it to yourself as you would tell it to a friend. This helps fix the information in your mental file drawer. Write down the various ideas you've discovered, if you have to. Some brilliant conversationalists actually keep little notebooks in which they jot down notes about interesting happenings so that they can quickly refresh their memories if they find themselves forgetting an important aspect of a good story.

If you know something about art, literature, music, and world history—the makings of culture—you will not only have a rich background on which to draw but you'll also have good protection against self-consciousness. You needn't be an authority on these subjects. Even a slight acquaintance with them gives you added polish and enables you to hold your own or at least to understand what others are talking about.

B. D. Unsworth

236

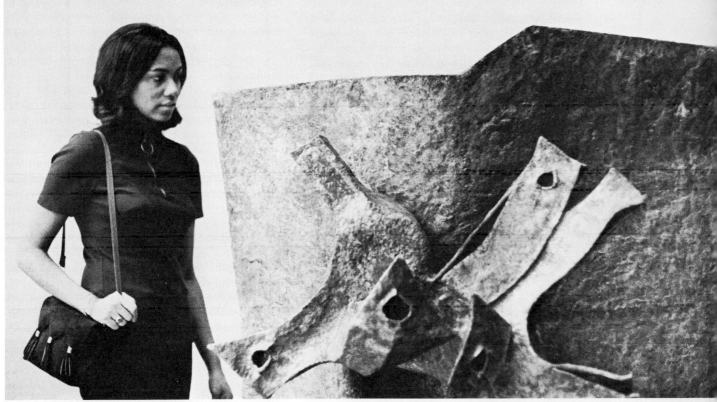

B. D. Unsworth

Improving your cultural background can be inspiring and thrilling. A slight taste usually makes us want more. The paintings, books, and music that are classics have withstood the test of time—they have been favorites down through the years. They have entertained, amused, and exhilarated all kinds of people. If you haven't already discovered their magnificence, you owe it to yourself to do so.

When you listen to good music or study a great painting, approach it with an open mind to discover what it can tell you. Look for the beauty that others have found in it, and let this beauty touch your emotions. Try to imagine what the artist was attempting to say. Look for the rhythmic sweep of lines and the interesting perspective in a picture, the ingenious blending of harmonies in music, the truthfulness of the characterizations and the splendid choice of words in literature. Your life will be fuller and richer for the new joys you will discover.

One of the most delightful ways to learn about earlier times is to read historical novels and biographies of famous persons. They give us a deeper understanding of the past and are fascinating reading.

And remember, the good worker with a rich background and observing mind rates Highly Desirable on any employer's list. There's always the day when some tidbit she learned will be mighty helpful to her boss or her work. And what girl isn't considered more valuable when she can hold an intelligent and interesting conversation with an important visitor!

❧ Party Talk

Prime yourself. Before a party we devote a good deal of time to perfecting our appearance. A little time spent in polishing up our conversation is also good preparation for poise. Are there subjects you might brush up on so that you can discuss them or at least ask intelligent questions? You may want to investigate your date's favorite hobby, the developing political situation, or the afternoon's major sports event. The object is not to become an expert yourself so that you can show off your knowledge, but rather to become familiar with the topics so that you can enjoy and participate in conversation about them—and can direct conversation to them when the party talk lags.

Check over the conversational subjects you've gathered to see what might be most appropriate. You might also want to run over the names and interests of people you expect to meet if you haven't seen them for some time.

If you're plagued with any inferiority feelings—and most of us are occasionally—stamp them out quickly. They do nothing but cause trouble. By now you have progressed far enough in this course to take pride in your lovely appearance. Your posture is improving, you are becoming more graceful, developing a better figure, and you know how to dress and to use cosmetics to bring out your best. Forget yourself. You can take pride in your accomplishments, so don't let your charm leak away in wasteful worry. It's time to stop wondering what others think of you. Realize that others have had—or still have—the same self-consciousness that bothers you and have overcome their fears so that they seem assured and poised. This should prove to you that you can do the same.

You won't, however, want to go to the opposite extreme, where you seem too cocksure. The least little slip such a person makes becomes a loud kerboom. Instead, concentrate on helping others have a good time, and you will surely have one, too.

At the party. As you arrive at the door, pause a moment to take a deep breath. This allows you to collect yourself, perks up your circulation just a bit, and gets you off to a clearheaded start. Then go first to greet your hostess. She will introduce you to someone if you are a stranger to the group and may say something like, "Ann Murray, this is Jim Brown. Jim's home from Purdue for the weekend. He just finished his exams." This gives you material for opening a conversation that will set you off to a good start.

When you are attending a meeting or other

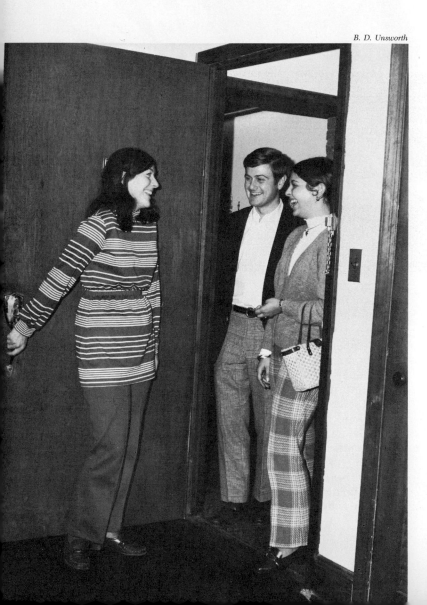

B. D. Unsworth

238

large gathering alone, don't slink into the nearest vacant chair. You will show more poise if you walk calmly well inside to select a seat. Then instead of sinking into yourself, look around you and smile. If you can't get into the conversation of those immediately around you, perhaps you can spot someone else who seems alone. Here is your opportunity to make a friend, and one friend quickly leads to another.

Men. Back to Jim Brown—and men in general. When you meet a man at a party, don't cling. Men are a wary breed, always expecting a girl to try to put her clamps on them. You will be considered far more poised if you can invite others into your conversation or if, after you have talked with him for a while, you can leave to help your hostess pass refreshments or to talk to another friend. You can always come back later, you know. And you will be far more welcome than if you had overstayed. Some clever girls manage to depart so that a conversation is left unfinished—the perfect excuse for returning to resume it.

A man usually prefers the girl who lets him do the active pursuing. Her part is to let him know that she is interested. Play it subtly. Your happy manner, your kindness to everyone, and your manner of gently boosting his ego by being an encouraging and responsive audience will charm him. Of course, you will enter the conversation frequently too. But if you hog the time showing off what you know, he'll think you're not interested—and you won't learn anything about him. The greatest success comes by giving him plenty of scope to display his own knowledge and opinions.

Pest control. Occasionally at a gathering you may find that you are stuck with someone who is definitely a pest or a bore. You, as a lady, will not want to be rude to anyone. Your charm rating will continue to be high if you can involve other people in the conversation and then exit inconspicuously. Treat even the most undesirable individual kindly. You can't go wrong by

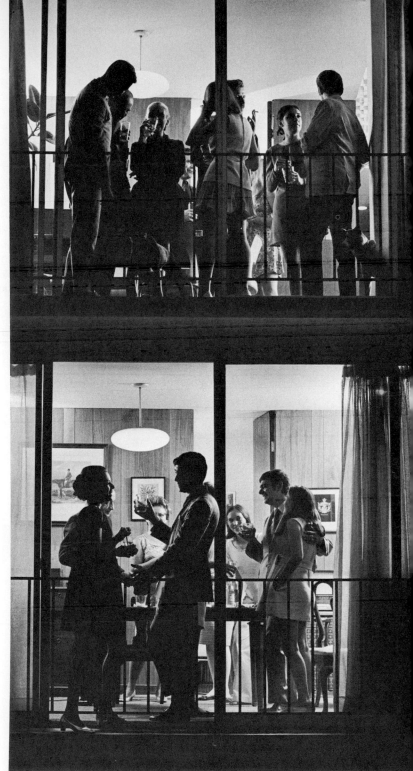

Courtesy of INA

239

being kind. The rough diamonds of the world are noted not for their high social gloss but for other more exciting qualities. Take the matter lightly, maintain your friendly manner, and you are likely to discover that he is not quite as dreadful as predicted.

Taking your leave. When it's time to go home, announce your intention, seek out your hostess to thank her for a pleasant time, and then go. The person who prolongs his leavetaking is a burden to the hostess and a drag on the party. If you become intrigued by something and change your mind, say that you intend to stay a while longer so that the party can get back to normal.

When you want to see someone again, Jim Brown, for instance, you might subtly suggest

B. D. Unsworth

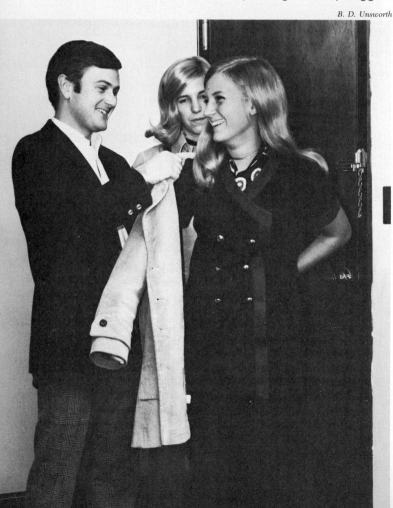

a possible further meeting by some such parting remark as "Let me know how your (history paper, tennis match) turns out." Then it is up to him.

❧ *Smooth Talking*

Here are some suggestions that will help keep the conversation running smoothly. They're as applicable to a day on the job as to a night on the town.

• Keep your voice up when you finish speaking. This adds a note of continuity that invites the listener to go on with the subject. It's as if you said "Don't you agree?" If your voice drops, the effect is one of finality, as if you said, "Well, that's finished and nothing more can be said about it."

• Keep in tune with the conversation. If everyone is being light and gay, don't plunge in with a heavy topic. If the conversation is a serious discussion, be serious in your contributions, although an occasional light touch— appropriately offered—is often refreshing and welcome.

• Keep an open mind. Even though someone is expressing an opinion that you disapprove of deeply, listen to what he has to say—you will at least gain insight into why people hold different opinions, and such understanding is part of sophistication. When you express your opinions—in turn with others, of course—be careful to state them in a way that leaves the door open for others to add their thoughts, conflicting or not. If you explain why you have an opinion, don't attempt to persuade others to your point of view unless you're certain that they are equally interested in such a debate.

If you know there are topics that one or more of those present can't discuss maturely, steer clear of such subjects and deftly direct the conversation to less controversial matters.

• Keep your poise at all times. If someone disagrees with you or belittles your opinion, don't take it as a personal affront.

• Emphasize the positive. The friend who can share your occasional gloom is a good friend indeed. But for other friends and for most social occasions, you're far more pleasant company if you can sidetrack unhappy moods and

240

discuss enjoyable things. You don't need to be Pollyanna, but neither do you want to criticize or complain so much that you are tagged as a sourpuss who can't appreciate anything. Others can't respond to you unless your generally happy, accepting attitude tells them you're likely to appreciate what they say.

• Be enthusiastic whenever possible. Enthusiasm is appealing. Overenthusiasm, however, tends to sound gushy. You need never fear letting your enthusiasm get out of bounds if you do not let it go beyond the point of sincerity.

• Never be catty or engage in gossip. You may think you're being witty, but even though others laugh, they'll wonder when your claws may be turned on them. Frankness and wit play important roles in conversation, but both are fragile instruments that should be handled with care. Brutal frankness or jokes at someone else's expense can be cruel. The person who can be completely candid, witty, and even sarcastic without offending others may be highly entertaining—but he is also extremely rare.

• Watch your timing. When you are speaking, say what you intend to say and stop. Some speakers nervously drag on and on, talking long past the point where the listener was stirred to add something to the conversation. They seem afraid of allowing a pause. This type of speaker takes the words out of his partner's mouth, then wonders why his partner is so silent.

• Include everyone in your conversation. If someone makes a school or office joke in a group with outsiders who might not understand, courtesy demands that you offer a brief explanation. Don't let the conversation dwell overlong on ''inside'' talk.

• Don't try to seem important. We all know we're important to ourselves. The appreciation freely given by someone else means much more than self-praise or an unwilling compliment wrung out of a listener besieged by another's recital of self-merits. Instead, raise your charm rating by showing that you appreciate others. Give them a good opinion of your heart, and they'll want to appreciate your mind.

• Don't belittle yourself. This tends to sound phony, especially if your listeners feel called upon to come to your defense. In some cases you might even point out flaws that otherwise would go unobserved.

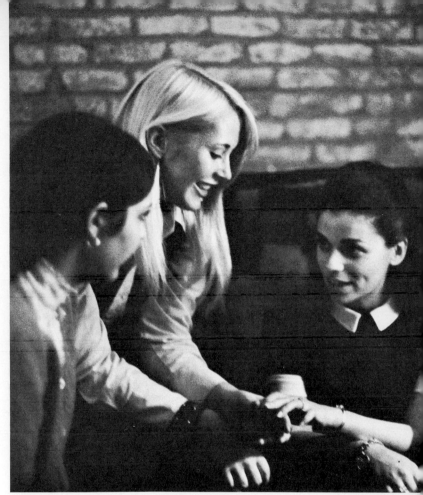

B. D. Unsworth

• Accept compliments graciously. A warm thank-you and a friendly smile are all that are necessary. Don't protest that you don't deserve the compliment or, worst of all, expound on your virtues. You will always appear self-possessed and charming if your reply reflects the speaker's kindness and generosity or the value of his opinion. You can say something such as ''Thank you, I'm so glad you enjoyed it. That makes me very happy,'' or ''It's good of you to say so. You're very kind.'' If the compliment is a gay, extravagant one, your answer should be in keeping: ''Now I can simply float through the rest of the day!'' After acknowledging a compliment, casually switch the conversation away from yourself.

• Don't exaggerate. Guard against the temptation to overemphasize or to exaggerate by either tone or word. Give a word credit for its

241

full value. Don't say *marvelous* if you mean *good,* or *horrible* if you mean *fair* or *poor.* Such overstatement undermines listeners' confidence and leads them to underrate what is said.

• Encourage your listener to talk about himself. Give him such tag lines as "Did anything similar ever happen to you?" or "Perhaps you've felt like that, too, sometimes?"

• Credit others. Help your friends feel clever and important by repeating their amusing remarks to others and always giving proper credit. If someone has just told you a good story and others join you, ask him to repeat the story for everyone.

• Keep personal matters personal. While you have some leeway with your close friends, it is never good to air the family wash in public. This is particularly true at work. The girl who discusses her romances, her father's faults, or other personal matters embarrasses her listeners and loses their respect because of her lack of discretion. By the same token, you will, of course, want to avoid asking others any questions that sound prying and might possibly offend.

❦ *Everybody Loves a Listener*

From the boss to your beau, you will be highly appreciated if you can be an attentive listener. A good listener often performs a valuable function—she inspires the speaker and helps him clarify his ideas. Numerous executives have come up with brilliant solutions to vexing problems while talking it out with their girl Fridays. And you know how often a problem seems to shrink in proportions when you can talk freely to an understanding friend.

The main reason we fall short as listeners is that we're too busy thinking ahead to what we will say next. Once you have directed the conversation to the other person and set him going, then you must perform one of the most difficult of conversation tactics—keeping quiet. Ninety percent of being a good conversationalist is being a good listener. Many people, women particularly, have wonderful reputations as charming conversationalists and yet actually say very little—they listen. There seems to be an almost universal need to talk, and since we are all essentially egotistical, we love to talk about ourselves.

Being a good listener is not easy. It requires complete attention, some prodding now and then with good questions, and the ability to direct a conversation well. Comments like "Isn't that interesting!" encourage the conversation. Give it your best tonal quality and be sure to sound sincere. How do you sound sincere? By being sincere. By making an attempt to be as alert as possible and by following closely what is said.

Other keep-the-show-going comments might be: "How did you happen to learn about that?" "That's the first time I ever heard about such an idea." "Where were you when you ran across that?" "How did you happen to be there?"

You also convey your interest by your physical reaction—perhaps by leaning slightly forward in your seat or by shifting your hand slightly in response to what is said—by the expression on your face, and by looking directly into the eyes of the speaker. If you are genuinely sincere, you won't overdo.

Great restraint is sometimes required to refrain from telling one of your favorite stories, which might divert the conversation to you. Of course you should take part in the conversation and share your experiences, but hold your big fire until the conversation lags. If the speaker is talking enthusiastically, let him enjoy telling his experiences—and you enjoy your reputation for charm.

❦ *How to Tell a Story*

Some storytellers can make an ordinary experience sizzle with excitement, while others kill even the best tale. Sizzle or fizzle—it depends on the skill of the speaker. While there are some raconteurs who seem to be naturally gifted, good storytellers are *more often* made than born. They've studied the techniques and they've practiced until they have achieved a polished style. Here are some points that help make a story a success.

• Make it easy to get the picture by stating the subject near the beginning of the story.

• Don't digress. Tell your tale in a clear, straightforward manner without bringing in extraneous details or haggling over whether it happened Wednesday at two or Tuesday at three.

• Use explicit terms. The person who says "it" or "thing" or "this fellow" is likely to lose his listener. The experts learn to be as exact as possible and to substitute a specific term for a general one whenever possible. How much more colorful a picture is created by saying "the smell of roast beef and apple pie" instead of "the smells of dinner."

• Keep it brief. Most stories are strung out too long.

• Once you have told your punch line, stop. Some people enjoy their own stories so much that they like to repeat the ending so that they can laugh all over again. Maybe they can laugh twice, but chances are their listeners can't.

The most successful stories are told with a light touch. Some girls with reputations for humor have developed such a sense of fun that they can find something entertaining in what others would consider pretty tame stuff. They regard the world as a very amusing place, and since they look for fun they can usually find it and can project it to others.

The best way to improve your storytelling technique is to practice. Try jokes and funny stories at first. These must be kept going at a fast pace and are good discipline. Try them on your family and friends. To get a laugh, you must put a joke across well.

A good way to improve your ability to tell a serious experience is to select a brief newspaper story. After you have read it carefully, put the paper aside and write your own version. When your words are put down in writing, you can judge them more easily. Compare your version with the original to see where you are weak, where you may have digressed, or where you could have used more forceful or colorful words.

Practice telling stories aloud to yourself. Then practice telling them to your friends. The more you keep at it, the smoother your delivery will become. Make yourself tell at least three different stories to friends each day. Soon you'll be able to shine with the best of them.

---

1 *In all your conversations for an entire day, practice directing the conversation away from yourself. Aim for the other person's interests and activities. See how long you can keep others talking about themselves or about impersonal subjects—not you.*

2 *On another day choose five topics that you would like to discuss with someone. In your conversations throughout the day, see how subtly you can lead the talk from one topic to another. This is excellent practice in directing the conversation and will stand you in good stead when you wish to divert the talk from unsuccessful topics.*

3 *Take a fifteen-minute walk, and see how many conversational ideas you can discover. You should be able to find at least eight.*

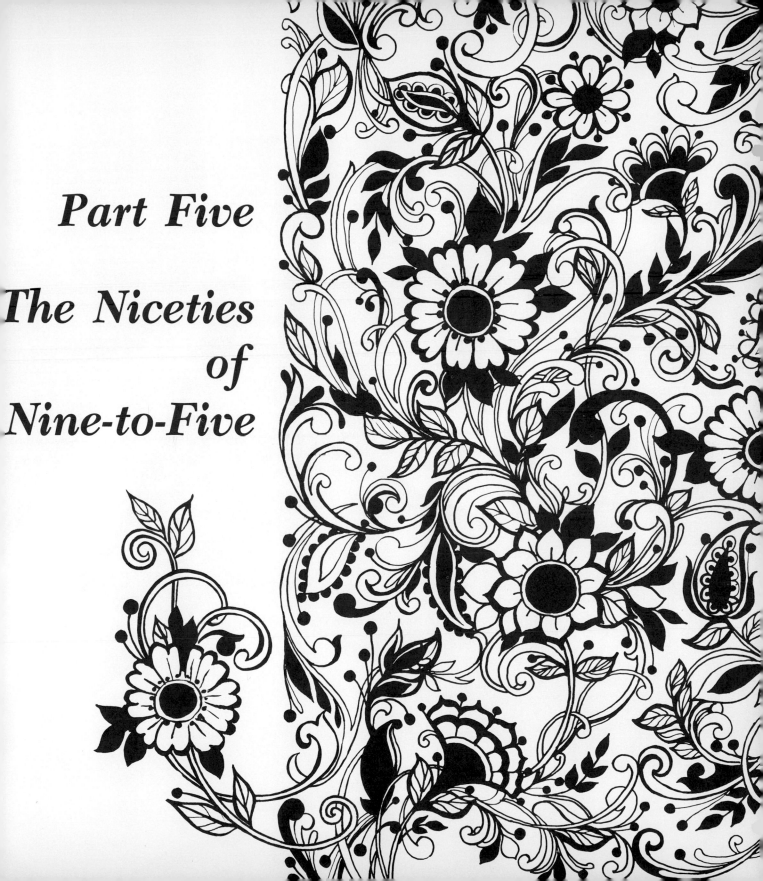

Part Five

The Niceties
of
Nine-to-Five

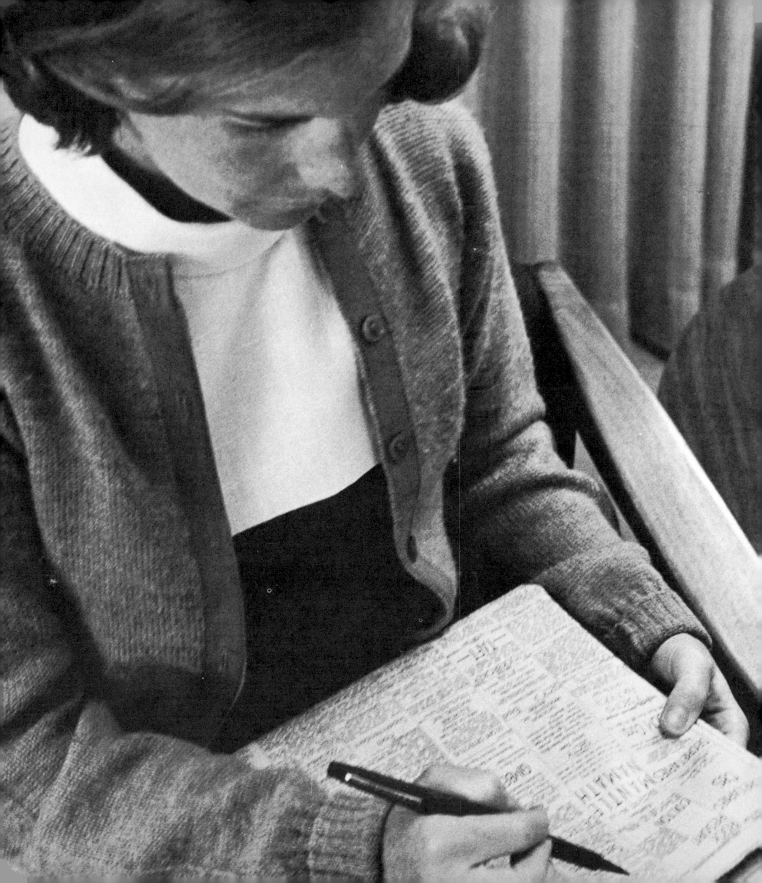

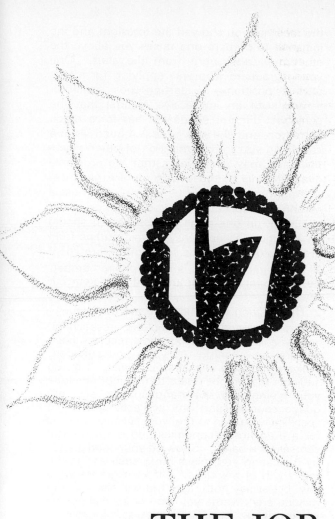

THE JOB CAMPAIGN

Your success in learning and applying your lessons in charm is put to a crucial test when you apply for a job. In this situation first impressions are all-important. You must give a good selling presentation on the first try because you seldom get a second chance. The best strategy is to plan each step of your job campaign in advance. You will need résumés and letters of application, and neither of these items can be well done in haste. Your interview outfit also deserves thorough consideration, for it will demonstrate your business taste—or your lack of it. Perhaps the most forethought should be given to the interview itself, because the poise, confidence, and grace with which you conduct yourself can make the difference between landing a so-so job and being offered a top-notch position. Most interview questions are routine, and you can think out ahead of time what answers you should give. But you must also be prepared to handle calmly any questions you have not anticipated. The technique is really little different from the way you respond to ordinary conversation. Naturally, an interview is somewhat more formal, and you must also speak up on your own behalf. But, for the most part, you will simply be applying the know-how you've already learned in this course. The rest is a matter of letting yourself relax so that you can be your usual charming self.

When you begin looking for a job, check with friends. They may know of openings in their companies. Read the classified ads in the newspapers. If you have a definite idea of what you want to do, write to companies that would be likely to have such jobs.

The Letter of Application

If you are using the help-wanted ads to obtain job leads, you will probably find that some of the most desirable positions request that you write out information about yourself and mail it in. This is done not only to help the busy employer sort out the applicants he considers unqualified but also to provide him with a sample of your work. You will therefore want to make your answer as complete and as concise as possible and as beautiful a specimen of your typewriting talent as you can create.

The most generally approved technique involves a brief covering letter plus a detailed résumé in outline form. Your letter should contain the following information.

1 The title of the position for which you are applying.

2 The reason or reasons why you are interested in this particular position—you want a job that lets you meet people, you are intrigued by the firm's products, and so on.

3 A reason why you feel you could contribute something to the business. For example, you've been told you have a knack for dealing well with people. Or, if the ad indicates that transcribing or letter writing is part of the work, you might mention that you have a sound background in English grammar or have won awards for your shorthand or typing skill. If the ad lists "good at figures" as one of the requirements, emphasize your mathematical ability. Ask yourself, "What is this employer looking for? What abilities would be helpful to someone in his business or profession? What qualities do I have that he would value?"

4 A mention of your résumé.

5 A closing sentence concerning your availability for an interview.

The Résumé

Whether or not you apply for a position by mail, you will be wise to compile a résumé. Many of the top-quality jobs, for which the competition is stiff (and which bring higher salaries), require a résumé. Even if none is requested, the fact that you showed the foresight and the initiative to prepare one raises you above the other applicants right from the start. One young graduate who was applying for a low-paying position—a starting position—presented such an impressive résumé that the personnel director suggested her for a much better job, and she was hired. A good résumé can bring you to the attention of other executives and may open doors that are ordinarily available only to those with more experience.

Your résumé should be typed—never use a carbon or duplicated copy of any sort—and should fit on one page if possible. It should be arranged in neat, easy-to-read outline form and should provide the following information.

1 Your name, address, and telephone number. Be sure to include your area code and your ZIP Code.

2 The position for which you are applying.

3 Your education (high school, business school, and/or college). List your most recent schooling first, mentioning the years you attended. Indicate the type of course or major. List the subjects that might relate to this job. Include your typing and shorthand speeds, any language courses, and any subjects that might specifically pertain to the work (science courses for a drug firm, economics and mathematical courses for a bank). Show off your good grades by indicating your class rank, such as "in the top fourth of my class." If your grades were low, better say nothing. You will also want to include any awards you won or special honors you received. In addition to awards for specific business subjects, you should also include citizenship or language awards. What activities did you participate in at school? Were you an officer of any organization? Any such information helps the employer sift you out from the rest of the beginners. It shows him that you possess leadership ability, have varied interests, and were well liked by your schoolmates. Your résumé is your personal advertisement and should include any information about yourself that proves you are an intelligent, responsible person with initiative and ability.

4 Experience. Include any previous employment, beginning with the most recent. Give the dates of employment as well as a brief description of the type of concern you worked for and the kind of work you did.

If you have never worked in a business office before, don't sell yourself short and classify yourself as having no business experience. Did you work on your school newspaper or year-book? Were you secretary or treasurer of your class or of some other large organization? Did you ever relieve the switchboard operator, help with the mimeographing jobs, or do filing or clerical work in the school office? Perhaps you helped in your father's office or in a local store on Saturdays and holidays. Work as a camp counselor, hospital volunteer, or baby-sitter should also be mentioned, because they show your initiative and responsibility and your ability to get along with people.

5 Personal information. Include your date of birth, general health condition, marital status, hobbies or interests, and any other pertinent personal information that will help the employer get a better insight into your talents and abilities. You can put your vital statistics and special interests near the end.

6 References. Include names of three or four adults who know you well and will speak favorably of you—perhaps a teacher, a clergyman, and a professional or business man. Give the addresses of references. You will, of course, obtain permission in advance from these people before using their names.

An example of what a good application letter might say is shown on page 250.

When your letter and résumé have been completed, rush them to the mailbox. Good jobs always go fast—and those first in line are sure to receive most attention.

❦ *Your Interview Outfit*

The girl who knows the importance of a smooth start on job-hunting day makes complete preparations the night before. She plans her outfit carefully and completely, down to the earrings and nail polish she will wear. She checks each item to see that it is sparkling clean, fresh, polished, or pressed and that no loose buttons or weak straps will cause last-minute emergencies.

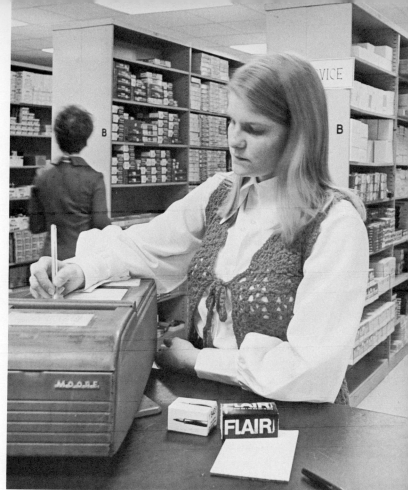

Courtesy of The College Store Journal

Remember to include any summer or part-time jobs in your resume. They show that you have had business experience and a certain amount of get-up-and-go. Such experience can make a good impression on employers.

She chooses a well-cut suit or a smartly tailored dress to impart the businesslike air of efficiency so dear to the heart of employers. She realizes that her outfit must be fashionable but that it should not be too high-style or too exotic. Prospective bosses scare all too easily. Color? A quiet, subdued shade bespeaks her business know-how. Although almost every hue of the rainbow is seen in the apparel of business girls today, the dark or muted shades are still favored and should be chosen for job-hunting outfits. Accessories can be gay and bright, of course, and should be carefully coordinated to show good taste.

7 Hamilton Terrace
Crestview, Illinois 60625
August 20, 197-

The Crestview Courier
Box 421
Crestview, Illinois 60625

Gentlemen:

Your notice, advertising a secretarial position
in a pharmaceutical laboratory, sounded very
interesting to me.

Science has always been my favorite subject,
and I received the Thomas J. Palmer Science
Award at high school. I attend Mercer Business
College, where I take many courses, including
business arithmetic and typewriting.

Enclosed is a complete résumé of my background
and qualifications. If they are what you have
in mind, may I speak to you about the position?

My telephone number is (312) 555-8767. I would be
happy to come to your office whenever it is
convenient for you.

Sincerely yours,

Joanne Burnell

Joanne Burnell

```
                          RESUME

Joanne Burnell                      Date of Birth:  January 25, 1950
7 Hamilton Terrace                        Height:  5 feet, 8 inches
Crestview, Illinois 60625                 Weight:  135 pounds
(312) 555-8767                     Marital Status:  Single


POSITION SOUGHT:  Secretarial

EDUCATION:       Mercer Business College, Crestview, Illinois
                 Year of Graduation:  197-
                 Specialization:  Executive Secretarial

                 Took courses in typewriting (65 net words a minute),
                 shorthand (120 words a minute), secretarial procedures,
                 and office machines.  Also had courses in general business
                 and liberal arts.  Was treasurer of the Student Government
                 Council, assistant business manager of the college news-
                 paper, a member of the Red Cross Council, and was graduated
                 in the top tenth of the class.

                 Crestview High School, Crestview, Illinois
                 Year of Graduation:  1968
                 College Preparatory Course

                 In addition to the standard courses in English and mathe-
                 matics, took courses in history, biology, chemistry, and
                 Spanish (four years).  Was a member of the Honor Society,
                 the Spanish Club, and received the Thomas J. Palmer Science
                 Award.

EXPERIENCE:      Brooks and Co., 109 Main St., Crestview, Illinois 60625--
                 (312) 555-7000 September, 1969, to present.  Part-time sales-
                 girl.  I have consistently had one of the highest sales
                 tallies in the departments in which I've worked (costume
                 jewelry, toys).

                 Dr. Howard Dean, 42 Tall Oaks Drive, Plainfield, Illinois 60626--
                 (312) 555-0303 June, 1968--September, 1969.  Receptionist in
                 office of dermatologist.  Through greeting patients and
                 answering telephones, I learned to deal with many types of
                 people.  I also was responsible for sending out bills, for
                 keeping office accounts, and for filing patients' records.

HOBBIES:         Outdoor sports, painting

REFERENCES:

Mrs. Hannah Rowe            The Rev. William Schwartz    Mr. Robert Holmes
Dean of Instruction        1 Trinity Place              109 Briant Street
Mercer Business College    Crestview, Illinois 60625    Crestview, Illinois 60625
90 Superior Boulevard      (312) 555-0972               (312) 555-8926
Crestview, Illinois 60625
(312) 555-8240
```

251

Although many women seldom wear hats, a job applicant will make a better impression if she wears a simple, tailored hat—one that is fairly small and not extreme in style. Although a hat is not essential, many personnel directors are impressed if a prospective employee has the good business sense to wear one.

The same reasoning applies to hosiery. Although many fashionable women go bare-legged in summer once they've acquired a good tan, many employers consider stockings essential to business formality.

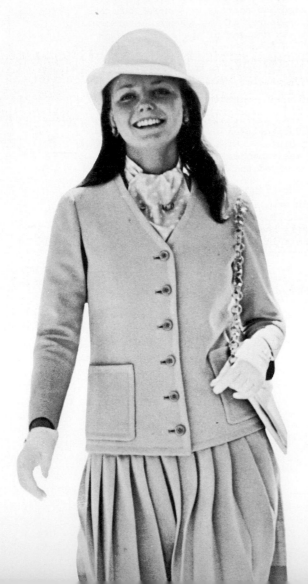

If the job seeker is lucky enough to own a fur coat or jacket, she wisely leaves it in her closet. A simple cloth coat does more to further the impression that she knows how to dress appropriately on the job.

Her makeup and grooming are the epitome of perfection. Her gloves (a must in summer as well as winter) are clean and fresh. Perhaps she carries an extra pair in her handbag in case her first pair becomes soiled. She's also sure her bag is in good condition with no unsightly bulges to ruin its trim lines. Shoes are simple and suitable, passing the test for even heels, unscuffed tips, and a high polish.

Appearance is such an important gauge of personality that you should be sure every detail is in order and that you look your best. Then you will feel confident and can devote complete attention to the interview.

❧ Be Prepared

Like a good Girl Scout, you owe it to your job future to be fully prepared for any emergency. Because the pens in personnel offices are usually a haphazard lot, you'll do well to take along a good pen of your own, plus two well-sharpened pencils, an eraser and an eraser shield—all of which may be valuable in filling out applications neatly or in taking tests. Remember, too, to include your social security card and perhaps a small notebook for jotting down addresses, directions, and other information.

When an employer is interviewing an applicant, he has so little to go on that he may attach undue importance to minor slipups. He might be quite willing to give a second application form if the first is spoiled or to lend a pen if the applicant's gives out during a dictation test, but this may make him wonder about her thoroughness and efficiency.

❧ Extras That Impress

What can you do to make you stand out above the others trying for the job?

• Offer a copy of your résumé. Even though you may have sent a copy of your résumé along with your answer to the ad, it's a good idea to bring another copy to the interview. When an applicant is being considered for a job, her résumé may be passed through several hands and may not have been returned in time or, worse yet, may have been lost in the shuffle.

• Obtain a letter of recommendation. If possible, get one from a previous employer or from someone for whom you did volunteer office work. Glowing praise from a past employer can strongly influence a prospective one.

• Learn all you can about the firm. This most impressive extra depends on whether you know the name of the firm in advance. If you have obtained your job lead through an employment agency, you will most likely be sent directly from the agency to the company with no time for checking. If, however, you have time to do a little investigation before the interview, by all means do so. Try to bone up on the firm's services or products so that you are aware of its needs and know what qualities the employer is looking for in his personnel. Your local chamber of commerce should be able to help you. Perhaps your library has material about the industry that you could skim. Ask your father and teachers for imformation about the concern. A knowledge of the firm's reputation, expansion plans, and new products will all be good background information. Another advantage of such investigation is that you will probably also discover anything undesirable about the company that might make you hesitate to accept the job.

❦ Passing the Preliminaries

You're there. You've found your way to the office of this marvelous-sounding firm. As you step off the elevator a few minutes before the appointed time, you may suffer a few butterflies in the tummy—it's natural! Now's the time to quickly bolster your poise by reminding yourself of your perfect grooming, your careful planning, and your success in winning an interview in the first place.

A self-assured manner is a most important sales technique. If you don't feel as brave as

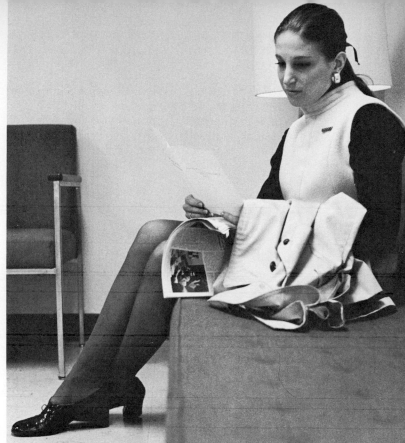

B. D. Unsworth

you wish you did, call forth the actress in you to make yourself appear assured and at ease. Not only will this little pretense help you to relax and actually develop the confidence you are portraying, but it will also pay off in its impression on others. A self-confident manner shows that you have faith in your ability and consider yourself worth hiring—a recommendation from the one who should know best!

The receptionist will probably ask you to be seated for a few minutes. Don't be impatient or feel put out if the "few minutes" grow longer and longer. Perhaps your prospective boss is tied up with *his* boss. After all, businessmen *are* busy and their time is worth money to the firm they represent. As yet, yours is not.

You'll want to maintain your best manners while you wait. Even now, you may be under inspection. Smoking and gum chewing are, of course, taboo. Some girls find that it helps them feel more relaxed to bring a newspaper or book to read. Make sure, however, that your choice is of a high caliber, because an employer will certainly notice it and will weigh it as a clue to your interests. You may also find it helpful to look and listen to what is going on about you. Try to get the feel of the company and its personnel.

✽ Top Form for Applications

Even though you may have sent a résumé ahead of time, you will probably be asked to fill out an application form. Most firms like to have employment records on their own forms so that they can more easily spot the information they want. Read all the instructions carefully before you write anything. If the instructions tell you to print, be sure to print. The ability to provide all information correctly, completely, and neatly will give a good impression of your work habits. Cross-outs, blank spaces, and vagueness are minus factors. A personnel director once confided to an interviewer that he always checked carefully to see if the applicant included her ZIP Code number. "If she is thorough and accurate, she'll put it in," he claimed. Because little things mean so much when there are so few clues to what you are like, you must take special pains to see that everything is done to the best of your ability. Check carefully to see that all information has been filled in, that any dates and all the names and addresses of references are correct.

✽ Charming the Interviewer

"Mr. Employer will see you now," the receptionist says, nodding to you. Take a deep breath as you follow her to his office. Let your posture and your poise show the confidence and self-assurance that he is looking for.

If the employer is on the phone or busy as you enter, wait quietly at his door until he finishes or looks up and motions you to a seat. You will, of course, keep your bag and any other belongings on your lap—not on the interviewer's desk. Don't light up a cigarette. Even if he offers you a cigarette, it is the better part of wisdom to refuse politely.

During the interview the employer must evaluate you to see how you will fit in with the requirements of the work and with the office personnel. In return, you will want to evaluate him to see what type of answers he is searching for. Mentally put yourself in his place, and try to emphasize the assets you can offer and the qualities that would be helpful in this particular position. The clever girl tailors her answers to show an employer that he will benefit from hiring her.

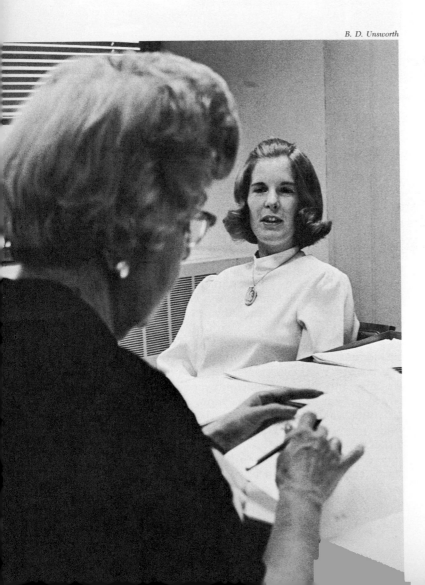

B. D. Unsworth

254

Some of the employer's questions may have already been answered in your application form, which he has before him. This repetition needn't be attributed to careless reading. His purpose may be to get you talking and to see how you express yourself. In your replies try to give all the pertinent information he desires without unrelated chatter. For instance, if he asks what type of work you did in your father's office, you won't boost your score any by merely saying, "Oh, anything that needed to be done." How much better a sales technique you'd use if you answered, "I typed letters and bills, did the filing, and greeted visitors. I often described our service and prices over the telephone, and I ran errands." Thoughts of the magnificent luncheons Dad treated you to, crotchety Mr. Adams, who always had one more job for you just at quitting time, or your father's handsome young assistant may whiz through your mind, but since these have no relation to the matter at hand, you will wisely avoid them.

Allow the employer to lead the interview conversation as much as possible. Applicants who talk too much or who overpower the conversation may be considered unlikely to get along well with other employees. If you don't get a chance to mention an important point, wait until the interviewer asks you if you have any questions. Then you can slip it in like this: "Yes, but first I'd like to mention . . ."

Most employers will ask such questions as, "Why do you want this particular job?" and, "How long do you intend to work?" Be sure you can come up with a good answer by giving these questions some thought before beginning your job search. Some interviewers may also ask what your ambitions are, what you consider your greatest assets, what hobbies you have, and what books you've read recently. If the interviewer should ask what salary you expect, mention a figure that is just a few dollars higher than the going rate for this type of job. You don't want to sell yourself short, but neither do you want to price yourself so high as to appear ridiculous.

If you have worked before and are asked why you left your last job, you will want to

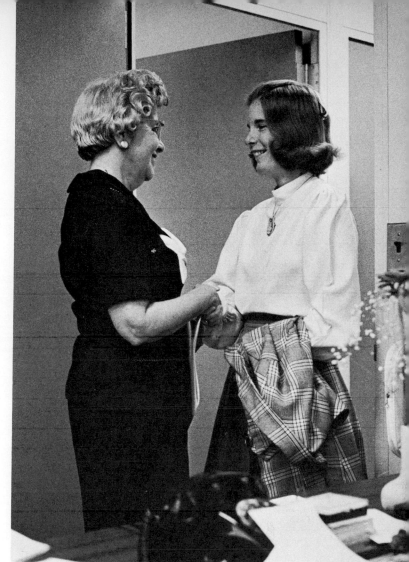

B. D. Unsworth

proceed with caution. Remember, the best psychology is to accent the positive, never the negative. For instance, say that there was not enough opportunity for advancement. *Never* that you couldn't stand your boss. No matter how unbearable a former employer was, you'll be wise not to criticize or complain.

In all your answers try to appear as alert, polite, and capable as possible. Show by your attitude that you intend to be a good worker and that you are seriously interested in this job.

255

Even if you don't think it is the job for you, be courteous and attentive. The cocky or too-good-for-this-job attitude that some job hunters display might boomerang some day when there is a really exceptional opening in the same concern.

If the interviewer considers you at all qualified, he will probably give you a good picture of the work and will explain hours, company benefits, and other aspects of the job. If you are not certain about any important phase of the work, such as the duties, opportunities for advancement, or the salary, don't hesitate to ask a few polite questions. You should have as clear an idea of the job as possible. However, the applicant who asks how soon she will get a vacation, how many holidays are observed, and whether coffee breaks are permitted will hardly convince a boss that she wants to *work*.

Regardless of how the interview went, you will have some thinking to do. Did you present yourself in the best light? Did you answer the questions well? Would you be happy in the job?

B. D. Unsworth

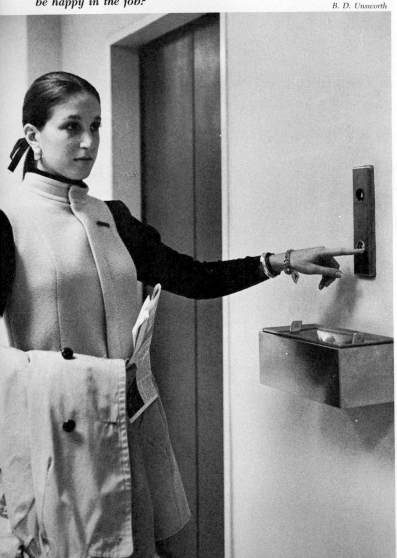

❧ Is the Job Right for You?

If you gave some careful thought before you began your job hunting, to the type of work you want, you should be able to decide easily whether this is the job for you.

• Is it a type of business that will be interesting to you?
• Aside from your business skills, can your other talents (artistic ability, writing ability, or other proficiency) be useful here?
• Will you be happy in an office of this size?
• Do the personnel seem to be the type of people with whom you want to work?
• Will the fast pace and excitement (or the quiet, calm atmosphere) be to your liking?
• If the work is detailed and requires careful attention, are you emotionally equipped to handle it?
• If it requires dealing with the public, does this appeal to you?
• Does this opening offer prospects of a bright future?
• Can you learn and grow on this job?
• Does the salary compare favorably with that offered for similar jobs in your locality?
• Is it a good location? Is the office convenient to transportation? Is the neighborhood safe to walk in after dark?

Your answers to such questions will determine your decision. Many beginners feel they should jump at the first job that offers the right salary. Careful, selective job shopping is more likely to result in a happy future.

256

❧ The Job Can Be Yours

If you are offered the job and are sure that this is the one for you, an enthusiastic ''yes'' should be given immediately. Don't let the good one get away. If, however, you don't want it, thank the interviewer and refuse kindly, perhaps explaining that you are considering another opening for which you feel you are better suited. Any remark that might seem to belittle the job you are offered should be avoided. Let your good impression remain in the interviewer's mind so that he may contact you at a later time if something more desirable should arise.

Perhaps you are a bit uncertain about the position and want time to think and to get a better perspective. Or perhaps you want to check other openings. Politely explain that although you are definitely interested in the job, you have some other interview appointments that you would like to keep before making a decision. Offer to let the employer know by telephoning him by a certain time.

❧ If the Interviewer Is Uncertain

If the interviewer wants to consider other applicants before reaching his decision, don't give up hope. Perhaps he, too, wants to be sure that he is making the best possible selection. To help sway him, why not make one more final sales appeal in the form of a brief thank-you note? Just a few lines, thanking him for his time and expressing your interest in the job, will bring you to mind again and do much to please the employer and to impress him with your capabilities.

1 *Learn as much as you can about the job opportunities in your area. What types of businesses are there? What specific products or services do they offer? Are any new firms planning to open offices? When you know something about the companies for which you could work, you can aim for the one that will be most interesting to you.*

2 *Ask your employed friends about their jobs. Try to get a picture of what it's like to work for their firms. Urge them also to talk about the work of their departments and the duties that their specific jobs entail. (One department of a firm can be very different from another.) In this way you can learn what departments might be most in line with your interests and abilities.*

3 *If you will soon be looking for a job, advertise this to your uncles and your aunts, your parents' friends, your employed friends. Job openings have a way of popping up unexpectedly, and someone just might happen to hear of one that would be right for you.*

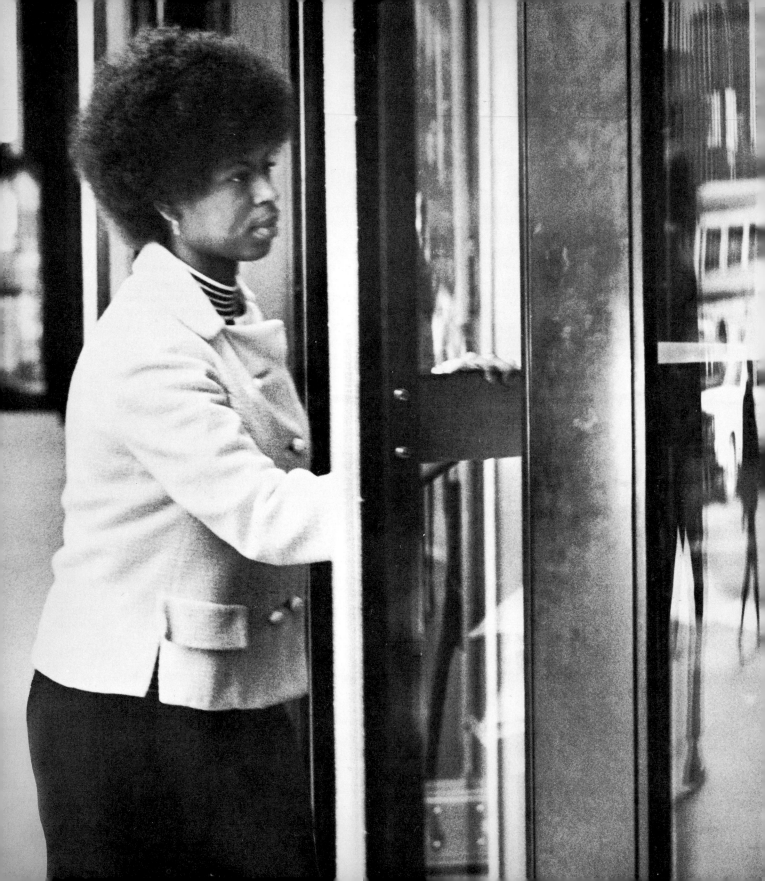

A CHARMING
BEGINNING

A new job is an exciting opportunity, a new and thrilling beginning. What lies ahead may be wonderful new friends, interesting accomplishments—even adventure. There will, of course, be many challenges—new skills to master, new routines to learn, perhaps strange customs and peculiar personalities to adapt to. A new job is an opportunity that deserves all you can give it. A beginner is in the spotlight the first few weeks. Her virtues and failings are carefully and curiously inspected. Your good beginning will encourage the staff to expect the best from you and will give you a bonus giant step in your climb to bigger and better things.

It is pretty much taken for granted that a new employee will arrive bright and extra early on her first day on the job. To forestall any unforeseen mishaps, allow yourself a good deal more time than you think you could ever possibly need under normal circumstances, particularly if the commuting is unfamiliar to you. If you haven't timed your trip during rush hour, remember to allow for traffic tie-ups. No matter how legitimate an excuse may be, it won't go over well. And the girl who arrives panting and in a guilty state of jitters is hardly able to apply the concentration that a new job demands.

Even before you begin work you should read any pamphlets or booklets that your company may have given you. These will save your asking unnecessary questions about hours, time off, insurance, and benefits. The booklets may also tell you something about the company's history and policies. A booklet may also contain an organization chart, which will show how your work will relate to that in other departments.

❧ Getting Your Bearings

If you are working in a large office, you will probably be introduced to many people during your first few days. Listen carefully so that you get each name straight the first time. Then repeat it to yourself and try to use the name in your conversation to help fix it in mind. The person who actually makes an effort to remember names usually finds it's quite easy to score a good average.

Once you are back at your desk and have a free moment, go over the names of those you have just met and try to attach them firmly to the proper faces. Some newcomers find it helpful to fortify their memories by devising a floor plan with the names and locations of the people with whom they will come in contact. Then when the boss booms, "Please rush this to Jenkins in Accounting," there's no need to falter, because even if your memory lapses momentarily, a quick check of that handy floor plan will show you the right direction.

Learn as much as you can about your firm. Study the company manuals and advertising material so that you will know about its products and services. The girl who is familiar with the background of her company soon develops the understanding and insight that makes her an asset to the staff.

Take notes, notes, and more notes. Sound advice for the beginner! Listen as carefully to all instructions as if you were hearing the greatest suspense thriller, for in fact you are. The instructions are the buildup. The will-she-make-it-or-won't-she outcome is up to you. So many things must be crammed into your cranium the first few days that it will be helpful to jot down notes about any instructions, procedures, or operations that might possibly be confusing. Some of your notes may seem trivial, but if they prevent an embarrassing slipup, they will be invaluable to you.

Ask questions. Don't be afraid to ask questions when new work is being explained. You aren't expected to know everything right away. And many an experienced staff member is so familiar with the work that he unthinkingly omits details necessary to your proper understanding of the job. Asking intelligent questions when the job is first given often helps prevent confusion and mistakes later on.

Do it yourself. The time will probably come, however, when you will be quite baffled by

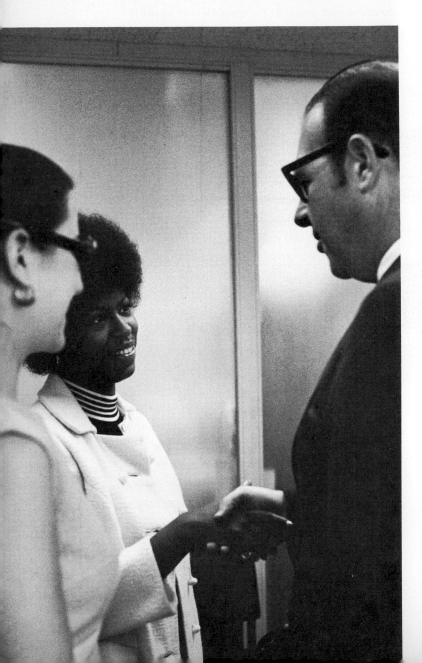

some aspect of the work you're doing. Although your first impulse may be to run for help to your boss or to the person who is training you, sit tight for a moment and see if you can possibly figure out the answer for yourself. If it's a matter of making extra carbons, you'll always be safe if you make the extras. If your question is about some sort of monthly or weekly report, perhaps you can check the files to find the last report to use as a guide. The files often can prove extremely helpful. They can rescue you when the spelling of a name is in doubt and can provide a great deal of information about the business and its operation. A company manual might give you a clue, too. If you still can't find the answer, then don't hesitate to ask someone. Most people are glad to help, particularly if they feel your questions are warranted and you aren't badgering them needlessly.

Learn from experience. If you are lucky enough to be broken in by the girl whom you are replacing, you have a golden opportunity to learn all the quirks of your boss's personality as well as of the work. Make careful note of how he likes things done and also of his pet peeves. Do everything you can to make a friend of this girl and to keep her from feeling "pushed out." If you must share the same desk with her, don't usurp her private drawer or in any way try to take over while she's still there. This may be ticklish, but you can't go wrong if you are thoughtful and considerate. Her friendship is well worth cultivating because she can save you from many a pitfall.

❦ Learn the Rules

If you want to be appreciated by the rest of the office team, you've got to learn the rules right away and play the game straight. The quickest way to arouse resentment is to break office rules or precedents. Don't take it for granted that certain privileges are just naturally given. Find out for sure. Are coffee breaks permitted, grudgingly tolerated, or forbidden? If rest periods are permitted, find out how much time is

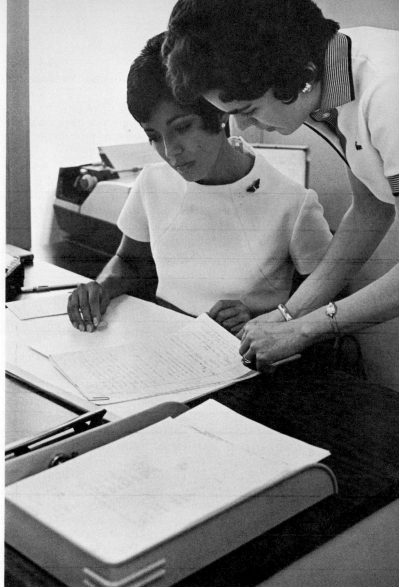

B. D. Unsworth

allowed so you won't overstay. How about lunch hour—is there a specific time you're expected to take yours, and is it actually *one* hour? Is smoking at your desk approved? If there is any doubt about any rules, check with your supervisor. The fact that others smoke or take breaks doesn't mean their acts are approved. They may be violating a rule that is not strictly enforced—but is a rule nonetheless. You don't want to be classed with those the boss growls about—merely because you didn't know the rules.

Be especially cautious in regard to smoking. Although some companies have no objection to employees' smoking at their desks, your particular boss may be annoyed by it. In one office where smoking was permitted, a supervisor was allergic to smoke, and out of consideration for her none of those who sat nearby would have thought of smoking at their desks.

If smoking is permitted and you do indulge, be careful that your smoke isn't continually wafted in one person's direction. Smoke and smoldering butts can be very annoying to a nonsmoker or to a person who has a cold. And overflowing ash trays have no place on your desk; they give a bad impression.

What about personal phone calls? In some offices personal phone calls are definitely prohibited. In others there are no set restrictions. If you are lucky enough to work in the latter type of office, be careful not to abuse this privilege. One of the most frequent complaints of bosses is that employees waste too much time with personal phone calls. It's a good idea to do your own telephoning on your own time whenever possible—during lunch hour or breaks—and to keep your calls brief. Your phone call, you must remember, is tying up a business line. There's always the possibility that your company may lose business or irritate a customer because he can't make contact. And woe be unto the girl who ties up the phone when her boss's boss is calling! Be considerate about making personal calls after closing time when only a few night lines are available. Try to limit your calls only to very urgent needs that can't be taken care of at home. The girl who holds long telephone gabfests with one friend after another during the working day may strengthen out-of-office friendships, but only at the expense of in-the-office relations.

❦ The Rules That Aren't Rules

When Amy started in her new job, she arrived so early that only a few members of the staff were present. She had been shown her desk the day before, and so she hung her coat on the coat rack beside her desk and sat down to await the arrival of the others. She noticed that her employer's assistant hung her coat on the same rack and so did one or two others. When her boss came in, he attempted to hang his coat on the rack, made a few blustering noises, and handed his coat to his secretary, saying, ''Here, do something with this.'' It wasn't until later that Amy learned, much to her embarrassment, that the coat rack, although right beside her desk, was reserved for her boss and his assistants.

Incidents such as this are sometimes unavoidable, but you are likely to skirt most pitfalls if you ask first and try to be as considerate as possible. When you see a special broad wooden hanger in a closet full of wire ones, you can be pretty sure it is somebody's private property—and that he will feel annoyed if you use it.

In matters involving the office hierarchy, a newcomer is wise to tread lightly. Why is the dictionary kept on Ellen's desk instead of on the window sill between you? Why is Connie allowed to cut in at the head of the line when the coffee cart arrives? Why does Miss Priddy keep her overshoes in the catalog file drawer? Why? Because that's the way it's done, that's all. Bit by bit over the years, special privileges have been carefully garnered along with seniority. Trivial as they may seem to a newcomer, they should be respected. Perhaps you may even learn later that there are reasons for some of these sacred rights, but, reason or no, sacred they are, and they should not be trifled with.

Such innocent acts as opening windows, adjusting the radiators, or moving the shades are also likely to disturb someone. Until you can determine the feelings of others on these matters, you may be wise to keep hands off. If you feel you absolutely must make some such change, be sure to ask first if anyone would mind. Your thoughtfulness and graciousness in these little matters will do much to charm the staff and win friends for you.

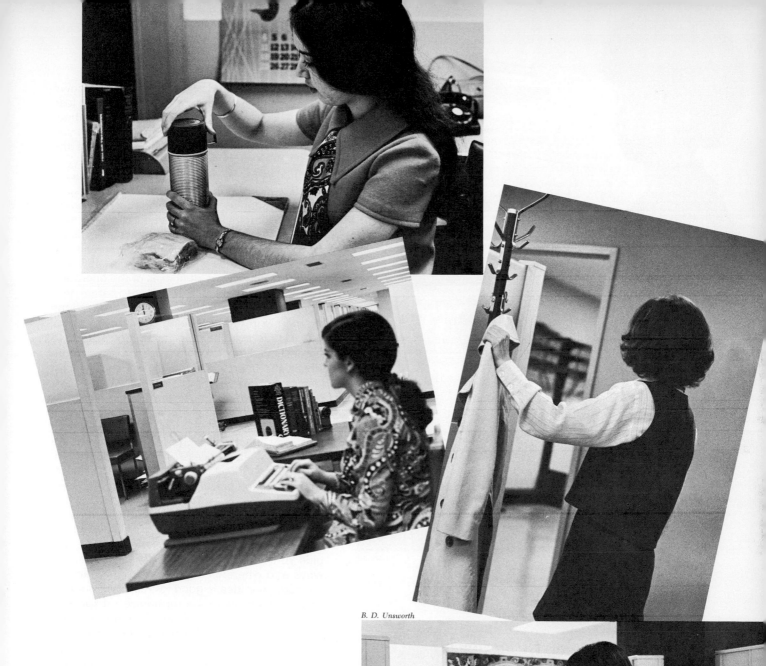

B. D. Unsworth

Actions that would be perfectly acceptable most places may be frowned on in
some offices. Find out if it is all right to
eat lunch at your desk, to take your lunch
hour when you wish, to decorate your
office, or to hang your coat in a certain
spot.

263

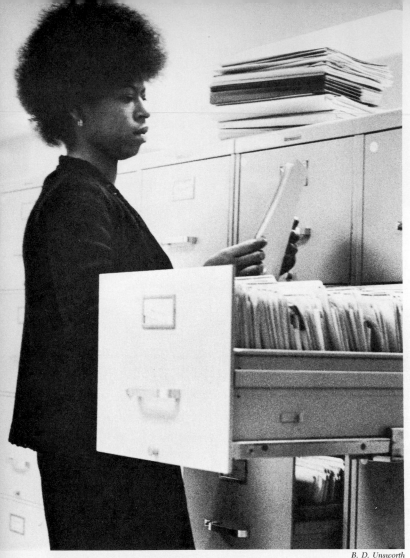

B. D. Unsworth

You may get a good idea for reorganizing the company files or simplifying an office procedure, but make sure you have all the facts before you present your idea.

❦ Reform Them Slowly

As a newcomer you have the advantage of being able to look at things with a greater degree of objectivity than those who have been doing the same work in the same way week in and week out. Perhaps it will occur to you that certain procedures seem needlessly involved or have no reason for being done at all. Keep your bright eyes open for ways in which you might improve the methods. Write your ideas down and keep them someplace where you won't lose them. Then say nothing and do nothing about them. At least not for a few months, until you are thoroughly familiar with all aspects of the work.

Any smart employer is eager to receive sound suggestions from one of his workers. Some companies even post suggestion boxes in which employees are invited to place suggestions for improvements and give awards for usable ideas. You will want to be sure, however, that your idea is *completely* workable and that you know about all phases of the operation that might affect such a change *before* you mention it to anyone. Half-cocked suggestions are merely irritating. Being creatures of habit, office staffs seldom react favorably at first to suggestions involving change. Before you whack the beehive, be absolutely certain your idea is holeproof. Probably the work is performed this way because that's the way it has always been done and nobody has bothered to change it. But perhaps there is a subtle reason that may not be obvious at first. Perhaps a more involved process in your department makes the work easier for another department. Or perhaps the present method is the pet brainchild of your boss—or his boss—and must be continued at all costs.

Write down your idea so that it won't become submerged in the inertia of routine, and bide your time. Meanwhile, try to learn all the whys and wherefores of the work. When you are sure your idea is good, phrase your suggestion as if you were asking advice. Express it in constructive terms of how it might improve the work, being careful not to cast aspersions on the old process and on those who have been blindly performing it. If your idea is accepted, you will be one charming lass whose business future will become beautifully rosy.

❦ Play It Smart

One of the first days that Lucy was on her new job in a leather goods manufacturing firm, her boss took her to the reception room and asked her to clean out the display cases, wash the glass counters, and rearrange the display samples. Lucy was horrified. She had just graduated from a prominent business school with top honors, was one of the fastest typists in her class, and had been trained to do better things than wield a duster and scrub cloth. But being a clever girl, Lucy swallowed her pride and obligingly set in. It wasn't until she had finished that she learned that she had been selected because the boss had been impressed with her good taste and felt that she could handle the job of creating an attractive display better than anyone else on the staff. Her cheerful attitude and willingness to work soon won her a promotion.

As a new and inexperienced worker, the beginner is likely to be the low man on the office totem pole. It's unfortunately true that in some cases the more tedious or menial jobs may be pushed off on her. Someone has to do them, and since the other employees have passed their fledgling period, these chores are dumped on the novice. If such is the case in your first crack at the business world, you'll be wise to accept the lowly job cheerfully and pleasantly. Never let yourself feel that any work is too belittling for you. The private secretary to a world-famous author and lecturer told how she once literally waded in and cleaned out his goldfish pond. The girl Friday to a noted decorator has often wielded a paint brush to convert some bit of gadgetry to the exact blue the client is searching for.

Many secretaries to famous personalities think nothing of preparing lunch for their bosses, taking suits to the dry cleaner's, walking the dog, or even baby-sitting with the children. No matter what comes your way, accept it with good grace. The day will soon dawn when you will no longer be the lowliest, and the less glamorous chore will be shifted to someone else. The cream naturally rises to the top. The girl who plays it smart by doing her best on *every* job will soon be accepted as an important member of the team, capable of handling more responsible work.

265

❦ Choosing Friends

Although you will want to be friendly to everyone in the office, as a newcomer you will be wise to take a bit of time before aligning yourself with any one group. You don't want, by mistake, to get in with what may turn out to be a clique. This may mean lunching alone the first few days and keeping to yourself slightly more than usual. But soon you'll be able to size up the staff. You won't swallow all the gossip you hear, and you'll be able to see who has the right attitude and who will most likely be your kind of friend.

You'll get ahead more quickly if you do even unpleasant tasks, such as cleaning up after a conference, as efficiently as possible.

B. D. Unsworth

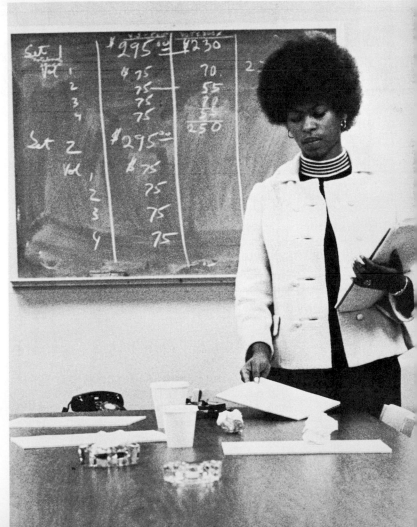

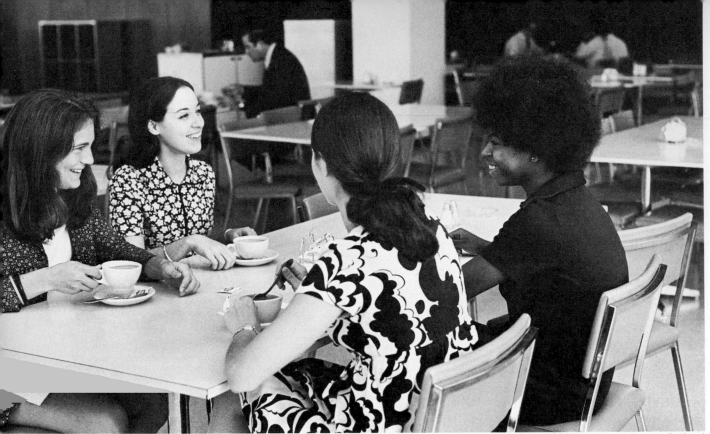

Joan Menschenfreund

When you're new on the job, try to get to know your co-workers at coffee breaks or over lunch. These people can be a big help in explaining office procedures.

Some girls quickly latch on to a couple of close friends and pretty much ignore the rest of the staff. On the whole, you'll be much happier if you have as many friends as possible. Lunch with different girls, and try to make friends with those in other departments as well as in your own. You'll not only have more fun, but you'll also learn more about other parts of the company and other work in case you should ever want to make a transfer.

❦ End of the Day

Amazing, isn't it, how many people survive the first days on the job! They may be a bit hesitant about them, but usually everything turns out pretty well—and may even seem fun in retrospect.

On your very first day begin the habit of organizing your work at closing time so that it will be easy to start on the next morning. Perhaps you can put all unfinished work together in a folder. As an aid to efficiency, leave yourself a note if there is anything that needs further attention in the morning. This is always a good practice, because if you are out the next day for any reason, someone else can follow through on your work.

As you tidy your desk, take a few moments to review what you have learned during the day. Are there any instructions you want to fix in your mind, any names or details you don't want to forget? If you made any mistakes, perhaps you can analyze them to see how they might be avoided. When we can learn from our mistakes, we run less risk of repeating them. Nobody's expected to be the expert her first day, but if she shows a willingness to learn and an eagerness to please, she'll make a charming beginning.

♨ Time of Departure

Promptness is a virtue appreciated much more at 9 a.m. than at 5 p.m. Even if everyone else begins an early cleanup as closing time draws near, the girl who is conscious of her good impression won't be eager to be the first one out of the office door. While your reputation is in the making, you should be especially careful that no one gets the wrong idea.

Many experienced workers have developed graceful leave-taking to a fine art. They wash up early enough to allow them to be back at their desks as the clock nears five. Although most of their work has been carefully organized and put away for next morning, one job is still out so that they can continue working until closing time or even a little beyond, if it means finishing a particular job. Although they depart a bit later than the girl who stands, hat in hand, foot poised to run, as she watches the clock tick from 4:58 on, these clever girls show a business-like sense of responsibility that pleases employers.

---

1 *The ability to remember names of new people you meet is largely a matter of concentration. Try now to develop the habit of listening for a new name and giving it your full attention. In the excitement of meeting someone new, our minds tend to leap ahead to all sorts of questions about the person. Train yourself to grab onto his name and to hold it fast in your mind before it is bumped aside by other onrushing thoughts.*

2 *The person who can control his mind sufficiently to concentrate well can often surpass the accomplishments of someone with superior intelligence. Those first few days on a new job, when there is so much to learn and remember, concentration is particularly important. Controlling attention is largely a matter of self-discipline and practice. If you have difficulty keeping your mind where it belongs, a little mental exercise will soon help. Practice confining your thoughts to just one thing for at least five minutes. Suppose, for instance, you choose a bird as your subject. Then force your mind to think only about birds and bird-related objects. You might think about birds in a nest, swans in the park, hard-boiled egg sandwiches, the feather trim on your new hat, the old-fashioned bird ornaments on a Christmas tree. Don't, however, let your thoughts squiggle away to the fun you had Christmastime at your tree-trimming party or to the scarf you want to wear with your new hat. Remember—birds, birds, birds. Keep your mind firmly under control. Practice this sort of thought direction at least twice a day for a week, more often if possible. The mind reacts like a muscle: the more it is exercised, the stronger it becomes and the greater the feats it can perform.*

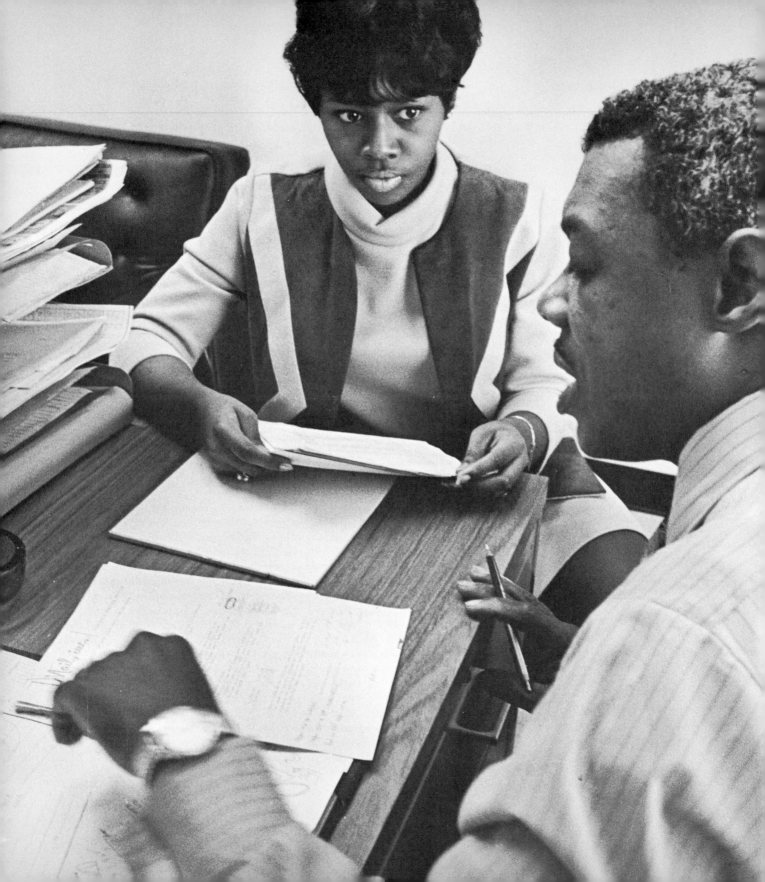

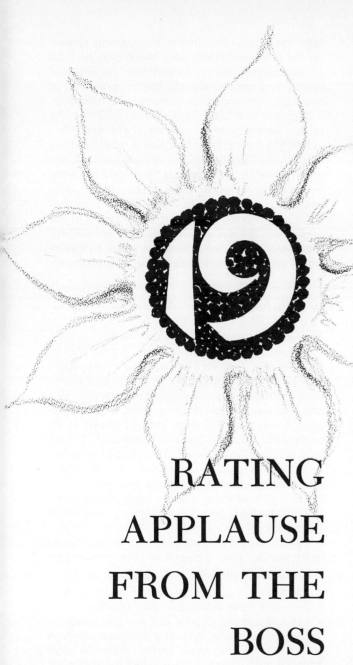

19

RATING APPLAUSE FROM THE BOSS

How to charm an employer is one of the lessons any would-be successful business girl must master at the start. Fortunately, bosses are people, and for the most part the same rules that work with others will win with your boss.

Try to understand your employer. How does he look at company problems . . . at your work . . . at you? Your boss knows that the only way *he* will get ahead is to do an outstanding job. In a large company an executive may be under considerable pressure to produce results. Office politics may be such that other young men on their way up are elbowing for his job. In such a situation he must turn out a stellar performance just to hold his niche on the promotion escalator. Even in a concern that doesn't have stiff internal competition, there are rival firms, rising costs, and operating difficulties to create pressure. It is essential for his department to do its best. This means that his staff must be efficient, must work together well, and must promote goodwill for the company. He is pleased when you fit into this plan and help further these goals. It is his responsibility to see that his staff operates smoothly. Any weak performance or clash of personalities among his employees is likely to disrupt the smooth functioning of the business and is, therefore, especially disturbing to him.

While it's true that he views you as a person in most regards, a businessman is also forced to look at you with dollar signs in his eyes. ''How well does she do her work? Does she fit in with the other workers? Does she possess a competent, polite manner that will help win more business for us?'' These are questions he must consider. The girl who can't measure up to the cold, hard requirements of business efficiency is out of luck. Attractiveness and charm go far and are invaluable assets in helping you work effectively, but alone they will not satisfy a businessman. They must be coupled with honest, hard work.

❀ Who's the Boss?

There's the distinguished gentleman in the tremendous office with the wall-to-wall carpeting. He's the head of the company. You can be sure

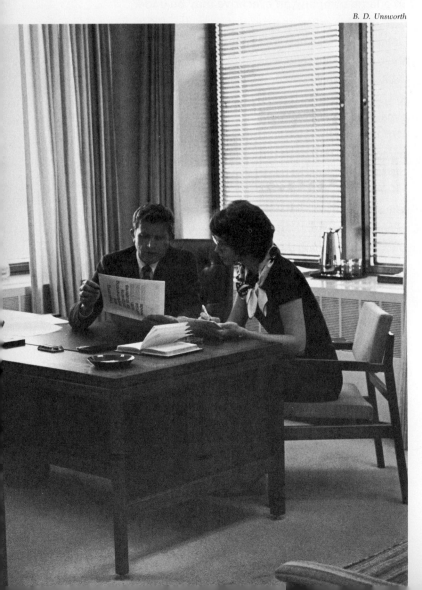

B. D. Unsworth

he's the boss. But in the intervening spaces on the company totem pole, there may be a lot of executives, minor executives, department heads, and individuals who have merely one or two workers responsible to them. Occasionally, a beginner is a bit dubious about who is "the boss," who should be catered to and given the velvet glove treatment. Actually, every person who is your superior deserves executive respect and deference, whether this be merely a private secretary or a higher clerk. The person who assigns you work and to whom you are responsible is your boss, regardless of his status in the company. Please and impress the person immediately above you, and the word will soon travel up and up to all the higher and mightier.

❀ Adjusting Your Attitude

Your attitude toward your boss can have a startling effect on your success in the job. When Mr. Sullivan, a rather bombastic sales manager, was looking for a secretary, a bright and promising stenographer was suggested to him. "But she's afraid of me!" he objected, and the job went to another girl who, though not quite so competent, had the poise and aplomb to cope with his harmless bluster. This type of boss can unsettle a beginner, but if she's smart, she'll make every effort to overcome her fears. The timid girl makes a man uneasy, for unconsciously he feels guilty about having caused her fear.

What should your attitude be? Bosses being quite varied, that depends on the person you work for. In general:

• Be friendly but respectful. A smile can hide—and help diminish—any timidity.
• Let him set the degree of formality; then, to be on the safe side, be just a bit more reserved than you feel you need to be. The girl who keeps a little distance usually has more chance for job happiness than the girl who is too chummy.
• Call him Mister unless he specifically tells you to do otherwise, regardless of how he is addressed by others on the staff. Most men prefer

to be addressed as Mister, even though they will probably call you by your first name. But if your boss suggests you call him Bernie, then by all means do so. Of course, whenever other executives or strangers are present, you will be careful to speak to him as Mister.

• Avoid wisecracks or personal kidding. Although many executives indulge in good-natured banter among themselves, they may resent it, as an affront to their dignity and position, if it comes from their staff. A smart girl will give thought to her chief's reactions before uttering her clever quip.

• Look for his good points. Overlook his bad ones. You'll enjoy working with him far more if you do. Be an appreciative audience, and a bond of good feeling will develop between you.

• Stifle any tendency to judge. One advertising executive complained that whenever he left early, his secretary's knowing little remarks—"Lovely weather for golf," or "It's a hard life!"—made him feel guilty, despite the fact that he was off to a grueling session with a client. A major portion of present-day business deals are consummated over the dinner table or on the golf course. Not only had his secretary no right to judge, but she should also have realized that an employee seldom sees the complete picture and is in no position to judge fairly.

❦ Aim to Please

The man behind your paycheck is pleased when you do a good job. Here are some work habits which concern him.

• Be someone he can count on. Show him that you are as dependable as you are charming. Let him see that you can be counted on to do a job right, that you are thorough, accurate, and careful in the many little details that are so important—spelling, taking messages, writing names and addresses, filing, dealing with figures, or handling money. If you are typing correspondence, check any dubious points —bosses can make mistakes, too, you know. If you must consult him about a correction, you'll want tactfully to avoid calling unnecessary attention to his error.

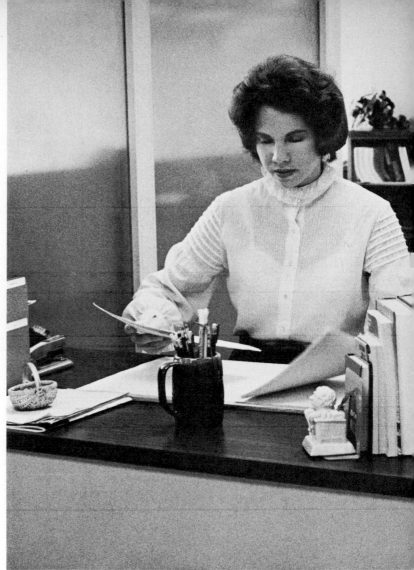

B. D. Unsworth

Keeping a neat desk is an indication to your boss that you are efficient and well-organized.

• Be neat in all you do. Such things as smudges, strikeovers, or sloppy erasures disturb the most saintly boss's disposition. And any boss is dismayed by the girl whose desk is a flurry of papers, carbons, and files. Perhaps she knows where everything is, but she's not likely to give the impression she does unless her desk has a tidy, businesslike order. If you smoke, be especially careful. An ashtray overflowing with lipstick-rimmed butts, smoldering remains, or spilled ashes is distasteful to most people.

• Be a self-starter. The girl who tries to find out what she can do to solve a problem, instead of taking a let-the-boss-worry-about-it attitude, will go far. Many a business girl has won her chief's appreciation by helping a customer herself, by gathering in advance information that her boss will need, or by composing answers to letters to save dictation time. You must, of course, be careful not to overstep your authority. You must be sure your employer would want you to act for him. If there is any doubt about your boss's attitude in such a case, submit your idea for approval first. The girl who

Sometimes a boss is in such a hurry that he has to dictate "on the run." Plan to take such things in your stride.

B. D. Unsworth

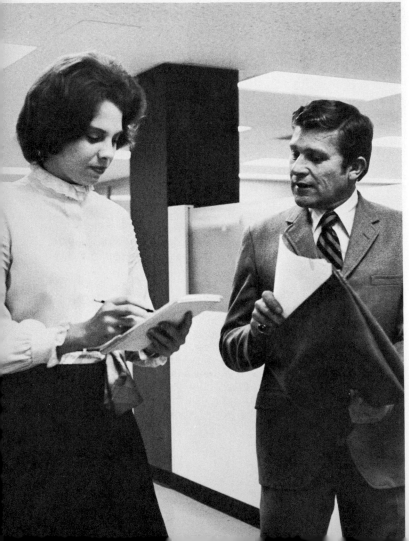

willingly takes all the responsibility her boss will give her shows that she is capable of handling an important job and quickly lines herself up for promotion.

• Be willing to work hard. Let your boss know that you are conscientious, that you care about doing a job right, and that you don't mind taking on the occasional extras that are sometimes necessary. If a task is tough or tedious, be a good sport—don't complain or make him feel like a slave driver.

• Be flexible. The girls who get to be private secretaries to top executives and famous personalities work under all conditions. They may take dictation in such strange places as elevators, subways, airports, taxis, or even beauty parlors as they trail their bosses through busy, exciting days. When a last-minute rush job arrives or a change in procedure or hours is called for, adjust to it easily and graciously. Occasionally you may be asked to do shopping for your boss or a personal favor such as a duplicating job for his wife's club. Take on these chores agreeably. Part of the job is making life easier for your chief, even to the extent of obliging his wife.

• Be well organized. Plan your work so that you do important jobs first. Collect everything you need before you begin a task so that you can work efficiently.

• Show your interest and enthusiasm. The girl who can adopt a "we" attitude in regard to the company and can develop the teamwork required to make it a success will please her boss and will get more satisfaction from her work as well. Try to learn as much as possible about your firm, about its products or services, about the various departments. Your work will become more meaningful, and you will be better informed and thereby better equipped to help your boss intelligently.

• Keep your mind on your work. No girl can keep her filing straight when she's deliciously reliving the previous night's date—or worrying why Rod hasn't phoned. She wouldn't waste her own precious lunch-hour shopping time on such unfruitful mental meanderings, and she most certainly should not squander the time that she is *paid* to think about business. Personal problems and daydreams are strictly for after-hours.

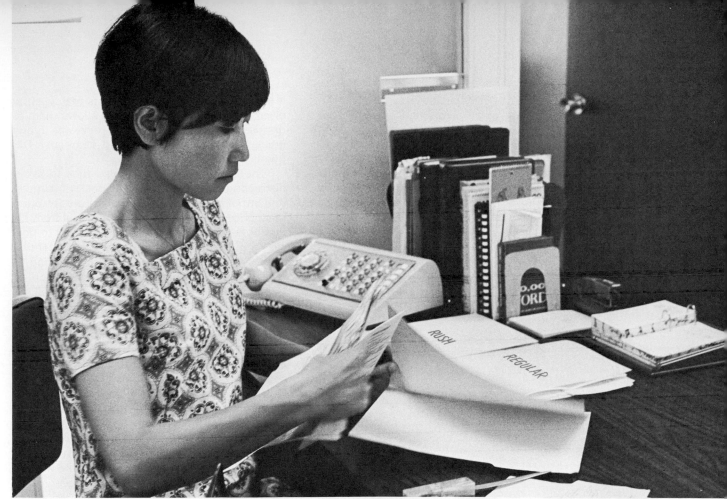

• Keep confidences. When your boss entrusts you with some confidential information, feel flattered and show that you can live up to his trust. Not only must you be discreet and carefully avoid mentioning the subject to others, but you must also be sure that your face and manner reveal nothing.

• Don't abuse his goodwill. The boss hires an employee to work a certain number of hours. He expects her to be at her desk (not in the ladies' room) at starting time. He expects her to limit her personal telephone calls and to save long personal conversations for lunchtime. Some offices operate like a classroom, with all but necessary conversation prohibited. Most companies are more lenient, but as one executive complained, ''Every day after lunch my girls waste a good part of the next hour comparing the bargains they got during lunch-hour shopping. The time they waste each day in personal chatter would easily add up to another full-time employee!'' Viewed from the boss's angle, it becomes apparent that such girls are a company liability.

ꙮ *Do Not Disturb*

Every boss has special ways of doing things. As early as possible on the job, you will want to find out his special likes so that you can cater to them. He'll probably have his own peculiar peeves, too, which you will delicately avoid, no matter how trivial they seem. But the main irritant of most bosses is interruptions. The phone calls, the visitors, the executive conferences that eat away at his time are not your doing, but you *can* help by being considerate of his time in all your dealings with him. Although you will sit quietly—and interestedly—when he has a story to relate, you will be quick to sense his impatience if you are telling a story. Your business discussions should be as brief and concise as possible. Many girls find

A good secretary will plan her work so that she doesn't have to bother her boss every two minutes with questions. By organizing her work she can get many answers at one time and save the boss a great deal of time.

B. D. Unsworth

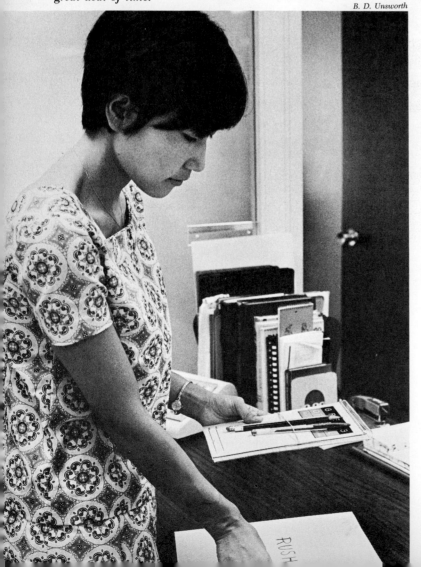

it helpful to keep a list of subjects they wish to discuss with their bosses. This allows them to dispose of all the accumulated problems in one quick businesslike session and eliminates frequent interruptions.

The considerate worker also tries to avoid distracting her employer. She doesn't barge in and out of his office every two minutes to bring mail, check his wall chart, get material from his file, or deliver finished work. She tries to possess a quiet manner that doesn't call attention to her presence. When someone is trying to concentrate, slamming drawers, noisily ripping paper from a typewriter, tapping a pencil, or uttering exasperated sighs when an error occurs on the bottom line can be sufficiently disturbing to shatter his thoughts completely. Other irritants: loud talking, singing or humming, gum chewing (loud or otherwise), a heavy walk, and distractions during dictation. A dictator has enough trouble trying to compose a coherent message without having to contend with a squirming stenographer, a footswinger, a hair fusser, a jewelry twister, or a girl who makes diverting doodles. Obvious boredom or a superior attitude that implies he is not the world's greatest literary light gives him a feeling of inferiority that quickly douses all inspiration.

❦ The Boss Is Boss

Your employer wants all letters sent in large envelopes, even though you realize small envelopes would do just as well and would be more economical. He decrees that you get along with one less filing cabinet, although the drawers are bulging already. What to do? Do it his way, of course. Some men want pencils used down to one inch stubs. Others fuss if a slightly tarnished paper clip appears on outgoing mail. Trivial, perhaps. Unreasonable, perhaps. But because your boss likes things that way, you do it that way. Otherwise, he's likely to find himself someone else who will. *MORAL:* The boss is boss. Keep him happy.

Jane's employer quoted a price during dictation that seemed far too low. After she left

274

his office, Jane checked on similar work and found that the quoted price was considerably below the usual figure. When she called this to her employer's attention, he said he was aware of the lower price but had his reasons for this. Unsatisfied, Jane continued to press the issue, pointing out the work involved and the foolishness of not allowing for sufficient profit. Although her boss seemed to want to drop the subject, she continued to argue the matter until finally he had to tell her that that was the way it was to stand and she should do as she had been instructed.

Although Jane was wise to check the unusual price and to confirm it, she should not have questioned her employer's judgment and argued with him. When a boss makes decisions, we must accept them and let them go. Jane was sincere in thinking she was right and that she was protecting the best interests of the firm, but she should have done as she was told without further protest. There are often considerations that influence an employer's thinking that he may not care to reveal to others. *MORAL:* The boss is boss. Don't argue.

You cannot go wrong if you remember that you are hired to help your boss do *his* job better. His idea of how work is to be performed may not be the same as yours, but because his is the hand that sways your future, his is the idea that counts.

❦ Changing His Ways

The exception to the previous advice is the case where the boss in unaware that he is sabatoging your efficiency, as when an employer unthinkingly leaves important dictation or rush orders until late afternoon. If this is his habit, a girl should have a heart-to-heart talk with her boss, tactfully explaining that when she must rush important work out so fast, she doesn't have time for the careful checking she feels the work deserves and is afraid some error may slip through. When faced with the prospect of better job performance, most executives will gladly rearrange their schedules.

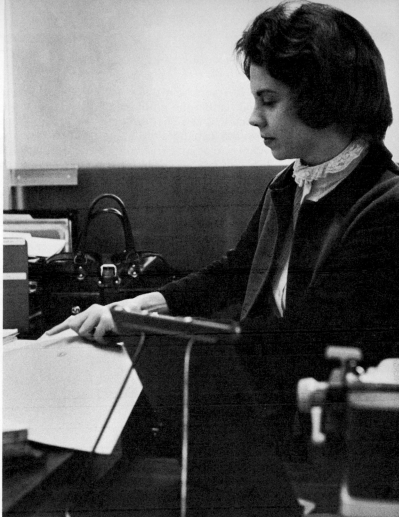

B. D. Unsworth

You will sometimes have to take work home, but your boss will probably reward you with extra time off.

❦ How Big a Load?

Occasionally a worker is so efficient that her boss loses track of how much work she is accomplishing. He merely knows that everything that must be done Meg does—quickly and well. When another involved task looms before him, he unhesitatingly turns it over to Meg, confident that she can be depended on to handle it properly and accurately. But eventually Meg reaches the point where her day becomes a hectic race with the clock and the need for frequent overtime or taking work home is too much of a burden.

275

How should a girl who is genuinely over-taxed handle the problem? Before raising any objections, she should see if there isn't some way she can possibly handle the extra work. What she definitely should not do is bewail her fate and tell her hard-luck story to every handy ear in the office. Neither should she continually complain to her boss in vague terms about the ''tremendous amount'' of work she has. Frequent complaints lose their effectiveness with even the most sympathetic ear.

When you find yourself overloaded, you may be able to get the receptionist or another secretary to help you.

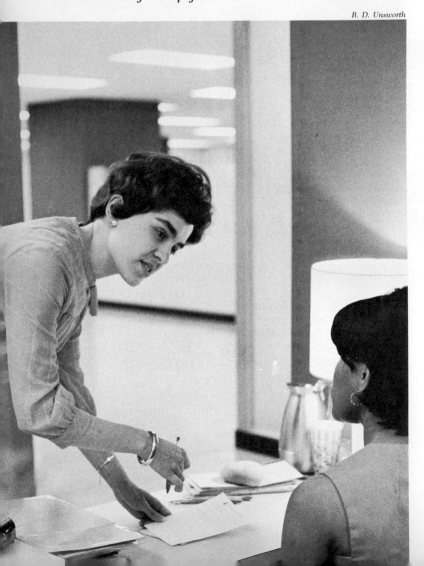

B. D. Unsworth

Instead, Meg should analyze her problem as objectively as possible to see how the overall work picture could be improved. Perhaps there are some shortcuts she could try. Possibly some of her more routine work could be taken over by a less skilled worker or by the receptionist or the office boy. Would a copying machine, a dictating machine, or some other equipment pay its way in saved time and improved efficiency?

Occasionally, a worker with a good record is reluctant to surrender any of her duties for fear of losing status. As a result, she is so burdened by unimportant routine details that she denies herself the opportunity to look up and ahead, to display the foresight and initiative that would make her stand out as an exceptional, creative worker who is more than just a good workhorse. Any girl with glowing aspirations owes it to herself to keep her eye on the future, to grow with the job. She cannot let herself stagnate either through her own inertia or her reluctance to pass off routine work so that she can help her boss with more involved tasks.

In Meg's case she would be wise to make a list of all the duties she now performs. (Often a busy boss is unaware of all that an employee handles for him.) Next she should list all additional duties or responsibilities she could take on if she had more time—duties that would relieve her employer of some of his load. Then she should indicate which routine jobs could be delegated to someone else or, perhaps, to a machine. Such constructive thinking impresses an employer that she is not merely attempting to shirk work but is sincerely concerned with helping him more effectively.

❦ Chain of Command

Kay worked in a large department. The procedure for choosing vacation time was to send around a chart on which each employee indicated his preference. If there were no vital conflicts, each person was allotted the time he had chosen. Shortly after the schedule had been made up, Kay learned that the friend with whom she'd been planning a vacation trip would have to postpone her vacation two weeks. Kay envisioned all their wonderful plans spoiled. She rushed down to the department manager's office and asked if the last two weeks in August were available. They were. With her spirits soaring high, Kay returned to her desk.

The next day Kay's boss approached her looking quite annoyed. "Why didn't you tell me you wanted to change your vacation?" he asked. "This morning I promised Ann that time. We can't get along without both of you, so I'm afraid you'll have to make other plans."

If only Kay had gone to her boss in the first place, he would have been aware of her desire to switch her weeks. Once he had approved Ann's time, he would not ask Ann to change.

The executive chain of command is a hallowed business tradition that no employee can afford to ignore. One of the unwritten rules of business is that whenever an employee has a request to make or a suggestion to offer someone outside the bounds of her immediate working group, she must first consult her own boss and work through him. Her immediate superior will be annoyed if he is bypassed, and, moreover, he can often smooth the way for her when he knows her plans.

It's always advisable to keep your employer informed of your plans, even of matters that would seem to be of little concern to him. When the gang is planning a luncheon for one of the girls, the boss may want to be one of the first to know about it—if only as a matter of pride. Bosses usually appreciate being in the know about department activities and may even be a little put out if they are not told first.

❧ Handle with Care

Mr. Ames was notorious among the staff for his temperamental disposition. His was a creative job, and he was often under considerable pressure to turn work out fast. The list of girls he had tried and rejected was as long as his temper was short. When Alice had stayed with him

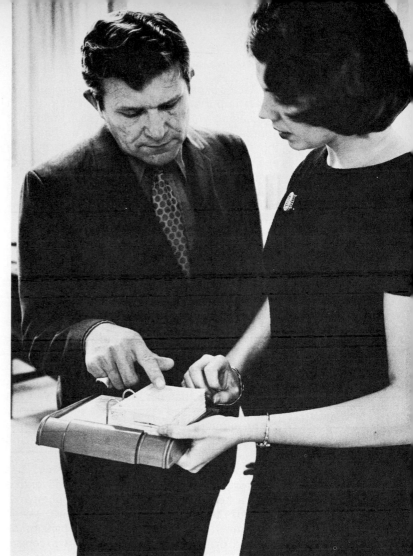

B. D. Unsworth

Make sure you keep your boss informed well ahead of time about your vacation plans or when you need to take time off for something special.

for three months, the staff was astounded. The explosions from his office were less and less frequent, and Alice seemed to be holding up remarkably well. "How do you do it? How do you stand him?" she was asked. "Oh, he isn't half bad once you understand him and realize what he's up against," Alice replied. "He's carrying a terrific load, and he really turns out some excellent material."

Alice's experience with Mr. Ames taught her a few important lessons that will help her in succeeding with any type of boss. Instead of approaching the terrible Mr. Ames as if he were the most unpleasant creature on earth, she decided to accept him as he was and to do her best to put up with him. She made up her mind to look for whatever good points she could find in him—which were many, she discovered—and to make every effort to please him.

Putting up with a difficult person is much easier when you take an objective point of view and realize that often there is nothing personal in his annoyance. Frequently his temper may be aroused by something that has nothing whatever to do with you. Alice was aware of this, and Mr. Ames was grateful when she overlooked his flare-ups. Alice's lack of condemnation had a calming effect in itself, whereas the other girls' show of disdain had provoked him to take out his wrath on them. Alice realized that her boss's nerves were on edge, and she had learned that serious family problems added to the pressure he felt. She endeavored to be as calm, as unobtrusive, and as quietly efficient as possible.

That was six years ago. Mr. Ames has overcome his jittery nervous condition and is now a top executive of a larger company. Needless to say, Alice is still with him. When Mr. Ames was offered the new position, he insisted on bringing Alice along (at a considerably higher salary), because he knew how valuable she had become to him.

If you are confronted with a difficult boss, allow yourself a six-month trial period to win him around. Try all the cajoling refinements of diplomacy, subtlety, and tact. Make an honest attempt to like him. Usually this treatment wins.

Even if it doesn't, fate may step in and give you a hand if you allow a little time. Because there is continual change of personnel in every office, it sometimes happens that the disagreeable boss leaves or is transferred to a branch office. Perhaps some other girl will quit, and your good attitude will bring you to the attention of her boss. Don't jump at the first snarl from

a nasty boss. Give him a full-fledged try before you cancel out.

If all your efforts are to no avail but you like the company, perhaps you can find a job in a different department. Learn as much as possible about the various departments of the firm and then ask the personnel manager if you can be considered when an opening occurs in the department of your choice. You'll make a better impression if you phrase your request in terms of your interest in the work without admitting any inability to adjust to your present boss.

🌷 If the Boss Wears Lipstick

Perhaps your boss is a *she,* and not a *he.* Then it's just as important to show the right attitude. Give her your best, and a woman executive is usually most appreciative. The tattered old prejudice against working for a woman is quite unfounded. Business is very wary of the woman who displays feminine wiles or temperament, and she is not likely to be chosen for a post in which she has responsibility over others. To reach a position of importance, a woman executive has had to prove her stuff against severe masculine competition—and often opposition. She has had to be better than the average male even to win an executive spot. You would expect to be able to respect a male boss, and there's even more reason why you would have the same expectation of a woman boss.

Naturally, no woman boss is faultless—just as no male boss is. It would be unfair to be more critical of your boss simply because she is a woman—you owe her the same willingness to look for good and overlook bad points that you would give a male executive.

Working for a woman boss may even have special advantages. Many female executives have traveled the secretarial route to the top, and they know far better than any male boss the complexity and problems of the job you must do. And if you merit promotion, you'll know for a certainty that your boss will not hesitate to advance you because you are a woman.

☙ *Loyalty*

Loyalty is one of the most valued business virtues. Many a boss is so wonderful that you automatically want to gild his reputation at every opportunity. But even those not-so-wonderfuls deserve—and respond beautifully to—the person who glosses up their reputation for them.

As an employee you are, perforce, your boss's publicity agent. Whether he is heroic or horrendous, nothing but the best publicity should emanate from you. His clients, his superiors, his staff, even the girls at the luncheon table should hear nothing but words of praise. When the office staff resorts to the insidious pastime of let's-pick-the-boss apart, loyal girl that you are, you can deftly change the subject.

Granted, bosses being individuals, there are bound to be a few bad ones. Some may not deserve loyalty and respect. An employee who lacks loyalty loses the respect of others, and her attitude reflects adversely on herself and her work. If you find yourself in a situation where, after considerable effort, you cannot respect your employer, you had better find yourself another job.

Not only do you owe your employer loyalty, but you will find that the benefits of loyalty are multiple. From a purely mercenary point of view, the faster you help your boss get ahead, the sooner you'll advance, too. No man will want to leave so valuable a champion behind. But for the sake of job satisfaction, nothing improves a relationship more than loyalty and joint respect. You know how a friend's esteem helps bring out your best. Employer-employee esteem is a winning combination that can make a job a joy and can help both live up to the gleaming reputations they make for each other.

---

1 *Analyze your employer (or if you are not working, pretend your father or some man you know well is your employer). What are his special preferences and dislikes?*

2 *Survey five executives of your acquaintance. Ask them what qualities they like most in employees and what qualities they find most annoying. Most employers are delighted to have a chance to air their feelings, and you may be surprised at how much you will learn.*

3 *Interview a woman executive. Ask her how she got her start and how she has risen to her present position. Does she consider her experience typical of other women executives? What advice can she give you to help you reach the executive level?*

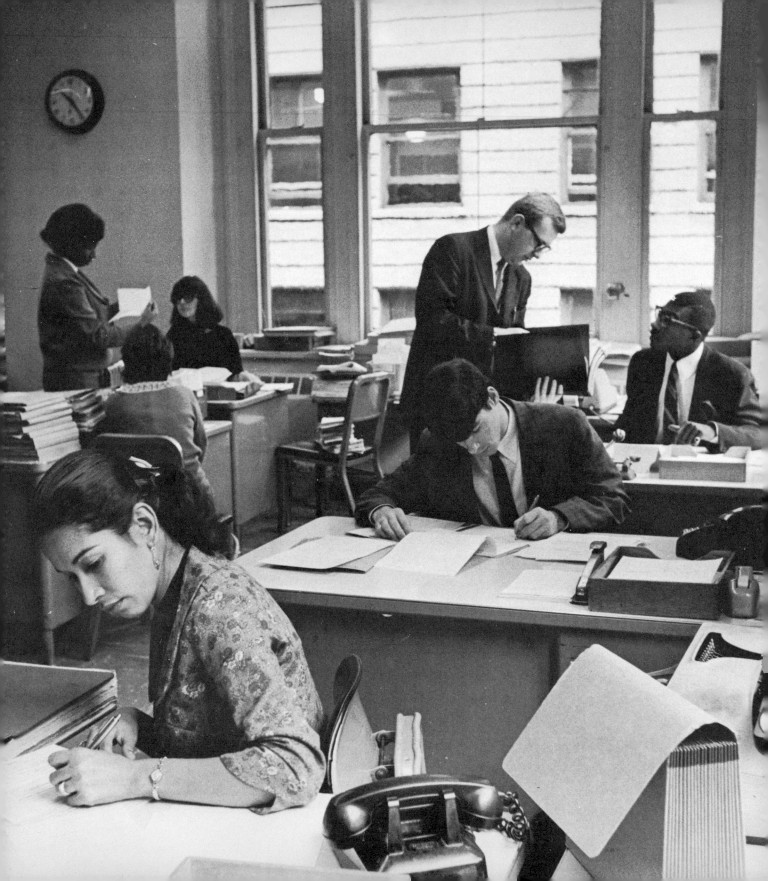

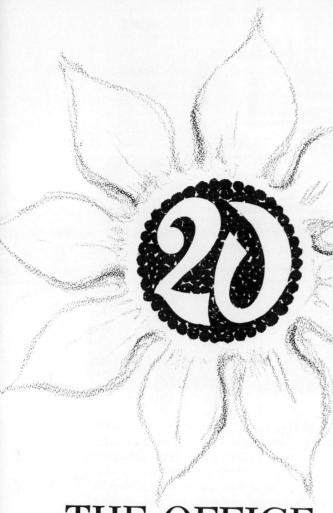

THE OFFICE STAFF

The business girl who endears herself to the rest of the staff finds her working hours pleasant and exciting. Her job becomes more than so many hours on the timecard at so many dollars a week. It becomes an interesting and rich experience in which friendship and the satisfying bond of joint accomplishment play an important part. Management is forever on the watch for a girl who can win friends and influence the staff. She is the one they want for supervisory positions and for important roles that involve interesting contacts. In the office it is particularly true that the lass who can get along is the one who will get ahead.

Conversely, as the director of a large employment agency in Chicago put it, ''More people lose their jobs because of personality difficulties than for any other reason. Many an extremely capable worker becomes classified as unemployable simply because she has not learned the importance of good relations with the office staff.'' An employee who is disagreeable and ill-humored has a hard time obtaining cooperation. When her sales report gets lost, it's likely to stay lost. When she has a rush job, she rushes alone. Few favors are offered, and her work becomes increasingly difficult when the staff refuses to cooperate. Management can ill afford to have such a misfit hampering smooth operation.

Tops on the list of those we appreciate are the girls who work both fast and well. If a worker keeps on schedule, no one is inconvenienced. But let that report be late for Accounting, and listen to the wails of woe! If work isn't done on time, often others must rush or must

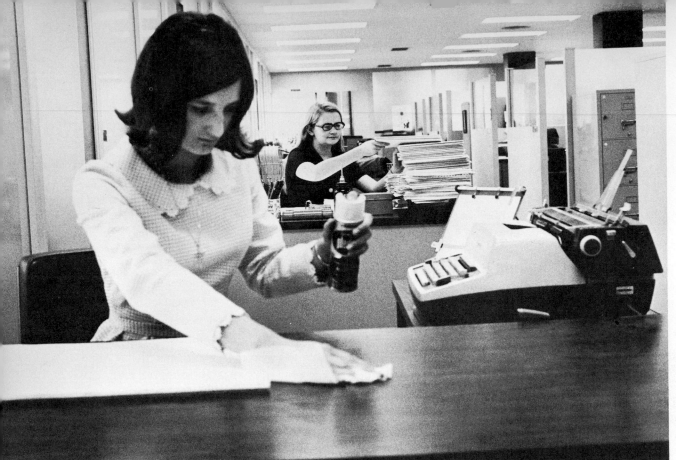

*Make sure you aren't doing "busy work"
when someone else is really overloaded.*

work overtime to make up for the slowpoke. Occasionally a beginner is so overly conscientious that she holds up work.

Myra had to compile and type daily numerical reports that were needed by the shipping department. Not being very good at typing figures, Myra made frequent mistakes. In her desire to be neat, she usually retyped the report before sending it on. A little lunch-hour practice would soon have improved her typing, but her policy of redoing work merely impeded progress and caused annoyance.

One of the most cherished employees is the girl who is willing to help when someone is busy. A secretary in a large department was so good a worker that she occasionally had free time. Often she used it to study trade literature so that she could learn more about the business or to discover additional ways in which she could assist her boss. But she also was the first to offer help when she saw someone in a jam. She not only won office-wide appreciation, but she also learned so much about the various jobs in the department that when an opening occurred for a supervisory post, her knowledge of all the work made her the ideal choice.

Another girl in the same department was also a skilled worker—far better than most—but when she finished her work, she was content to loaf. "I still turn out just as much as anybody else," she rationalized. "Why shouldn't I take time off when I feel like it?" If someone asked help on a special job, she would object, claiming that she wasn't hired to do that work. She hadn't learned one basic fact: no one can play it solo in an office. Prima donnas soon find themselves out in the cold.

One of the fastest ways to be blacklisted is to take advantage of other members of the staff. So Sorry Susie assigned to help cover the

282

phones is consistently late returning from lunch. Edna the Excuse Maker always has a terribly important appointment when she's asked to relieve someone at lunch time. Rubber Band Rosey stretches lunch hours and rest periods but is aghast at the prospect of overtime. And Nettie the Nail Polisher believes manicures should be done only on company time. These girls may think they are getting away with something, but their few extra minutes are dearly bought. It may be possible to fool the boss for a while, depending on how watchful and trusting he is, but it is never possible to fool the rest of the staff, who are everwatchful and far less trusting.

How do you win? With the virtues every business girl should have: cooperation, consideration, and tact. This means being diplomatic and pleasant to those below as well as those above you. Perhaps this may be difficult when the office boy ruins *your* single-spaced stencil or when Slapstick Sally squirts Coke on *your* freshly typed letters. But it is essential nevertheless. Let your warmth and friendly manner be liberally applied to both the lowly and the high.

Often the way an employee treats the mail boy or the switchboard operator has more significance than her attitude toward higher-ups. Any rudeness detected in her treatment of a lower-level employee flashes a red light in the executive cerebral structure. How can more authority be given to one who doesn't know how to use what she now has?

When someone ruffles you, do your best to put up with him. If the order clerk has made an error, discretely show it to her in private. Then call her attention to the need for a correction as diplomatically as you can—avoiding any "*you* made a mistake" emphasis.

The Golden Rule—treating others as you'd like to be treated—has been a standard of conduct down through the ages, and it works as well as ever today. Put into practice, it protects us from being inconsiderate. We remember to work quietly without disturbing or annoying others; we steer clear of gossip; we resist the urge to complain loudly when some-

one goofs or blunders; we're helpful to other newer employees. In short, we're nice to have around—we earn our laurels of praise.

❦ Maturity Value

One of the best investments a business girl can make is in habits of self-control. She can learn not to give vent to her emotions and to keep a firm and realistic grip on her vanity, temper, and tongue. In the office a girl just must act like a lady at all times, no matter how much she feels like slinging a stapler at someone. She

B. D. Unsworth

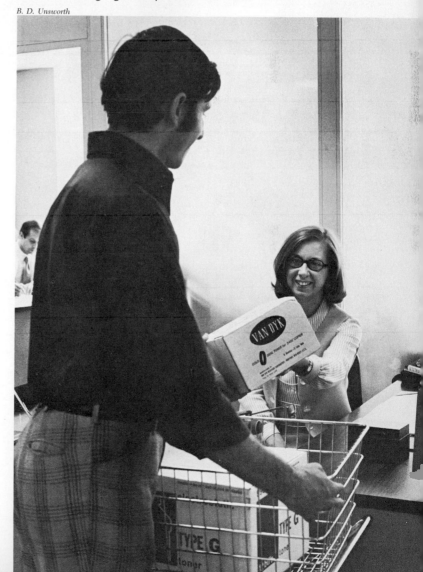

283

is expected to be poised and polite. This may involve keeping a near stranglehold on her emotions, forgetting the oh-so-deep sorrows of her current love life, and maintaining a pleasant disposition despite an onslaught of cranky customers. A big order, true, but one that when filled shows you have the poise to rise above day-to-day disturbances.

Women are often accused of being overly emotional and overly sensitive. Perhaps we

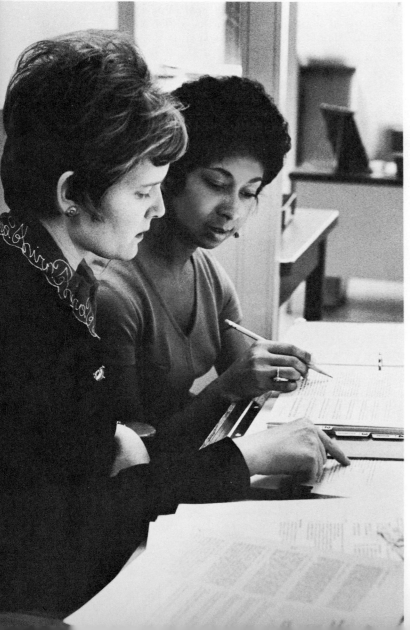

B. D. Unsworth

are, but it is the girl who keeps the damper on her emotions who fits in best in business—or in any social activity for that matter. The business world, particularly, is a rough-and-tumble place where sensitive feelings may be trampled on and where no one can afford the time or trouble to stop and soothe them. There will be occasions when someone else will get the promotion or be chosen for a desirable task such as modeling for the company magazine photos. Often nobody—but nobody—will compliment you on the outstanding piece of work you slaved over. But such is business life. If you accept it without sulking and apply a bit of good humor, you'll win respect and appreciation and be a lot happier.

Criticism may seem brusque at times, but we must be prepared to accept it cheerfully and thoughtfully. The girl who interprets criticism of her work as a direct insult had better head for the hills and take up a solitary career of basket weaving.

The best way to minimize trying times at the office is to balance work with outside interests. What seemed like such a mountainous misery at 3 p.m. slides down to molehill size after a happy evening of bowling—and, perhaps, becomes in retrospect just a hilarious anecdote to pass along to the gang. The person whose whole life is her work lacks such insulation and unconsciously tends to exaggerate the importance of every little incident that occurs.

Another quality that is used to gauge maturity—one that some young employees may forget—is dignity. Occasionally a beginner yields to impulse and shouts down the hall to a friend or runs lickety-split through the office. Eyebrows go up, a few frowns appear, and the other members of the staff hope their junior member will soon learn that business has a more formal set of rules than school or home. Pointless practical jokes and elaborate pranks, raucous laughter, and inappropriate schoolgirl clothing all act as a tag that reads, ''Do not promote until more fully matured.'' Most too-cute juveniles are unaware what annoying bores they can be to those who maintain more businesslike standards.

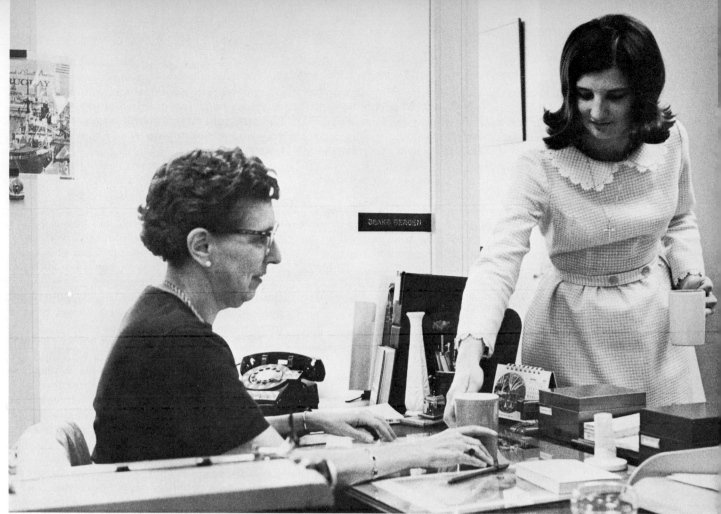

B. D. Unsworth

Saving a co-worker from a trip to get coffee will show kindness and consideration.

❧ Respectfully Yours

The office staff is a conglomeration of human beings thrown together by the accident of their having chosen the same place to earn a living. Many of them may be very different from you in educational background, experience, age, race, religion, politics, and general outlook on life. Perhaps you wouldn't have chosen them as the ideal set of daily companions, but associating with them can be a wonderfully rich and broadening experience. You will probably like most of them, but try to learn from them all and to appreciate their various points of view. Once you step out of the office door you aren't *forced* to have anything to do with those who don't appeal to you, but your nine-to-five hours will

be far more pleasant if you make a determined effort to like and respect everyone.

Of all the forms of intolerance that seem to be most prevalent in offices, the most frequent is lack of consideration and kindness for older workers. Perhaps elderly Mrs. Rae objects when someone opens the window not because she wants to be ornery but merely because she isn't feeling very well. When we're young and hale and hearty, we sometimes fail to realize that someone older may be tired rather than dull or bothered by arthritis rather than fussy. Age brings with it numerous aches and troubles, and many an older person who would be better off resting at home is forced to work because of financial conditions. Youth is a gift that is only loaned to us, and today's young people do well to remember that they may be in a similar situation at some later date.

An older worker may have set ideas—different ideas from you—about how work should be done. If this person is your superior, you should follow instructions even though the method seems old-fashioned. If the older person is not your superior, you will be wise to learn from her and to give any suggestions careful consideration. (Someone who has been doing the job for a number of years surely must know many worthwhile shortcuts.) If you

You may meet some people in your office who will become your friends for life.

B. D. Unsworth

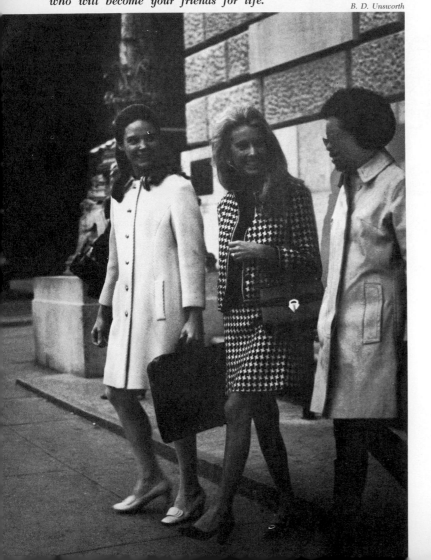

disagree with the suggestions, you won't want to cause hard feelings by raising objections. Perhaps you might unobtrusively check with your supervisor to see which method is preferred.

❦ Reserved—for You

While it is wonderful if you can find a bosom pal among those with whom you work, you should be careful about pouring out your heart to someone at the office until you are sure the friendship has a firm foundation. If suddenly the friendship should crumble, day-in-day-out association with this one who knows *all* can grate miserably.

The business girl who knows her way around wisely puts a "Reserved" sign on all her private affairs. She realizes that, on the whole, the best policy is not to become too involved with office associates. She keeps her relations pleasant but rather impersonal. Of course, she has lunch with the girls or may go to a show with some of them after work, but her family, her love life, her finances, her personal matters—these are strictly private. She doesn't try to delve into others' private lives either, and if someone is so thoughtless as to reveal something of too intimate a nature, she is careful not to offer advice and to remain as politely—and pleasantly—detached as possible. She doesn't bring up the subject again, knowing that the loose talker may have embarrassing second thoughts about her indiscretion. She also resists any temptation to pass the news along.

As for Chatty Kathy, who keeps the staff informed on all the "He said; I said," details of each date, and who discusses her family trials and tribulations—she seldom realizes that her stories aren't half as interesting to others as she thinks they are. Her lack of discretion quickly lowers her in the eyes of others, and in a short time she either bores everyone to tears or becomes a juicy subject for office gossip and ridicule.

The girl who maintains an impersonal attitude may miss the full gory details of a few little

286

dramas, but she will also avoid much unpleasantness and will keep herself above unsavory entanglements.

❦ The Sunny Side

In the office you know best the people with whom you work most closely, but you are observed by many more with whom you may be merely on a "Good Morning" or "Good Night" basis. They may not know that you saved the day for your department by making what seemed an impossible deadline or that in yesterday's storm you thoughtfully offered Shirley *your* umbrella to save her new Easter bonnet. But they do know that you have a happy manner and a gay sense of humor, that you smile often, and that you are quick to say thank you in return for their kindnesses.

The girl who keeps her sunny side on display is sure to attract friends—and keep them!

1 *List at least five helpful things you could do to make an office associate like you.*

2 *List five things you might find annoying in the behavior of fellow workers in an office.*

3 *When you are employed, what outside activities can you maintain to help balance the strains of your working day?*

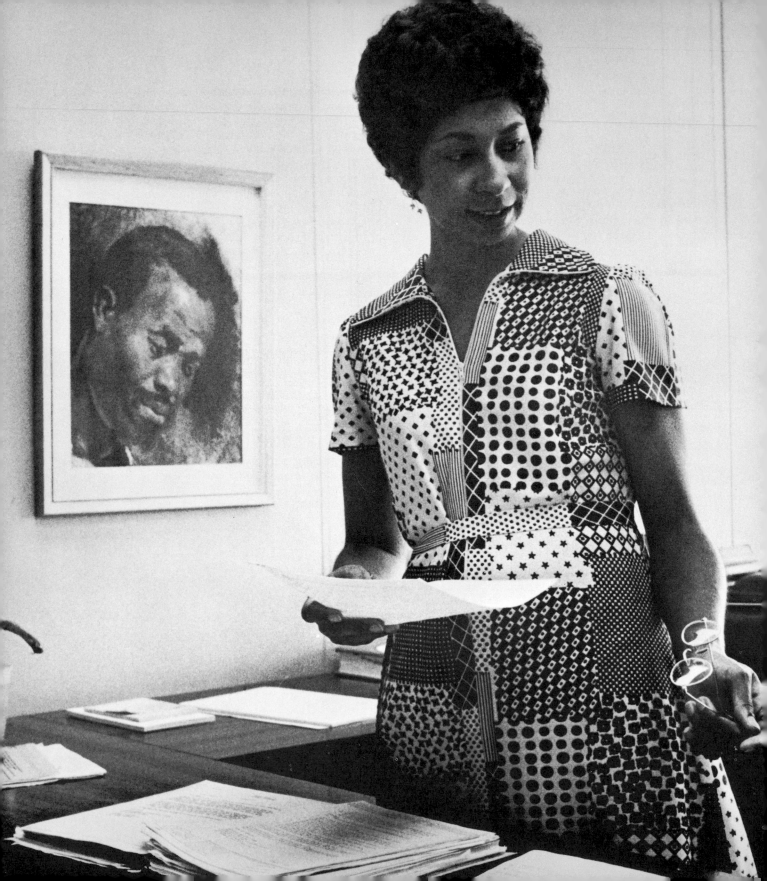

21

SUCCESS SIGNALS

How do you keep the green light beaming in your direction? It's one thing to get a job and to establish yourself as an accepted member of the staff, but the girl with charm and ability is looking ahead, too. She wants a chance at important, satisfying work with an important, pleasingly plump pay envelope! How can she set herself above the rest of the crowd so that management will take notice? Actually, it's not as difficult as it sounds.

In fact employers often have difficulty finding top-caliber material among the girls on the staff. If you earnestly try to do the best possible job, you will surely attract notice. To succeed, you need only keep up your good work. Everyone expects the new broom to sweep clean, but many new employees, once they have passed their trial period and feel somewhat secure, believe they can relax and go into a slump. All too many girls are content to park themselves in their swivel chairs from nine to five and, with a minimum of work, keep from being turned out in the cold. They just want to get by with as little effort as possible; they are not interested in contributing the little extra that could enable them to get ahead. But the business girl who consistently turns out top-quality work and who seeks out the helpful extras she can do stands out head and shoulders above all the rest of the crowd—she can't help calling attention to herself. Likewise, your good work and gracious manners will automatically publicize your ability to all those you come in contact with. And, bosses being prone to brag about their exceptional employees, the word spreads fast when plaudits are due.

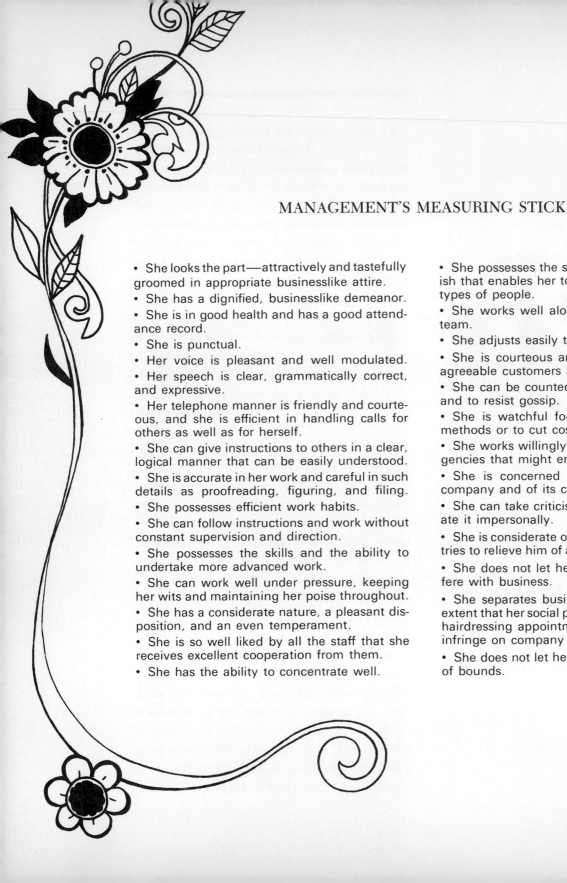

MANAGEMENT'S MEASURING STICK

- She looks the part—attractively and tastefully groomed in appropriate businesslike attire.
- She has a dignified, businesslike demeanor.
- She is in good health and has a good attendance record.
- She is punctual.
- Her voice is pleasant and well modulated.
- Her speech is clear, grammatically correct, and expressive.
- Her telephone manner is friendly and courteous, and she is efficient in handling calls for others as well as for herself.
- She can give instructions to others in a clear, logical manner that can be easily understood.
- She is accurate in her work and careful in such details as proofreading, figuring, and filing.
- She possesses efficient work habits.
- She can follow instructions and work without constant supervision and direction.
- She possesses the skills and the ability to undertake more advanced work.
- She can work well under pressure, keeping her wits and maintaining her poise throughout.
- She has a considerate nature, a pleasant disposition, and an even temperament.
- She is so well liked by all the staff that she receives excellent cooperation from them.
- She has the ability to concentrate well.

- She possesses the social and intellectual polish that enables her to associate easily with all types of people.
- She works well alone or as a member of a team.
- She adjusts easily to her superiors.
- She is courteous and tactful even with disagreeable customers and callers.
- She can be counted on to keep confidences and to resist gossip.
- She is watchful for ways to improve work methods or to cut costs.
- She works willingly despite occasional emergencies that might entail overtime.
- She is concerned with the welfare of the company and of its customers.
- She can take criticism calmly and can evaluate it impersonally.
- She is considerate of her employer's time and tries to relieve him of any tasks she can handle.
- She does not let her personal troubles interfere with business.
- She separates business and pleasure to the extent that her social phoning, shopping sprees, hairdressing appointments, and so on, do not infringe on company time.
- She does not let her office socializing get out of bounds.

The page at left shows what management considers when evaluating personnel for promotion. Ask yourself if you are preparing yourself properly and are building habit patterns that will enable you to make a good showing.

A large order? Hardly. If you want to do your job well, you'll follow most of these criteria without having to give them a thought. They're a problem only for the person who doesn't care, who wants only the easy way out.

❦ *Efficiency*

One of the business traits that is most attention-getting is efficiency. It is also one that is most essential for promotion. The person who flounders through her work can't even carry a full load, let alone the larger load a promotion might entail. Unless a girl is efficient, she needs constant supervision and can't possibly be counted on to direct others.

Perhaps you are naturally efficient and well organized, but even the girls who do not consider this one of their strongest points have been able to develop reputations for remarkable efficiency by following these suggestions.

• Plan your work. At the beginning of each day, make a list of the important jobs that you want to accomplish that day—not every job that's hanging over your head, but the necessary tasks that should be accomplished right away. With such a list to guide you, you'll be sure to tackle the important work first and will be less likely to let trivial matters take too much time.

• Do important work when you're most alert. Many people have a low ebb period just before lunch and again in the late afternoon. Others are slow starters in the morning. Do your most important or difficult jobs at periods of peak efficiency, leaving chores that require less concentration, such as tidying your desk or filing, for the end of the day.

• Make a note of all instructions. Lorraine's boss asked her to make a luncheon reservation for him at the Town House. As she approached her desk, her phone jangled urgently. Next came a special-delivery package that required immediate attention. Then a visitor arrived.

When her boss returned from lunch and asked what had happened to the reservation, Lorraine was horrified. In the rush of little emergencies she had completely forgotten about the reservation. If Lorraine had quickly jotted down her boss's instructions before she answered the phone, she would have been saved. There are times when you just can't afford to let yourself be interrupted until you jot down a quick reminder.

• Use a dependable reminder system. Since memories are fallible, many clever girls leave themselves reminder notes where they are sure not to be overlooked—pierced on a desk pen, clipped to a mechanical pencil, rolled in the typewriter—or, if it concerns an after-hours

B. D. Unsworth

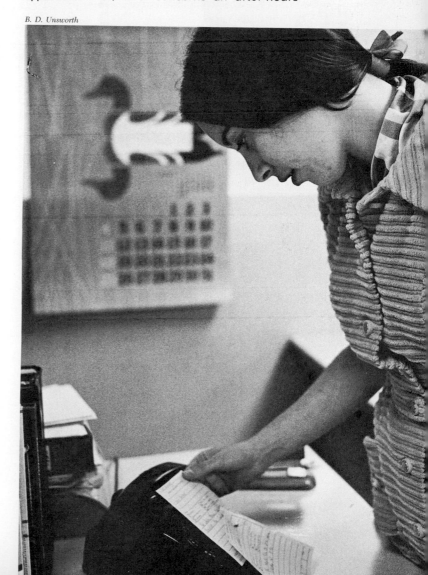

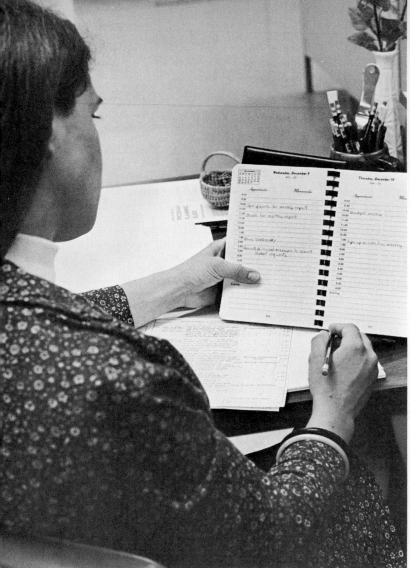

year when you get your new calendar. You can also include any birthdays or other events during the year that you will want to remember—for yourself or your boss. If your calendar is the loose-leaf type, where the pages are not thrown away, it can prove valuable as a diary if you need to check back to a particular meeting or appointment.

• Finish one job before you start another. The girl who has everything at hand before she starts and then works steadily until she completes the chore accomplishes much more than the girl who jumps from one half-finished job to another. If we stop in mid-letter to order more carbon paper or to check on train schedules, we lose time getting reorientated. If something important comes to mind in the middle of a job, make yourself a note and attend to the matter as soon as you finish. Of course, the telephone or a visiting customer can't be kept waiting, but there are many times when you can postpone interruptions.

• Look for shortcuts. Whenever you have an involved chore, ask yourself if there isn't an easier way to handle it. Perhaps you send out weekly schedules. Would a duplicated form that could be filled in quickly eliminate work? Or, if this isn't practical, could you save time by marking an old copy with tabulator settings and keeping this for reference so that you won't have to refigure each time you make out a new schedule? Perhaps you could compose form letters for replying to common situations. Or would a printed note do just as well? It makes good sense to cut down routine work as much as possible.

• Arrange your desk efficiently. A desk that is neat and well organized looks businesslike. In addition, there is little danger of losing something when everything is in its proper place. An efficient way to keep specific jobs together is to use folders. A folder of work always looks much neater than a lot of loose papers. Any pile of papers that must be kept on your desk while you work should be weighted down so that nothing is blown away by a stray draft. Other little efficiency ideas that save time: tying an eraser on each side of your typewriter (one for carbons, one for originals), keeping carbon erasure slips under the left edge of your typewriter, always keeping a pencil and telephone message pad beside your phone, making a list

matter, tucked into a hat band or glove cuff. Many girls use a tickler file (a file with a separate section for each day of the month) to remind themselves of upcoming jobs and chores that recur regularly. The hitch is, of course, that they must remember to look in the tickler file every morning!

Perhaps the least complicated and most valuable reminder system is the lowly desk calendar. On it you can note special work and appointments and can warn yourself a day or two ahead if advance preparations are needed. If you are responsible for once-a-month tasks, list reminders for each month throughout the of frequently used phone numbers. If you handle correspondence, it's also a great advantage to have your own copy of a dictionary and a secretary's handbook. If you must make frequent calls, obtain a phone book for your own desk.

• Check supplies frequently. Have enough supplies on hand to prevent your running out in the middle of a rush job. You don't, however, want to be so overstocked with any item that it clutters up your desk and your drawers and yellows with age before it can be used.

❧ A Growing Girl

One of the quickest ways to speed up the promotion process is to demonstrate how much you've grown (mentally, that is) while you've been on the job. Many a bright young miss has furthered herself by taking courses after hours. Such business courses as accounting, economics, letter writing, retailing, public speaking, or something specifically related to your firm's particular industry will give you a broader background for your work. An industry-related course also helps you gain the confidence and air of authority that comes from being well informed about your field.

Let your boss know about your courses. Perhaps you might ask his advice in selecting the best ones. If you have a report to make for school, try to do it on some phase of your own company's operation. Perhaps your boss

Taking a course that will help you with your job, or participating in a job-oriented seminar will show your boss that you are interested in your work and eager to get ahead.

McGraw-Hill News

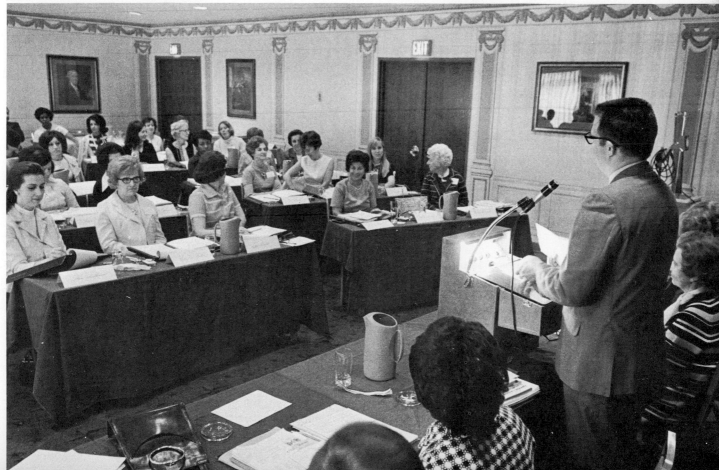

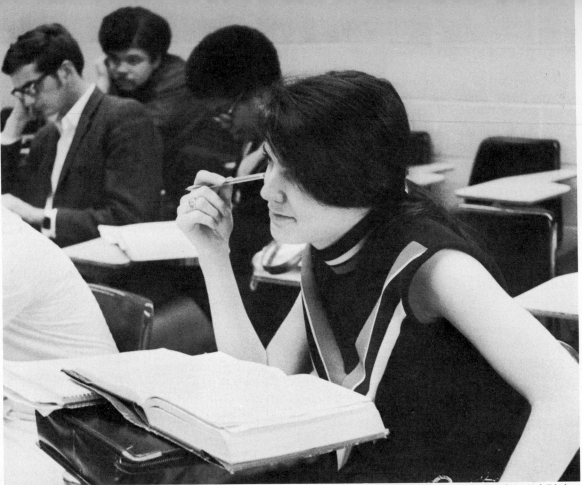

will set up interviews for you with other executives who can give you the information you need. Not only does this provide you with material for school, but it also helps you learn more about the company and, just incidentally, happens to bring you to the attention of other important people in the concern. The young person who sincerely wants to learn has a magnetic appeal. Human nature being what it is, we all seem to love to play teacher. Many a busy executive has been known to take considerable time and trouble to help someone who was genuinely interested in learning from him.

One additional advantage of your classes is, of course, the many friends you make among those who have interests similar to yours. You probably don't need to be told that many a marriage has blossomed from night school cultivation.

Even without taking courses, you can increase your knowledge of the business. You can learn as much as possible about the various departments of your firm and how they work together. Find out where and how the materials used in making your products are secured. What happens to the products after they leave the company portals? You might also learn how the company got started and what was responsible for its growth. Keep up with your company's new products and with those of its competitors. This is the background information that makes a girl more than a cataloger of thingamajigs. She may instead consider herself an authority on inventory for the control mechanisms vital to our newest space program.

You want also to improve your general knowledge. You want to be up on current events, important television shows, new plays, music, books, and all that is going on about you. Learn all the skills you can. Even such an unrelated skill as flower arranging helped one girl move up to become secretary to the top art director—he was impressed by her artistic ability.

❦ Be Promotion-Minded

We all know that it's easier to hit what you aim at if you keep your eye on the target. The same applies to your business future. Set a goal for yourself. Look ahead and try to decide the type of position you want to attain. Then go about learning as much as possible about it. You may never get this job—you may be selected for something far afield—but the fact that you are striving toward a goal will give you an advantage. Ambitious girls always keep an eye on the job directly above theirs. Volunteer to help or substitute for a girl in a higher-rated job whenever the opportunity presents itself. Your acquaintance with the work marks you as a likely candidate when a promotion or vacancy occurs.

But all promotions don't result from changing desks or bosses. Many smart girls have made themselves more important by taking on increased responsibility. One girl suggested an additional way for her company to profit by offering a supplementary service, and she was put in charge of the operation. Although the new service started out in a small way, she now has a force of twenty in her charge.

Other workers have advanced because their bosses were promoted. If you are the girl who helps the assistant manager, he may be moved up to manager and you may become the assistant manager yourself. Or you can advance without even changing your title. Suppose you are secretary to a department head who is appointed vice president. When he is promoted, you, as his secretary, go up a notch right along with him. By helping your boss do his job better, you are actually helping yourself. Keep this in mind and overtime seems less of a burden.

❦ Raise or Promotion Requests

The time may come when you feel your good works should be rewarded more fully than they have been. You believe that you deserve a raise or a promotion, and none has been forthcoming. How can you induce the powers-that-be to favor you?

Before you approach your boss, do a little clearheaded planning. When confronted with any sort of employee request, bosses invariably have the somewhat discomforting habit of wanting to know *why*. In the case of a pay increase, it's not that he wants to put you on

This secretary is looking over the job description of the position she hopes to obtain so that she can relate her qualifications to the job.

B. D. Unsworth

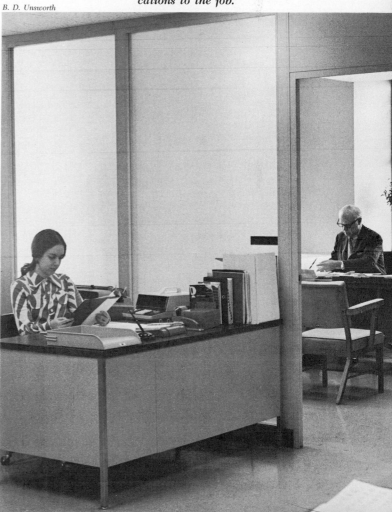

the spot. Most likely, higher approval is required for a raise, and your boss may want some reasons to substantiate his recommendation. You can't reply, ''Because I want more money.'' This he knows, of course. Wiser psychology suggests that to influence his decision most favorably you play up not what *you* want but rather how *he* has benefited by having you on his staff.

Suppose you want a raise and your company has no policy of regular pay increases for deserving employees. Or perhaps you have reached the maximum salary for your particular job. In such a case you'll want to prepare a sales talk that will show why you *deserve* more money. Here are some of the reasons you might offer to show that you are of greater value to your company.

• You have taken on more responsibility. Perhaps you've relieved your boss of certain tasks or enlarged the scope of your work.

• You handle more complicated work. Be sure to give specific examples. Perhaps you now handle alone certain jobs formerly supervised by someone else. Don't overlook them.

• You've increased your knowledge of the company. Its methods and its products are familiar to you, and, therefore, you can make more intelligent decisions about the work.

• You have helped build goodwill for the company. Can you name specific instances when you have pleased customers by giving them special help? Can you quote compliments received from customers? Any appreciative letters?

• You are familiar with the particular preferences of many customers. You can help provide the individualized service that they have come to depend on.

• You have made suggestions for improved work methods that have been put into practice. Or you have submitted ideas for obtaining more business, for pleasing customers, and so on.

• You have improved yourself. Can you cite any courses you've taken, lectures you've attended, or books you've studied—anything that has added to your business skills or personality development?

Your appeal for a raise will be more impressive if you type out your reasons in outline form. Every salesman knows that a written presentation enhances and emphasizes his sales pitch. A boss will also be impressed by your thoroughness and by the businesslike manner evidenced by a typed presentation.

If you are seeking a promotion, it is most important that you write out your qualifications. Perhaps you know the prospective boss very well—even to the point of exchanging daily comments on your favorite baseball team. Even so, it's advisable to prepare a résumé.

```
                    INCREASED RESPONSIBILITIES
                        DURING PAST YEAR




    1.  Supervision:  With addition of Patty D. to staff I have
handled her orientation, training, and the supervision of her
work, as well as the necessary rearrangement of paper work between
us.


    2.  Records Management:  When sales training was added to your
responsibilities, I set up new forms, procedures, and files for
our expanded records system.


    3.  Professional Associations:  During your travel absences
I have covered three monthly SAM meetings for you, reporting
activities and doing some correspondence for the Program Committee
on which you serve.  I have also joined The National Secretaries
Association and am serving on the Education Committee.


    4.  Secretarial Manual:  As a direct result of the secretarial
manual I prepared for my own job (and which Patty has found so
helpful), I have been asked by Personnel to head a committee of
secretaries to expand it for company-wide use.
```

In all probability he has only a vague idea of the work you do. In your résumé you can enumerate all the exact types of work you handle (transcribing, filing, record keeping), all the contributions you have made to your present job, and the ways that you can best help your prospective boss in his work. You also have an opportunity in a résumé to describe past experience and accomplishments and to mention other abilities that you may have no chance to use in your present position. You are able to bring to his attention many details he may not be aware of or may have forgotten. Also, since you may be competing with outsiders who are applying for this job, your neatly typed presentation will help you compare favorably with them.

❦ Popping the Question

Any girl who has approached her dad for an advance on next week's allowance knows that the best time is when he's in a good mood. The same applies to your boss. Watch for a time when he's been telling jokes to the staff, has just returned from a pleasant luncheon, or has received good news. If he's trying to get out a rush job, is troubled about difficult work, or is seething from some sort of annoyance, keep away from his door.

When you do confer with your boss, aim for the happy medium between overselling and underselling. A good salesman knows just how far to push so that he seems smart and ambitious without becoming annoyingly aggressive. He lets the facts sell for him and does not try to exert high-pressure tactics.

In the course of your conversation bring out the length of time that has elapsed since you received your last raise. (In most instances, an employee is not expected to look for a raise unless she has not had one for at least a year.) When you do so, state it without any sarcasm or complaining chip-on-the-shoulder attitude. This merely annoys a boss. The situation is difficult at best, and you want to keep relations as pleasant as possible.

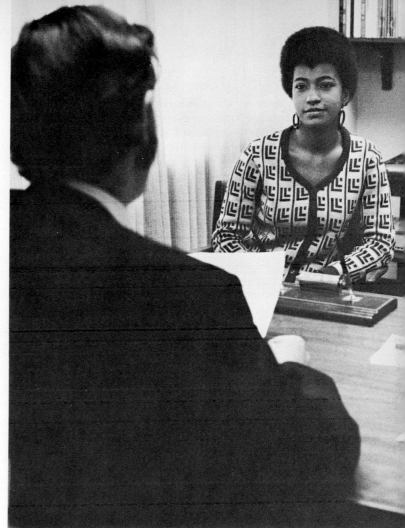

B. D. Unsworth

Occasionally an employee lets herself become so worked up over a promotion or raise that she threatens to quit unless her request is granted. Some bosses bristle at this type of ultimatum and are just likely to take the attitude, ''If that's all the loyalty she feels for us, let her quit!'' Although we don't like to face up to the fact, no one is so vital to a company that she can't be replaced. Sometimes the idea of getting a replacement may even have a certain tinge of appeal for an angry executive. A newcomer is usually someone who is eager to please, and, also worth considering, she is someone who will probably settle for a lower salary.

297

On the whole, bosses want to please. They want to grant raises, and they want their employees to stay around long enough to qualify for 25-year-award gold watches. There are times, however, when a slump in business or a squeezed budget may make a raise impossible. One girl who liked her job thought it would strengthen her case if she threatened to quit unless she got a raise. She didn't get the raise—and found herself backed into the position of having to resign because the company couldn't afford to pay her more. A few months later, when business had picked up, she was chagrined to learn that her former co-workers had all received salary increases.

If you find yourself spending several years going around in circles in a routine job, it may be time for you to move on.

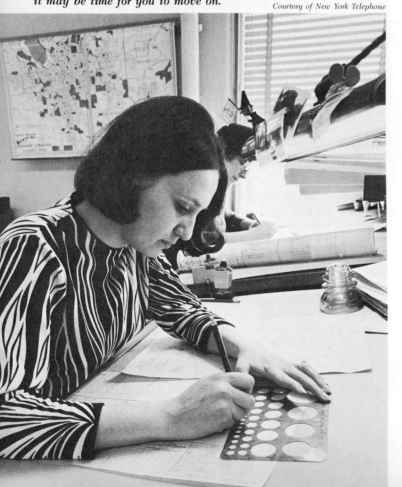

If a raise is refused, a worker is perfectly justified to turn the tables and ask why. She will inspire respect when she explains that she wants to know if something is wrong with her work so that she can correct it. There have been times when the refusal of a raise was such a jolt to the so-so worker that she snapped out of her lethargy and got down to business, soon deserving—and receiving—the raise she had been denied a short while before.

❦ Red Light Ahead?

There are jobs, of course, where nothing looms before you but a big red stoplight. It's obvious that you can't get ahead and that your employer can't afford—or won't pay—more money. You realize that your only course is to get another job. If this is your decision, by all means say nothing about it. Then quietly go about the business of hunting for another position. No matter how much you'd like to dramatically hand in your resignation, resist the temptation.

There are many advantages to holding on to a job until you have another. For one thing, you still have a steady salary rolling in and you can afford to be choosy about selecting the work you really want. A girl faced with starvation is likely to jump at any job, perhaps one even less promising than the one she has left. Another advantage is that you have an opportunity to survey the field. It sometimes happens that a job hunter comes to realize that she is a lot better off in her present company than she thought she was and decides that her own job is well worth holding on to.

Don't, however, be afraid to change jobs. Some girls who have the ability to go far stay in low-paying, unchallenging work year after year merely because the job is pleasant. There are many other pleasant positions to be had —and they become much more pleasant when accompanied by a promising future and a more substantial salary! Look quietly and choose carefully before you make the break. If you have high career hopes, a dead-end job is merely a waste of precious time.

298

Changing jobs too frequently, however, is also bad. The fickle job-hopper who flits from one position to another, never satisfied and never staying long enough to give the job a chance, soon finds herself blacklisted. Employers scare off easily when confronted with a job record of frequent changes.

❦ Finding Another Job

Hunting for a new job while you're employed is more complicated than when your days are your own. You don't want to annoy your present boss or arouse his suspicions by stretching lunch hours or taking time off. You can save much time and fruitless effort by working through an employment agency (though this usually involves a fee that may wipe out the advantages of a better salary for several paychecks to come). Many girls manage to follow up newspaper ads without too much difficulty. Most would-be employers are glad to set up lunch-hour or after-five appointments to accommodate working girls.

If there are certain firms in which you are specifically interested, don't just walk in cold. You can make a faster and more direct entrée by first sending a résumé and an application letter that requests an appointment. Aside from demonstrating your efficiency, a résumé is often very helpful in saving time for the job hunter with a job. It can sometimes eliminate the time-consuming filling out of application forms and can quickly emphasize your best selling points, thereby cutting down interview time.

❦ A Graceful Exit

After you've obtained a new job comes the problem of severing ties with your old employer. You'll want to do this in as graceful and as fair a manner as possible. Even though you might feel quite sour about your present job, you'll want to leave like a lady. Stormy tell-him-off scenes are never wise. They slam the door tightly behind you and leave an unpleasant memory that may still be there when recommendations are needed in the future.

Be fair to your present employer by giving him sufficient time to find a replacement. Two weeks' notice is customary. Even though your new boss may want you to start immediately, he'll respect your consideration for your present boss.

1 *Survey some of your friends who have been working a few years and have advanced in their jobs. Ask them about the types of promotions they received. Did they move up with their bosses? Did they change bosses or departments? Ask what factors they considered were responsible for their being selected for a promotion.*

2 *Discuss how you would go about finding a new job while you are still employed.*

Part Six

Making
The Most of
Five-to-Nine

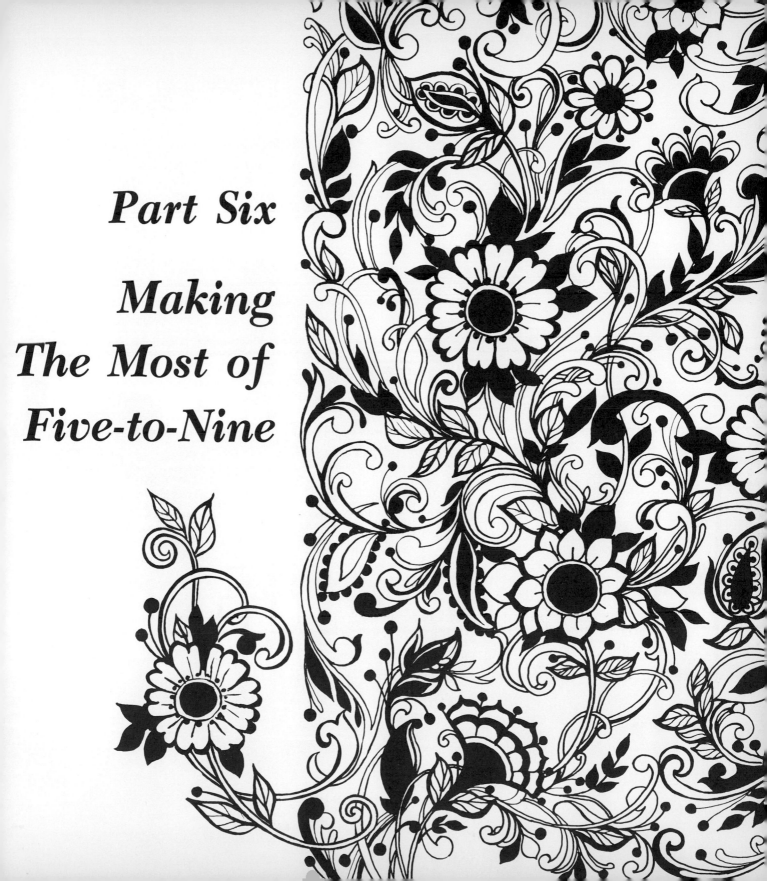

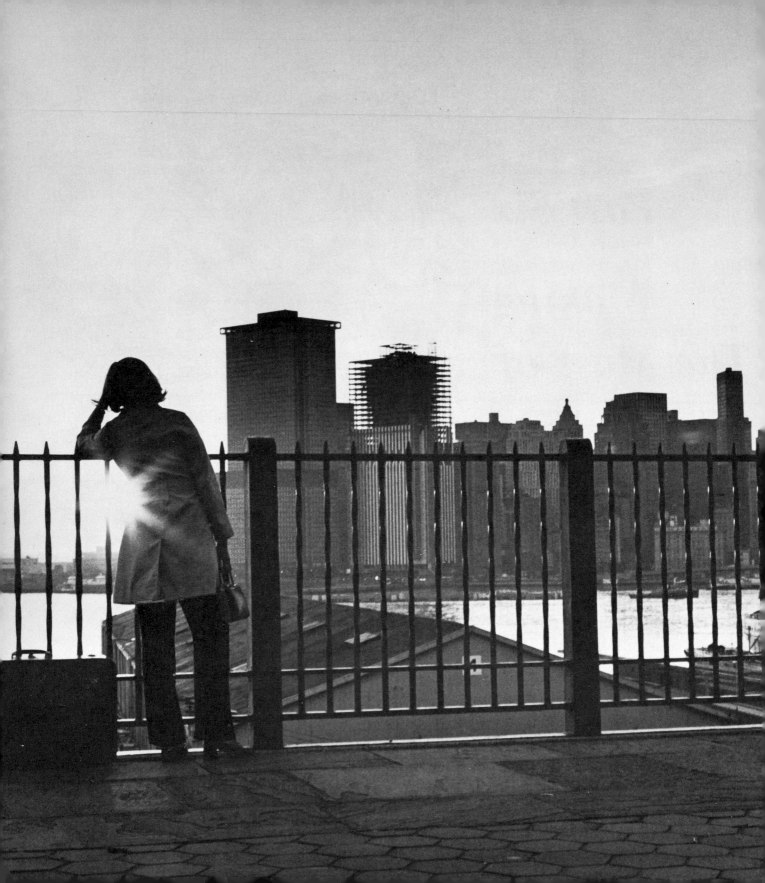

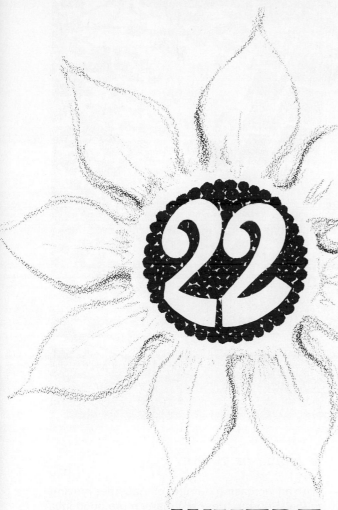

WHERE
YOU LIVE

The big city has a magnetic attraction for the small-town girl with the brains and the ability for a bright career. It's a place of varied opportunity, bigger salaries, glamorous jobs. And, of course, there's always the excitement of city life—fascinating places to go and things to do, more people, more parties, more frantic fun.

Many a graduate with her new diploma in one hand and a suitcase in the other immediately heads for the city, considering it the ideal place—the only place—to make her fortune. Perhaps it is, for living in a big city has many advantages—if you are the right type of girl.

The girl who has a loving family and a wide circle of friends whom she would miss might *not* be the type. And the girl who has grown up loving the beauty of the outdoors and the fun of outdoor sports may feel as deprived in the city as the stunted trees that struggle to grow beside the shadowed, unfertile, grime-laden streets. Another wrong-type girl might be the young miss who would find the fast pace of city living too hectic. Life on your own has many more problems than the one you lead when you're cozily ensconced in the love and comfort of your family home. There's no one to pass out the knowing advice a mother or father can offer, no one to cook or clean or mend for you, no one to soothe away troubles and to remind you that you've always been such a wonderful girl—no one who really cares as much about you as your family does. You have to be able to depend entirely on yourself.

One of the aspects of city living that bothers some transplanted small-towners is the contin-

303

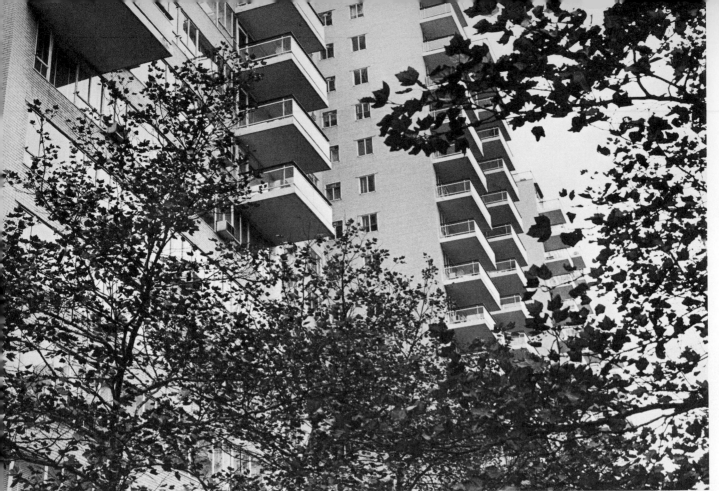

Living in the city has advantages—convenience to your job, shopping right around the corner, and a variety of cultural activities—but it can be impersonal.

❦ Home or Roam?

ual need to prove themselves. At home they've achieved their status. Everybody is aware of their virtues and accomplishments. Their family is known and respected, and they, in turn, fit into the town and are respected. A city is too big for this type of acknowledgment. There you can easily get lost in the crowd. You may have been a diving champ, the girl voted most likely to succeed, and a gold-medal shorthand winner, but to your city neighbors, you are merely the girl in 8A. To some small-towners, however, the opportunity to be judged solely on personal merit is one of the most appealing aspects of city living.

With an increasing number of industries moving to the suburbs, there are many more good jobs available within easy commuting distance. These deserve thorough consideration. Perhaps an interesting and exciting job can be found close to home, even right in your own town.

But if you long for city life and possess the independent spirit, the maturity, stamina, and ability to manage money that living alone requires, you'll probably have a marvelous time. And your business girl years are the time to try it. If possible, persuade one of your best friends to go with you. Someone else to share your adventures makes life easier—and more fun.

🌷 A Hole—or Heaven?

When you're city-bound, your first concern is a place to live. Before you make the move, try to learn as much as possible about the city of your choice. If you are not familiar with it, you may want to make a preliminary visit in order to become acquainted with the various sections. Can you consult any friends who live in the city and can advise you? If you're planning to enroll for courses in one of the schools or colleges in the city, you will probably be eligible for student housing or you may be able to obtain recommendations for other approved places. It's much easier to make the move when you have some idea of where you will live once you arrive. There are several types of nonschool housing found in most cities, each with definite advantages and problems. You'd be wise to check them against your own needs and desires before you leave the nest.

A hotel. On the plus side, a hotel offers you a place to park until you can get the lay of the land. It requires no furnishings, linens, or entangling leases that make moving away difficult. The cleaning, bedmaking, and cooking problems are nonexistent. However, hotel living is usually hard on the budget. Many cities have hotels that cater to women, such as the Barbizon in New York or those run by the YWCA, which are less expensive. But even if the rates are reasonable, eating out isn't. Some girls also feel that hotel living soon pales when they must make the effort to get dressed and go out for each meal. They are also faced with the problem of no place to entertain and no facilities for parties. And hotel living lacks the settled, homey feeling that gives a sense of stability.

A boarding or rooming house. These are usually less expensive and less elegant than hotels, but they offer the same freedom as hotel living. They also offer many of the same disadvantages. They vary widely from excellent to miserable and should be investigated carefully. Some are run specifically for young women and are managed by a housemother type of super-

visor. Some boardinghouses provide meals. Some have kitchen facilities where the girls can cook for themselves. A boardinghouse of this type enables you to make friends easily.

Rooming with a family. When you rent a room in someone else's home a great deal depends on the family you live with. They may be marvelous, a pleasant substitute for Mom and Dad, or they may be either of two extremes: ever-present, allowing you too little privacy, or ever-absent, letting you alone to such a degree that you almost feel like a trespasser. The life

In some cities organizations such as The Salvation Army have residence houses that can become "a home away from home" for a young businesswoman and provide her with a ready-made collection of friends.

Courtesy of The Salvation Army

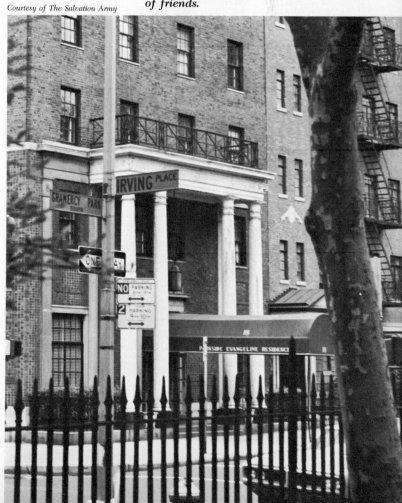

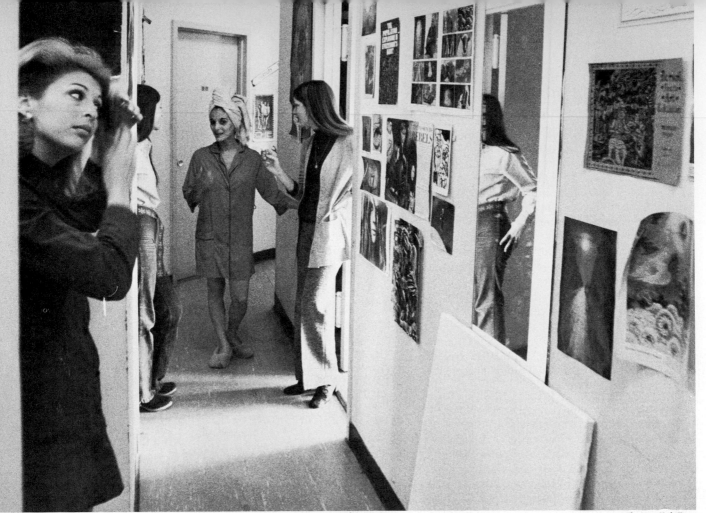

of a roomer can also be lonely if there are no other young people in the family or nearby. Living with the right family can be most enjoyable, but they must suit your needs and your temperament.

The advantages of this arrangement are similar to those of hotel or boardinghouse living. All the necessary furnishings are supplied, and usually the cleaning is done for you. In some cases meals are included. Rates are often quite reasonable.

A residence house. If you're lucky enough to get into one of the residences run for business girls, you'll have the fun of college dorm living at quite low expense. Because most such residences are run by religious groups or other nonprofit organizations, they are usually subsidized. Some have restrictions as to age (often under 35), salary (low), religion, education, and occupation (some are specifically for apprentices in art, ballet, music, or drama). The most desirable houses may have long waiting lists. It is usually advisable to apply well ahead of the time you expect to come to town and to make other plans to tide you over in case a vacancy doesn't materialize in time.

For the new arrival, the advantages of a residence house are many. They are particularly desirable as a first step because they allow you to gather the courage and the cash for apartment living. It's easy to make friends and to find a prospective roommate there. You are surrounded by girls who have the same interests and problems. Usually a happy community life prevails, with the girls finding dates for one another, swapping belts and jewelry, and pitching in when someone has a big job to finish. There's always someone who's good at setting hair or altering dresses and always someone who has plans for fun that can include you. A maid takes care of the cleaning, meals are usually provided, and often there is a recreation room of some sort in which you and the other girls may entertain dates.

On the minus side you may find that the setting isn't as homelike as you'd desire and that at times there are simply too many people around. Occasionally you may yearn for silence, for privacy, for the pleasure of enjoying a good black mood without having someone attempt to jolly you out of it. By the time these feelings take on any sizable proportions, a residence will have served its purpose. You'll no longer be Little Girl Lost in the big city. You'll have made a slight niche for yourself. You'll have a circle of friends and a job and perhaps a raise or two to make apartment living more feasible financially.

❦ Consider the Apartment

If you dream of having a place of your own, you must reckon with the cold, hard fact that apartment living, fun though it is, is usually more expensive and more time-consuming than living in a residence or other accommodation. Rents in the better locations are usually amazingly high. Most rents do not include gas and electricity. Some landlords even leave it up to the tenant to provide heat. A high rent can sometimes be offset by taking in one or more roommates, but the problems of cooking and cleaning and doing the laundry are ever present. You man the mop, lug the groceries, and wash the dishes. Usually, though, because it's a place of your own—a place to take pride in—

you don't really mind. You have every little girl's dream of a chance to play house come true, and you'll learn much from the experience.

Furnished or unfurnished? Will you want a furnished apartment or an unfurnished one? Rents are higher for furnished apartments, but all furniture and most necessary household equipment are included. This makes it easier to move, to give up the apartment, or to split up with an altar-bound roommate. Of course, a furnished apartment may not be a decorator's dream, but much can be done to give it a personal touch by adding a few of your own accessories and pictures.

No matter how highly the landlady extols the view, find out who will do the painting and make any necessary repairs.

B. D. Unsworth

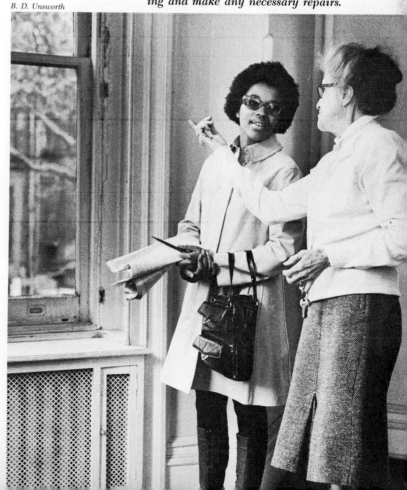

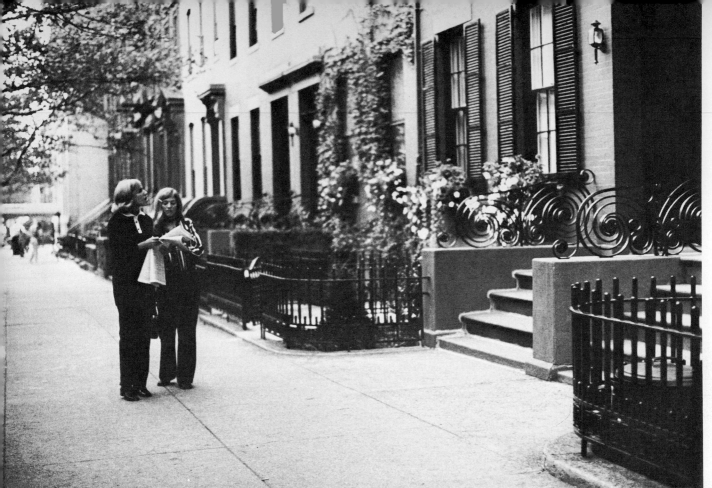

There are many considerations in choosing an apartment—among them, the neighborhood. Is it pleasant? convenient to your job? convenient for the activities you enjoy?

An unfurnished apartment is the choice of the girls who yearn for a chance to fix up their apartments in a manner a bit advanced for Mother's taste. It allows them to express their individuality—and to play with the puzzle of decorating on a budget. But your budget must include more than just the furniture. While the rent is lower than that of furnished rooms, an unfurnished apartment is merely bare walls with a ceiling and bare floor. You provide everything from spoons to beds, from scouring powder to vacuum cleaner. Possibly the family attic will yield a few treasures you can use, and maybe you can borrow some things from home, but there will be many things that must be purchased—a problem to finance and a problem to divide up should you and your roommate part. Tip: *Never* buy anything together, as *both* of you are sure to want it when the time comes to split up.

Tracking down an apartment. When apartment hunting, there are several methods you can try.

• Consult friends. When you've decided upon the section of town you want to live in, spread word of your search among all the residents you know. Many of the most desirable apartments pass from friend to friend and are never advertised.

• Go to a real estate agency. This is the quickest and easiest method, but in many cities it involves a fee, which is often substantial.

• Follow the real estate ads. The newspaper ads supply many good leads—especially those in the Sunday section. When you find something that sounds right, go after it as early as possible. Good places go fast. Perhaps you can even obtain the classified section of a morning paper the night before so that you'll have a head start on other apartment hunters.

• Scout the area. Since many of the best apartments don't need to be advertised, you may be able to find what you want by walking through desirable neighborhoods and watching for vacancy signs. This can prove tiring and time-consuming, especially for a girl with a busy workday schedule.

• Leave your name with the superintendents of several buildings you are interested in. In any large apartment building the turnover is fairly frequent and superintendents are often glad to have a waiting list of applicants. If you are anxious to move in, don't just list your name and then forget about it. Call up frequently to remind the superintendent of your interest. Another way to speed up the process is, of course, to use the mighty power of a tip, distasteful though it may seem.

It pays to look highly respectable on apartment-hunting expeditions. You want to convince the landlord that you are the type of tenant he wants. Many landlords are reluctant to rent to single women, and some won't consider renting to more than two girls. Some landlords even hesitate about two girls, fearing that if one marries, the other may not be able to pay the rent.

❧ Rental Technicalities

When you live in a hotel, a boardinghouse, a room in a private home, or a residence, you can move in with no more financial outlay than a week's rent in advance, and when you wish to leave, a week's notice or less is usually acceptable. Renting an apartment, however, can be much more involved. Usually a lease (see pages 310–311) is required.

A lease is a contract between you and the landlord, giving you the right to live in a specified apartment at a specified rent for a specified period of time. A lease for more than one year must be in writing or it is unenforceable. The lease lists the duties and responsibilities of both the tenant and the landlord. The landlord benefits by being assured of steady income for the period. In return, you are assured of having the apartment for the length of the lease at a fixed rent.

A lease usually requires that before a tenant takes possession, the landlord be given a certain payment (generally one month's rent) as security against damage to the premises or cancellation of the lease. Before you can move in,

Even if a building has no vacancies, it is a good idea to talk to the building superintendant. He usually knows a month or two in advance about tenants who will be moving out.

B. D. Unsworth

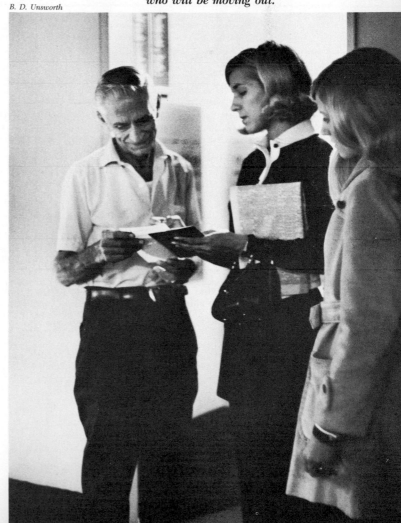

This Agreement, made the................................day of

....19......... Between...

....as Landlord, and

....as Tenant ;

WITNESSETH, that Landlord hereby LEASES to Tenant, Apartment No...........................

on the.....................................floor of the premises known as No...................................

....

City of.., for the term of...

unless sooner terminated as hereinafter provided, to commence...,

19......... and to end.., 19........., to be occupied as a strictly private dwelling apartment by Tenant and Tenant's immediate family consisting of only and not otherwise. And the Tenant hereby covenants and agrees to pay to the Landlord,

the TOTAL RENT OF $................................. in equal monthly payments of $............................... each, in advance, on the first day of each and every month during said term.

Tenant shall pay the said rent at the time and in the manner above provided without demand therefor.

THE SAID PREMISES ARE ALSO LEASED UPON THE FURTHER COVENANTS AND CONDITIONS:

1. Tenant shall take good care of the apartment and fixtures therein and shall at Tenant's own cost and expense make, when needed, all repairs, replacements and decorations therein and thereto, whenever damage or injury to the same shall have resulted from misuse, or neglect by Tenant, Tenant's family, employees, or visitors. Tenant shall not drill into, drive nails, install new locks or change apartment entrance lock or deface in any manner any part of the building, or permit the same to be done, and at the end or other expiration of the term, shall deliver up the demised premises in good order and condition. Tenant shall indemnify and save harmless the Landlord for and against any liability or any injury to person or property resulting from any negligence or improper conduct on the part of Tenant, Tenant's family, employees or visitors. Landlord is exempt for any and all liability for any damage or injury to persons or property caused by or resulting from steam, electricity, gas, water, rain, ice or snow, or any lack or flow from or into any part of said building, or from any damage or injury resulting or arising from any other cause or happening whatsoever unless said damage or injury be caused by or be due to the negligence of Landlord.
2. That any and all shelves, locks, plumbing fixtures, or any other improvements that Tenant may place or cause to be placed in the said apartment shall immediately become a part of the house and the property of Landlord.

4. That Tenant, and Tenant's heirs, executors, or administrators shall not assign this agreement, or underlet the premises, or any part thereof, or make any alterations in the

310

apartments or premises without Landlord's or Landlord's authorized agent's consent in writing, or to permit or suffer upon the same, any act or thing deemed extra hazardous on account of fire; and shall comply with all the rules and regulations of the Board of Health and City Ordinances applicable to said premises; and that Tenant will not use or permit the said premises or any part thereof to be used for any purpose other than above mentioned.

5. That Tenant shall, in case of fire, give immediate notice thereof to Landlord who shall thereupon cause the damage to be repaired as soon as reasonably convenient; but if the building or demised premises be so damaged by fire or otherwise as to require rebuilding, the term shall, at the option of Landlord, cease, and in case it so ceases, the rent shall be paid only up to the time of the fire, unless such damage be caused by the negligence or improper conduct of Tenant, or Tenant's family or servants.

10. That Landlord will furnish, without additional charge, hot and cold water; heat during winter months only. Neither Electricity, Gas or Telephone service is included in the rent, but shall be paid for separately by the Tenant. There shall be no allowance to Tenant for a diminution of rental value, and no liability on the part of Landlord by reason of inconvenience or annoyance arising from the making of any repairs, alterations, additions, or improvements in or to any portion of the building or demised premises.

21. That Tenant has this day deposited with the said Landlord the sum of $............................. as security for the faithful performance of and compliance with all the terms, covenants and conditions in the within lease. That if Tenant fails to comply with each of said terms, covenants, and conditions, or surrender said premises without the written consent of Landlord, or be dispossessed therefrom prior to the expiration of this lease, then, and in that event, the sum herein deposited aforesaid, shall belong to Landlord, as a part payment of the disbursements, attorney's fees, costs, and expenses that Landlord may undergo for the purposes of regaining possession of the said premises and preparing same for renting; and the same shall not be considered as payment for any rent due, or to become due by reason of these presents, or in any manner release Tenant from such rents herein reserved, or from any of Tenant's obligations. If, however, all the terms, covenants, and conditions be fully complied with by Tenant, the said security shall be returned to Tenant after expiration of the term.

IT IS FURTHER AGREED that the character of the occupancy of said demised premises as above expressed, is an especial consideration and inducement for the granting of this lease by Landlord to Tenant, and in the event of a violation by Tenant of the restriction against assignment or sub-letting, or if Tenant shall cease to occupy the premises or permit the same to be occupied by parties other than Tenant, Tenant's immediate family and employees, or violate any other restriction or condition herein imposed, this lease may, at the option of Landlord or Landlord's agents or assigns, be terminated in the manner hereinbefore recited.

In Witness Whereof, the Landlord and the Tenant have hereunto set their hands the day and year above written.

Signed and delivered in the presence of :

Witness ....

....

311

therefore, you must be able to pay the equivalent of two months' rent—a month's rent in advance plus an equal amount as security. The security payment is returned at the end of the lease. Some landlords will deduct from the security the cost of any damage done by the tenant—even such minor things as nail holes in the wall or a chip in the sink enamel. In most cases, however, the security is returned intact. (If you want a telephone—and most people do—you will also have to leave a sizable security deposit with the local telephone company.)

Most leases contain clauses that allow the tenant to sublet an apartment to someone else should she be forced to move. Usually the landlord reserves the right to approve the new tenant. Some leases, however, specify that the security is lost if the tenant moves out before a certain period of time has elapsed. The tenant is also expected to pay the costs of advertising the vacancy and of rerenting the apartment and of any redecorating that may be required.

Many leases contain clauses stating that if the tenant doesn't want to renew her lease, she must notify the landlord in writing a certain number of weeks or months before the expiration of the lease or it will be automatically renewed. Should a tenant forget to give such notice, the lease automatically renews itself for another term (not to exceed one year).

Sometimes you will have to do the painting and the fixing up yourselves, if you're going to get the right apartment for the right price.

B. D. Unsworth

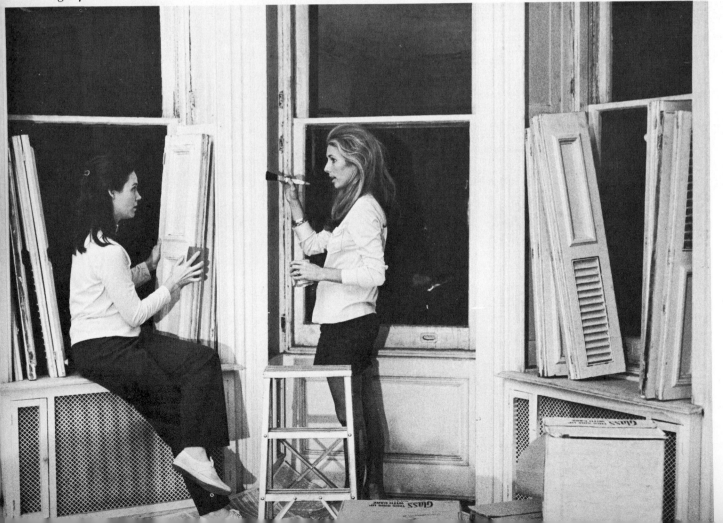

If the tenant overstays the time mentioned in the lease, the landlord can, if he desires, hold her to the lease for another term. One girl who planned to move out the last day of the month changed her mind because it was raining too hard. Although she moved the very next morning, she found herself faced with a lease for another year. (A delay is permissible only in extreme cases of serious illness or death in the family.)

If the tenant wants to stay on after the expiration of a lease and the landlord accepts the next month's rent, the landlord is considered to have renewed the lease and can't change his mind or try to evict the tenant, even though he may have others waiting to move in.

❧ Choosing Roommates

Much of the fun of sharing an apartment depends on your success in finding a congenial roommate. Ordinary activities become fun when shared with the right person, but a personality that grates will blight even paradise.

Two roommates, Joan and Barbara, who are an especially happy pair, summed up pretty well what they want in a roommate: "She should like the things you like—at least the big things—so that you have someone to share your interests," said Joan. "She should be considerate and fair," added Barbara. Both girls agreed that a sense of humor is most important.

The areas that seem to cause the most strife should be discussed between you beforehand. Do you *both* like to entertain? Do you enjoy similar types of recreation (theater and concerts or rock music and baseball games)? Is one of you a chatterbox, while the other prefers peace and quiet most of the time? Do you have similar ideas about money? Is at least *one* of you easygoing?

As Joan and Barbara agreed, you don't have to match up like two buttons on a blouse, but you should have somewhat similar standards and viewpoints on life. The serious-minded miss who wants a career had better not team

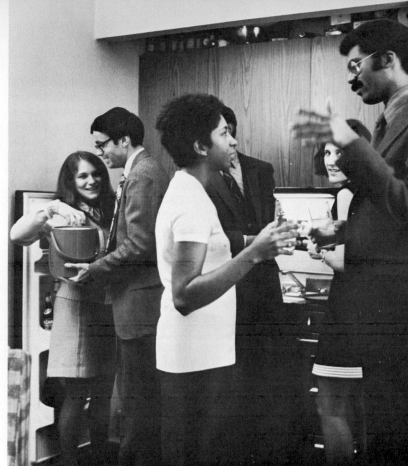

B. D. Unsworth

Living with a roommate can be fun when you have similar approaches to life. If you both like to entertain and you like the same things, you've got a good start.

up with the party girl who comes to the city for the sole purpose of tearing a few years into confetti. Similar standards about housekeeping, although sometimes hard to assess in advance, are important in helping a relationship click smoothly. Barbara commented, "I lived with one girl who left her clothes all over the place. Our apartment was always such a sloppy mess that I couldn't stand it. And my roommate thought I was unbearably neat!" But you can't be a perfectionist, the girls added, pointing out that sometimes you have to put up with an unmade bed or a less-than-gourmet dinner when the pressure of time or finances interferes.

Independence is another quality that roommates need. Occasionally there is a girl who

313

likes to play momma, but difficulties usually arise when one girl leans too heavily on the other. Often the stronger roommate rebels against too much responsibility, or the weaker objects because she feels stifled by being subjected to unwanted authority.

Most trivial differences can be *kept* trivial if you respect these differences and resolve to put up with them. Barbara goes to night school and must occasionally study late. Joan, who likes to go to bed early, has obligingly outfitted herself with an eye mask to keep out the light. On the other hand, Joan can't bear conversation before breakfast, so Barbara saves her thoughts until the morning coffee has perked up her roommate's sluggish spirits.

Most girls who come to the city alone seem to find roommates either in the residences or in other places where they live or work. Many also have found kindred souls among those they've met through classes they attended or through such activities as choir, hobby groups, or dramatic clubs. The consensus of opinion seems to be that if roommates work for the same firm, they'll be less likely to become oversaturated with each other's company if they work in different departments and have different workday experiences.

❦ Two for Company

Whether to take on a roommate or to live alone is a decision each girl must make. Living alone is considered peaceful by some, deadening by others. Those in favor like the freedom of not having to cater to someone else and of not having to compromise at every turn. You're your own boss, responsible only to and for yourself. No one can object to what you do or how you do it.

But lonely it can be. As it has been said, there's security in numbers, even if the number is only two. Another person to confide in, to help you out if you're sick or broke or don't know the ropes is mighty comforting. Needless to say, learning to live with someone else is excellent training for marriage.

Aside from the matter of compatibility, the big dark shadow that hangs over most twosomes is usually that of the man on the horizon. If one roommate marries first, quite an upheaval takes place—both emotional and financial. The girl who's left behind will certainly need a quick replacement unless she can swing both halves of the bills herself. For this reason, some girls prefer having more than one roommate.

❦ Three Is a Crowd

Four is more so, especially when it comes to roommates. Before you get involved in a three-or-four roommate deal, make sure you're the gregarious, flexible soul who can thrive on life *en masse*. Getting along with one roommate can sometimes be a strain—and each additional roommate can be just one more source of friction. Also, one less chance for privacy. But, on the brighter side, also one more source of close friendship. Many such relationships have been known to work out beautifully. Just make sure you're the girl for them and they're the bunch for you before you hop aboard the merry-go-round.

If there is a choice between having three or four roommates, often it's easier to be part of a foursome. Multiple roommate setups have a way of separating into groups. Threesomes sometimes split into a two versus one faction. When there is a division among four, it may not be even, but a two and one and one split is less uncomfortable.

❦ Rules for Roommates

If you want to foster a happy relationship with your roommate, you'll want to observe the following rules.

• Don't make a play for your roommate's date. She snagged him first, and you're honor-bound to direct your allure in some other direction.
• Don't poach on her preserves. Keep your belongings separate—separate drawers, sepa-

314

rate shelves, separate halves of the closet. Overflow into her premises will surely be resented. Just because she isn't using all her space doesn't give you the right to take over.

• Have equal facilities whenever possible. If there's only one comfortable chair in the place or only one good spot for writing, there's likely to be discord. Try to borrow or buy (secondhand if necessary) whatever you need so that you can both be comfortable.

• Be considerate of her sleep. Some people need more sleep than others. If she likes to go to bed early or snooze late in the morning, tiptoe quietly so that you won't disturb her.

• When there's housework to be done, pitch in. If one girl slaves while the other relaxes, there are likely to be hard feelings. For the greatest harmony, try to arrange your cleaning schedule so that you both work at the same time. One idea that has worked well is to assign each girl to a room or job and rotate on a weekly basis. This way, the cleaning gets done and you have clearly defined areas of responsibility. It saves trouble and tempers!

• Seldom a borrower be. If you've earned her devotion, she'll probably suggest that you wear her tangerine scarf with your beige outfit, but asking for it may not go over well. People usually lend you what you ask for, but often with a degree of resentment. Only borrow in real emergencies, and never ask for anything valuable or perishable; you'll worry so much that you won't enjoy it anyhow.

• Don't exude overmuch about the man in your life. She's glad for you, yes, but too much is too much. Also, if her life is a bit low on masculine affection at this point, someone else's continual man-prattle may make her feel just that much more dejected.

• Don't decide to throw impromptu parties. Check with her first. The one time you decide unexpectedly to invite the gang in she may have just washed her hair or may be suffering from a seething headache.

• Respect her need for quiet. If she's cramming for a course or is just in no mood for conversation, give her the peace she needs. Be judicious, too, in your timing of television.

---

1 *If you live in a small town, compare the good and bad points of local job opportunities with those of a city. Can you find the work you want near home? Will it have the type of future you want? How do salaries compare with those of city jobs? Check a city newspaper want-ad section to get an idea of the work available and the salaries offered. Would it be possible to commute to a city job or would the time and expense involved make it more advisable to live in the city? How much would commuting cost? How long would it take round trip?*

2 *Learn as much as possible about the housing available in the city you might want to work in. Study the real estate section of the city's newspaper and, if possible, the classified section of the city telephone book. What type of housing is available? Are there any places that cater to young women for which you might be eligible? Compare the rates for the various types of hotels, boarding or rooming houses, and residences. What prices are asked for a room in a family home? How do apartments, both furnished and unfurnished, compare?*

315

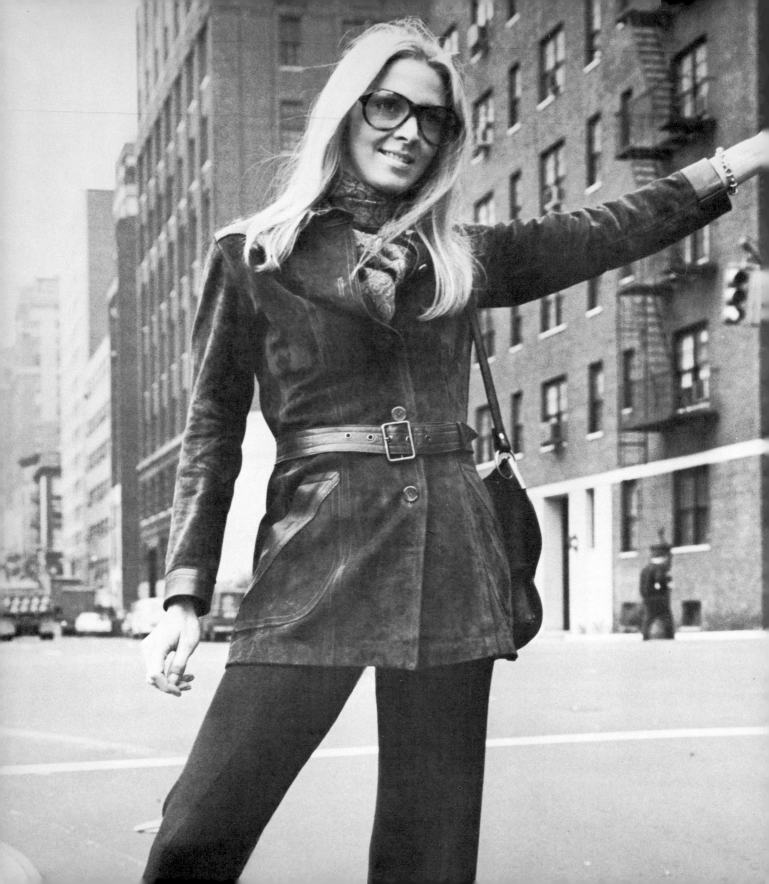

23

HOW
YOU LIVE

Charm grows most successfully when it is nurtured by a happy, well-ordered existence. If our lives run fairly smoothly, without hair-tearing emergencies and avoidable crises, we can devote our energies more fully to concentrating on charm.

The girl who never quite manages to get caught up with herself has too many distracting annoyances pricking at her poise. To make the most of the opportunities life offers, you must manage your energy, your time, and your money so that the routine matters of daily living quietly fall into line. Then you can devote full attention to the *big* things that make life worth living.

A lovely Southern belle came to New York a few years ago to have a fling at city living. Marylou was completely captivated by New York. She was fascinated by the plays, the opera, the ballets, and the continual round of activities available. She seemed determined to see and do everything that was going on.

Evenings after work found her dashing off to a box office for standing-room tickets (the only kind her salary permitted). Supper was often a drugstore hamburger or the meager nourishment of hors d'oeuvres at a cocktail party. Because she was well liked, weekends were equally hectic, with gala dates and parties that lasted until early morn. Marylou was in a gay, exciting whirl. She hadn't time to sleep. She barely bothered to eat. But as the year wore on, Marylou noticed that the big whirl was less and less fun. She found herself dragging through each day at the office and dragging even more through the evening. She no longer looked forward to big weekends. Of course, once she gave herself more rest and took the time to eat relaxed, nutritious meals, she quickly snapped back to normal. And she kept up these good health habits because she found both her job and recreation more fun when she felt her best.

Marylou's error of judgment is a common one. It's so easy to skimp on rest and food, but such punishment has its effect sooner or later. No girl can feel vivacious when she's short on sleep and poorly nourished. In fact, abusing one's health over a long period of time can result in serious illness, besides susceptibility to every minor sickness that makes the rounds. Why take the risk? Anyway, life is more fun if you always keep yourself at your peak of health. You may have to pass up some good times, but you'll enjoy those you do attend far more because you've been good to yourself.

❦ Be Good to Your Career

Being healthy has a lot to do with everything in life. When you feel below par, your whole outlook sours. It's hard to be alert and accurate at the office when you haven't had enough sleep, and it's hard to control your emotions when you're hollow inside because you've skipped a meal. Any job seems dull, any exertion too much, and no promotion worth striving for if you feel miserable. Maybe an extremely good-natured boss will put up with you if you have a low day now and then, and if there are no upsets, you can coast through safely. But, oh, how risky! There's always the unexpected to contend with—the really big job you might muff or the sudden promotion interview you might mangle. Opportunity doesn't wait until the morning after a girl has been to the beauty parlor, had ten hours sleep, and eaten a country-style breakfast. For business girls *any* day may be an important turning point, and you always want to be ready.

There's also the little matter of playing it square. It's hardly fair for an employee to overspend her time and energy on fun to such a degree that she must rest up on her boss's time and can't function efficiently. It's even more unfair for her to neglect her health to the point that she's forced to stay home. No one should come to work if she is seriously ill or has a bad cold that she might spread to others, but it is possible to work when you have a slight headache or a sore knee. Every worker who stays out not only costs the firm money but also puts an unfair burden on the rest of the staff. Many firms can't afford to carry someone with a high absentee record and are often forced to let such a person go. Your attendance and the state of your health are, of course, important considerations in evaluation for promotion. The more responsible your job, the more others depend on you and the more necessary it is for you to be at your desk, in top form, each day.

Being overly conscientious to a fault is unwise, however. No one should overspend her energy on work and office worries to such a degree that she overtaxes her nervous system and bankrupts her health. The girls who lead the happiest, best-balanced lives know the wisdom of leaving office problems behind them when they close their desks at night and of offsetting work strain with weekends of sports and relaxation. For the sake of your charm, your health, and your job:

• Resolve to get eight hours sleep at least four nights a week. Allow yourself no more than one wee-hours bedtime a week, and this on a Friday or Saturday.

• Resolve to eat three nutritious meals a day. Never skip a meal, especially breakfast. Stoke up on foods rich in vitamins, minerals, and proteins rather than "empty" calories.

• Resolve to get some exercise in the fresh air each day and to indulge in some active sport at least once a week.

❦ How to Find Time for It All

Probably nobody has found time for everything she wants to do. With most of us, "everything" is just too big an order for any measly twenty-four–hour day. But an amazing number of girls seem to pack a tremendous amount into each day. They're the ones who are never too

318

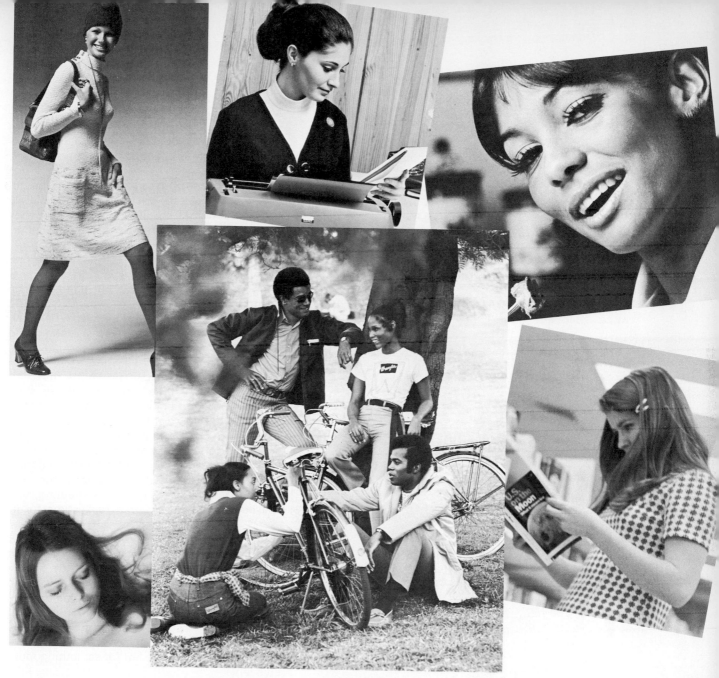

tired, never have a messy-hair day, a noth-ing-clean-to-wear problem, or any of the other troublesome trivia that interfere with important doings. They're the girls who lead busy, happy lives, dress with shopwindow perfection, and manage it all calmly and efficiently and eco-nomically. Regulate your time so that every day allows sufficient time for the following:

- A well-groomed appearance
- Doing a good job for your employer
- Leisurely meals
- Reading and learning something new each day
- Fun and relaxation
- Sufficient sleep

319

How can you streamline *your* living? Think about your own daily activities—what do you do? How do you do it? Which of the following time-savers can you use to help you get greater advantage from your free hours?

Decide what you want most to do. Part of the problem is that sometimes we try to do too much. We can't stretch time, we can only eliminate some of the nonessentials that are squeezed into our schedule. If you want to read some good books, for instance, but never can seem to get around to it, figure out what less

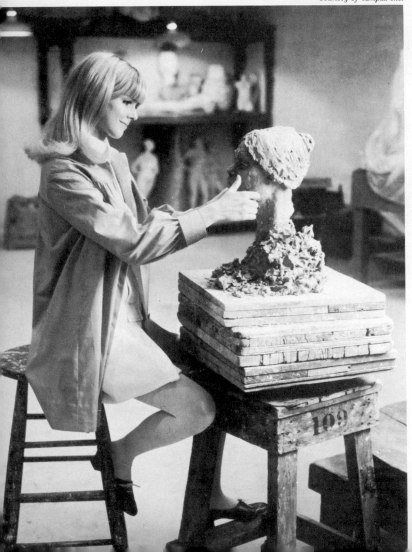

Courtesy of Tampax Inc.

interesting recreation is taking up your time. Many people spend more hours than they realize reading so-so magazine stories, watching mediocre television programs, or doing something else they don't really care much about.

Some girls get so wound up with trivial puttering that they miss half the fun. One girl who took a Western vacation tour completely baffled the rest of the group. Every time they returned from exploring some scenic wonder, they would be met by Ethel who would proudly announce, ''I feel so good—I just shampooed my hair'' or ''. . . did all my laundry'' or something equally commendable but tedious. The Grand Canyon, Yellowstone, Mount Rainier—nothing could divert her for long from her craving for cleanliness. While the rest of the group were a bit more grimy, they saw and did much more on this wonderful vacation.

Everybody has to decide what's most important for her. If it's super cleanliness, then be antiseptic and enjoy it, but make sure this is really what you want most out of life. More worthwhile goals for a young girl might be education for career advancement, cultural development, improvement of talents, preparing for marriage, helping those less fortunate, and so on. When you really want something, you will be able to find or even make time for it.

Get the necessary chores out of the way as quickly as possible. Because you must eat properly and look presentable and live in an orderly place, you can't skip chores. But some people tend to waste time trying to find excuses that enable them to avoid doing unpleasant things now. Instead, if they'd just do the chores *first* and get them over with fast, there would probably be time left for something more enjoyable.

Streamline your surroundings. Some time ago, in a TV interview, Elsa Maxwell uttered some sage advice that hits home for many of us. She said that her amazing ability to accomplish so much was due largely to not letting herself become overburdened by possessions. It takes a strong constitution to resist buying some fascinating little knickknack or to throw out an especially becoming but outdated dress. And how often have you bought two of something to save a penny, even though you wouldn't need the extra for six months? The nuisance value of such clutter cancels out thrift. You have to clean around it, find room for it, care for it. Such unneeded extras are permissible for women who live in roomy houses and have nothing more urgent to do with their time, but business girls are wise to simplify their lives as much as possible.

Parting with still useful possessions hurts much less if you can give them away. In one apartment house the tenants, mostly young office workers, made a practice of leaving on the newspaper pile any good items they felt forced to part with. This allowed other occupants free choice of anything of interest. Such a system seemed to be a much more satisfying solution than heartlessly dumping some charming but useless possession down an apartment incinerator. Many charity organizations are delighted to accept your castoffs. If you keep in mind that someone desperately needs an item you use once in a blue moon, it's much easier to discard intelligently. A good measurement for most items: if it hasn't been used in three years, discard it.

Don't clutter your life with too many activities. Some girls try to do everything at once— drive themselves wild with four night courses instead of two, feel compelled to accept every offer of fun, never say no to any appeal for assistance. Remember, there's next semester, next week, or tomorrow. It's good to be active, true, but some girls overdo to such a degree that nothing comes out right. Concentrate your energies on a limited number of worthwhile endeavors if you want to get the most enjoyment from them. A practical schedule to follow was devised by a group of big-city cliffdwellers for their weekly activities. They allowed one evening for a night course, one for a volunteer job, one night for washing and sewing, and one night free.

321

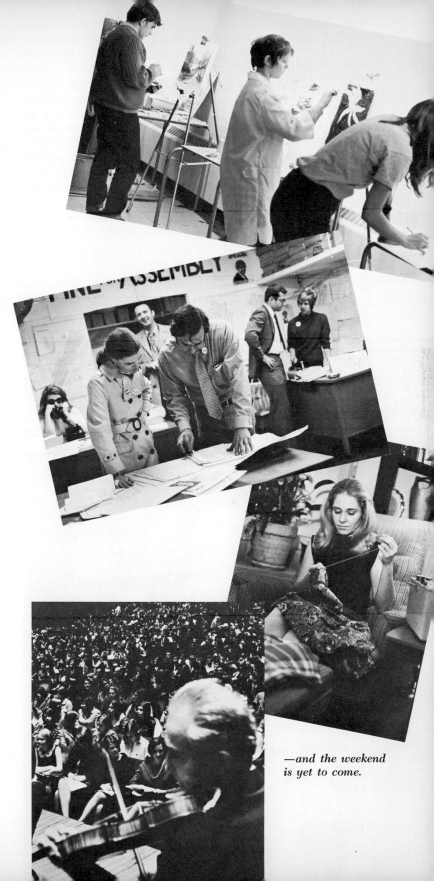

—and the weekend is yet to come.

Do it the easy way. Everybody must decide how important her time is. When you're pressed for time, it can be as precious as money. Then how wasteful extensive shopping for bargains, running to several stores to compare prices, or searching doggedly for just the perfect gift becomes. Sometimes you *have* to settle for something less than the greatest value or the very best choice.

Another way to make life easier is to use as many easy-care items as possible: no-iron and soil-resistant fabrics for clothing, curtains, and other household furnishings; no white collars unless the outfit can also be worn without the collar; dark shoes instead of white; no fussy fabrics. Perhaps each such special-care item takes but a few minutes extra work, but the total time lost can assume amazing proportions.

Don't make double work. When some girls come home after a busy day, they are tempted to throw their coat, purse, umbrella, and what-have-you on the nearest chair. As they change clothes, they may strew what they take off on the bed. Then, when they're all ready to relax, what happens? They're faced with the depressing chore of picking up everything and putting it away. Actually, it's a lot easier and quicker if you make a habit of putting away the coat, hat, and other clothes as you take them off—while they are in hand. This way, the room looks much tidier and you avoid an extra cleanup later.

Schedule your chores. Many girls find it helpful to have some sort of plan for the week's activities. If you live with roommates (or sisters), a work schedule simplifies the problem of who gets to use the iron, when to do the cleaning, and so on. Here is the schedule that two roommates, Lois and Julie, have worked out for themselves.

MONDAY. As this is a good TV night, the girls do chores that enable them to be home if they want to watch. Julie does her hand laundry, mending, and ironing while Lois gives herself a shampoo, set, and manicure.

TUESDAY. Lois has a class. Julie is a volunteer reader for the blind.

WEDNESDAY. Choir practice for both girls, followed by study or reading.

THURSDAY. Weekly marketing, followed by "TV chores"—shampoo, set, and manicure for Julie; hand laundry, ironing, and mending for Lois.

FRIDAY. Dates or "Y" activities.

When you're sharing an apartment, you also have to share the work.

B. D. Unsworth

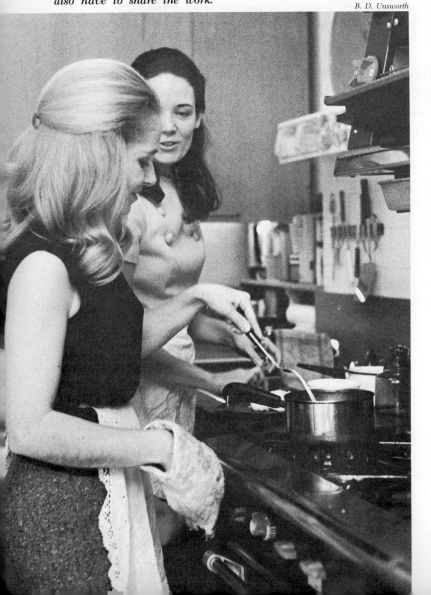

322

SATURDAY. Morning: cleaning and machine laundry; afternoon: shopping, errands, studying, or fun; evening: dates or parties.

SUNDAY. Morning: church; afternoon: if dateless, they try to plan fun (skating, bowling, bicycling, a walk; sometimes a trip to a museum, zoo, or art gallery); evening: devoted to special cooking—perhaps a small roast or chicken and a more elaborate dessert. Occasionally a casserole is made and stored in the freezer for week-night use. The girls often have guests for Sunday night dinner.

Since Julie and Lois are a very harmonious twosome, they usually cook and clean up together. Other roommates, especially if three or more girls live together, find it more convenient to divide up the work. One group of four, with a very small kitchen, worked out a schedule by which each girl shopped and cooked for a week and the others cleaned up.

In any event, it's important that each girl do her share. Many otherwise happy relationships are strained because one girl feels she is stuck with too much of the work.

1 *What timesaving suggestions could you initiate to make your life more enjoyable? For the next three days see how many spare moments you can save from mundane activities to put to use doing something you really care about.*

2 *Take a good look at the place where you live. Is it efficient and well organized? Or is it cluttered with good but unused items that use up precious space or that require extra care? See what you can do to streamline your surroundings.*

323

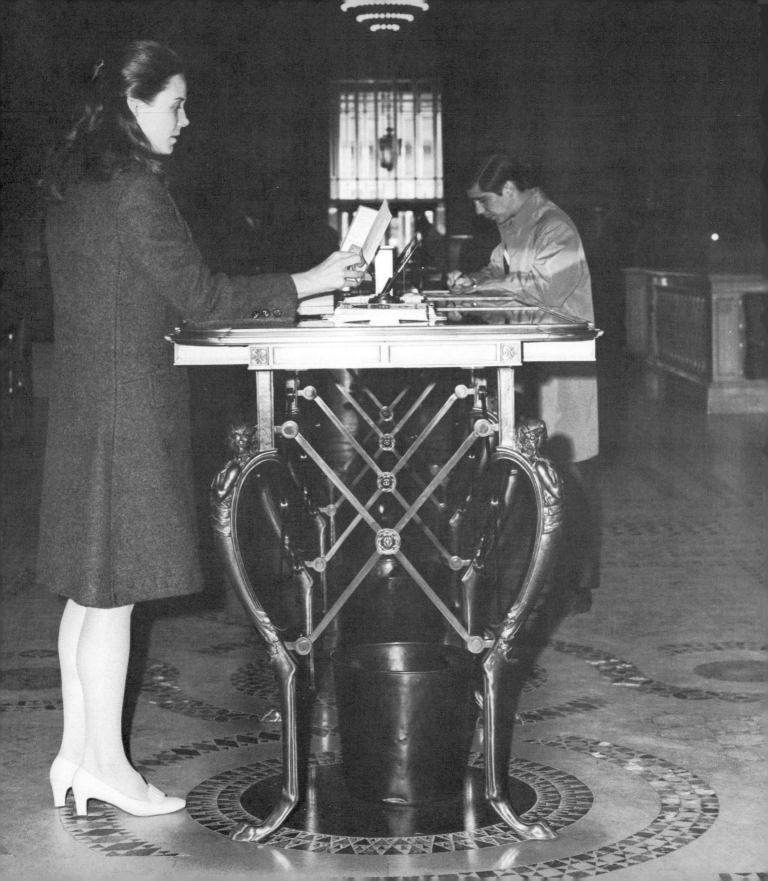

DOLLARS
AND SENSE

For any girl with fewer than six oil wells, money management is one of the most important skills to master. Your own peace of mind, your smart appearance, your way of life, and your future wedded bliss (money problems being one of the chief causes of marital strife) can be greatly influenced by your ability to handle money wisely.

You get a nice feeling when you're financially independent—when you know that your paycheck will stretch far enough to cover the necessities with, perhaps, something left over for fun. Some girls who have developed sound money habits through their school years have little difficulty living on their income, yet others seem to be continually broke no matter how large their salaries become. The secret? Those sound money habits. Like saying thank you, brushing your teeth, or keeping to the right, good financial habits should become an automatic part of your life.

You can easily be overwhelmed by your first salary check, particularly if it is for a two-week or longer pay period. How marvelously rich it makes you feel to have all that money in hand! But—how much it has to cover! For most girls, earning a paycheck brings with it several new obligations. Instead of receiving an allowance from Dad to cover your clothes and other necessities, you will probably not only pay for them yourself but will also contribute something to the family treasury to help pay for your room and board. If you live on your own, you will learn mighty fast how easy it is to overestimate your paycheck and how fast those dollars do a disappearing act. Those lovely, lovely dollars must cover a multitude of items, and only careful management will enable you to maintain the happy state of solvency from one payday to the next.

🌷 *Black Is Becoming for Budgets*

Two of the most important lessons any novice with a paycheck can learn are: (1) Live within your income, and (2) don't let yourself get into the red.

Having a budget is the best way to make sure you have enough money for everything.

B. D. Unsworth

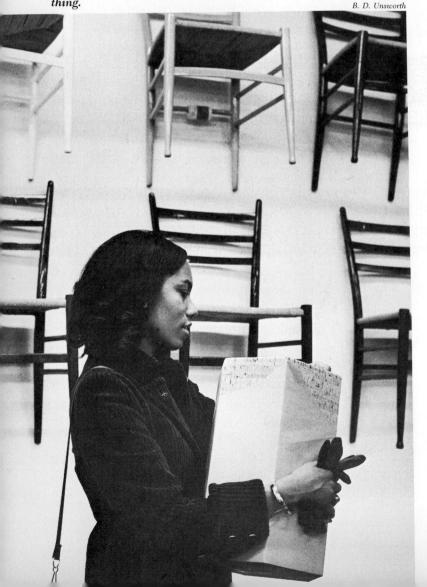

A beginner's salary is bound to be rather low, and it may not allow you to live as comfortably and as luxuriously as you are accustomed to doing, particularly if you have left the family home to seek your fortune. Your new dwelling may be a bit stark at first, and you may not be able to afford that darling suit with the steep price tag. If you embellish your living quarters and your wardrobe gradually, bit by bit as each paycheck allows, you will take special pride in each new acquisition. Every cash purchase will be a tribute to your earning ability and to your success in handling money.

From the day you receive your first paycheck, decide to keep your financial status in the black as much as possible. Liberal credit terms, generous charge accounts, and installment plans make it sound so easy to own anything you want merely by signing your name. But woe to the inexperienced miss who gets herself in beyond her means! Being in the red is far from rosy. Some girls find themselves in the miserable state of having each new paycheck already gobbled up by last month's debts.

🌷 *Beware the Debt Demons*

If you want to assure a safe start, avoid all types of borrowing and debt, which is what installment plans and charge accounts actually are. Many of the girls who've had financial difficulties feel that the biggest mistake they made was opening a charge account. A charge account can be particularly treacherous if it is the revolving credit variety that allows you a certain credit limit (usually $100) but charges $1\frac{1}{2}$ percent interest per month on the unpaid balance. When you stop to do some arithmetic (it works out to 18 percent a year), this can be a whopping bite unless you pay up fast.

Even a regular charge account, in which your bill should be paid in full each month, has its risks, because it's so easy to go overboard, so tempting to sign your name to the salescheck and walk out with your lovely purchase. When the time comes to pay up, the total bill may be something of a shock.

Installment buying is another unhappy system that is best avoided. Interest charges for items bought on the "easy payment" plan usually run a big fat 12 percent a year. Unless you absolutely need the item immediately, you'll do much better to save up the money first. After all, the person who can manage to pay installment payments after the purchase should be able to pay the same amount into a savings account beforehand so that she'll have the money for a cash purchase. *She who saves first, saves most.* Remember, too, when you are paying off a loan, the interest charges you must add on reduce the amount of money you have for other pleasures. Who wouldn't rather use her money for a weekend trip than for carrying charges!

A sound policy to establish: Never purchase luxuries unless you pay cash. Of course, there may be times when it is imperative to take out a loan, such as when you must have a car in order to get to work. If you merely want a car for fun, better pass it up until you have saved the money. Another reason to resist buying a car is the high upkeep and operating costs involved. These can be too much for a limited budget. If you must borrow, read your contract very carefully and investigate all the hidden charges before you sign on the dotted line. Usually it is advisable to go first to your bank—or to a couple of banks—when you need to borrow money. A bank is always reliable, but some finance companies may not be. And bank rates usually are lower than those charged by loan companies.

If you owe money, don't let your debts become overdue. Only if you pay your bills promptly can you establish a good credit rating —something very necessary if you ever expect to borrow money again, to obtain a lease on an apartment, or to take out a mortgage someday to buy a house of your own. When creditors go unpaid, they may also become so impatient that they take the matter to the indebted person's employer—all of which does nothing for her standing on the job. A person who can't manage her own money affairs will rarely be recommended for a more responsible position.

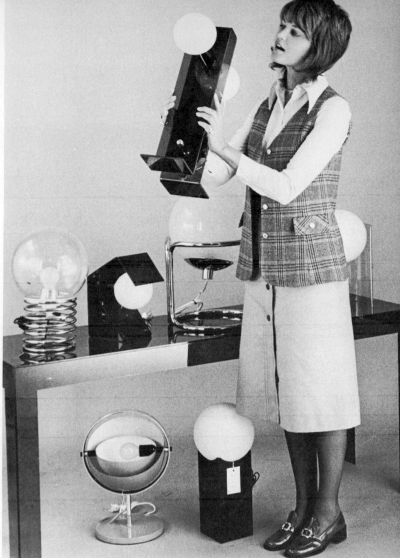

Courtesy of Macy's, New York

❦ Miser or Spendthrift?

We all know the girl who's paid on Friday and broke on Monday. She realizes money is merely a means to an end, but, unfortunately, her means always seem to end too soon. She blows it all on whatever whimsey catches her fancy, and then spends the rest of the week lunching on fingernails.

The opposite is the money hoarder, who considers money as an end in itself. She carefully stores it away, afraid to spend it and worrying over every purchase she is forced to make. She may even lose friends because she

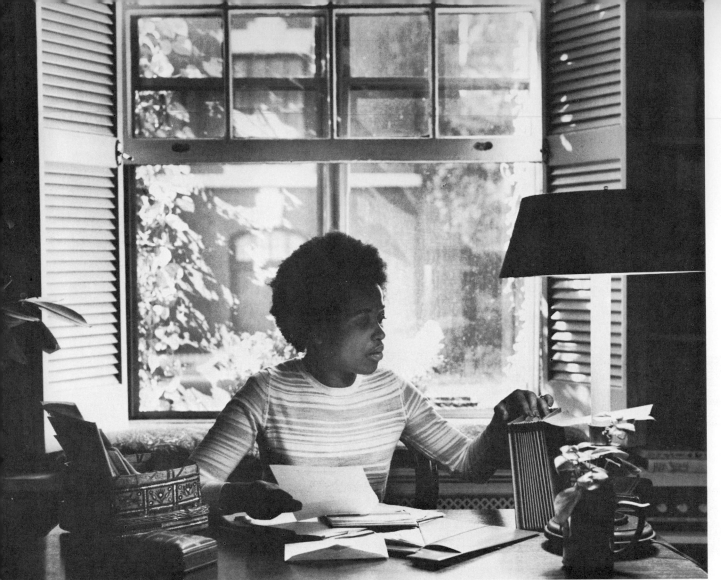

can't help being a tightwad with others as well as with herself. She causes herself much unhappiness because she has completely lost sight of the fact that money is meaningless except for what it will buy.

Somewhere between these two extremes is the sensible approach—that of the girl who knows how to make her money work for her. She is the girl with the clear-eyed view of what she has to use, the well-thought-out plan for spending it, and the self-discipline to follow through.

❧ A Budget Will Help

A budget is simply a plan for using your money. One of the chief virtues of a budget is that it helps you keep track of where the money goes. When you know what your expenses will be, you can see how much money will be left for fun and can plan intelligently how best to use it.

A budget needn't be adhered to as a matter of life or death. It shouldn't oblige you to keep each sum strictly quarantined for the sole purpose it is set aside for. A budget is merely a guide, and it should be flexible. There should be enough leeway so that you can occasionally skimp a bit here to splurge a bit there. The value of budgeting is that it gives you a clear picture of exactly where you can skimp and of how much you can splurge.

Most important of all, a budget shouldn't be grim. It should be realistic and should allow room for at least a few minor indulgences. The girl who lives a Spartan existence so that she can save an exorbitant amount may soon make herself miserable. Better a more normal amount saved and a little extra allowed for fun if the budget is to be practical and workable.

❦ Budget for a Working Girl

Here is how a typical young secretary might spend her money if she lived according to the budget shown. Our Wilma the Working Girl earns $110 a week and has planned her budget so that she has a little leeway in most categories.

BUDGET

Expenditures	Week	Month
Rent	$20.55	$88.60
Phone and Utilities	2.15	9.25
Food and Household Items	19.80	85.80
Clothing	11.00	47.65
Clothing Upkeep	2.50	10.80
Personal Care	3.00	13.00
Medical Care	2.50	11.00
Transportation	4.70	20.35
Recreation and Reading	8.00	34.65
Gifts	1.65	7.60
Incidentals	6.15	26.65
Hospitalization	1.25	5.50
Insurance	1.17	5.00
Savings	5.83	25.00
Taxes	19.75	85.80
GROSS SALARY	$110.00	$476.65

Wilma shares a three-room furnished apartment with another girl. She pays half the costs for rent, phone, utilities, and household expenses. The roommates usually cook their own breakfasts and suppers and buy their lunches on work days.

The *clothing upkeep* figure covers laundry, which the girls do in coin-operated washers and dryers. It also includes laundry supplies, dry cleaning, storage, shoe repair, and any clothing repair or alterations.

Personal care includes such items as Wilma's cosmetics, toothbrushes, toothpaste, shampoo and hair supplies, deodorant, soap, tissues, manicure supplies, haircuts, sets, and permanent waves.

The *medical care* figure covers doctor bills, dental care, eyeglasses, and all the cough drops, aspirins, and other medications Wilma buys.

The *transportation* figure includes not only Wilma's fare to and from work but also covers extra trips for shopping, church, or entertainment.

The amount for *recreation and reading* covers half the cost of newspapers because the roommates share this expense. It also covers Wilma's share of TV, radio, and record player repairs, plus all the magazines, books, records, and sports equipment she buys. Wilma is on a weekly bowling team; she's taking a course in ceramics and likes to go skiing occasionally. In summer she belongs to a community swimming pool, which costs $60 a season, and plays tennis at city courts, which require a $10 permit. Because the girls' recreation is often paid for by their dates, Wilma can stretch her budget further.

The estimate for *incidentals* includes donations for church and charity, films and camera supplies, stationery, postage, and an occasional sundae or soda.

Some of the items not provided for in Wilma's budget: further education, cigarettes, operation of a car, a vacation, travel expenses for visits home, weekend jaunts, purchase of furniture or appliances.

✿ Planning a Budget

When you begin planning a budget for yourself, you will follow these steps:

1 Estimate your monthly income. If you are not working, find out what salary you can expect in the job for which you are preparing. (Keep this estimate on the low rather than the high side.)

2 Estimate your fixed monthly expenses. These are certain expenses—rent, carfare, taxes—that occur regularly each month. If you

In your budget you must set aside a sum to cover your medical expenses. Medical insurance will usually not cover regular check-ups or dental work.

Authenticated News International

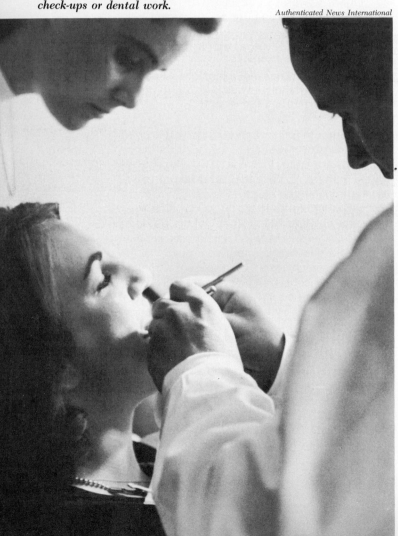

will have any additional large occasional expenses—such as tuition for schooling, insurance premiums that are paid quarterly, automobile license and registration fees, or other similar costs—you should break these down into average monthly figures and add them to your fixed expenses. Then subtract your total fixed expenses from your monthly income.

3 Next take a look at your flexible expenses—those such as food, clothing, and personal care that can vary from month to month—and see just what you are spending for them. The best way to get a good picture of these costs is to keep track of them for a month or two by keeping a tally in a little notebook that you carry with you. Use a separate page of the notebook for each of the flexible categories in your budget. These would probably be Food and Household Supplies, Clothing, Clothing Upkeep, Personal Care, Medical Care, Recreation and Reading, Incidentals, Gifts, and Savings. Then jot down every expenditure you make under the proper category heading. Such a record gives you a good idea of how those dimes and quarters actually disappear.

At the end of the month you will add up the figures in each category. The totals for some categories may be a bit surprising. Then add up all the categories to find what your flexible expenses total. Subtract this figure from the money remaining after you deducted your fixed expenses.

Then comes the big question. Surplus? Deficit? If you're lucky enough to have a little money to spare, you will have a cushion for the extra expenses that crop up. If, however, your expenses tower above your income, you'll need to revise your spending habits or see how you can adjust your budget so that it is better suited to your needs.

If you are not familiar with the prices of foods and household items, accompany your mother on shopping trips and note how much she pays for the soap, facial tissues, shoe polish, and other supplies that you take for granted. Note what the food bill comes to. (Even if you have no intention of taking yourself off to live in an apartment, you'll find this sort of investigation quite valuable and revealing to you as a future wife and homemaker.)

❦ Tailoring Your Budget to You

There will undoubtedly be many personal factors that will influence the budget you make. Costs and salaries vary considerably in different parts of the country. The climate you live in and the type of job you have will also affect your needs. You will want to analyze each category of your budget to see how you can adapt it to best suit your way of life.

Rent. If you plan to live away from home, you will not capsize your budget if you heed the advice of the financial experts. They say that your rent should not exceed one week's salary. Sometimes a more desirable location is important enough to make you choose living quarters with a higher rent, but you must then be prepared to trim other budget allowances.

If you live at home, you will probably want to contribute something toward your keep, but this is likely to be a nominal figure.

Food. What you spend for food will depend on where you live and on whether you eat at home, cook for yourself, or buy some or all of your meals in restaurants. Your social life will also affect your food budget.

If you cook for yourself and are inexperienced, invest in a good cookbook that will help you plan economical meals. Some basic cookbooks are available in inexpensive pocket editions, and you can borrow some of the well-known standard cookbooks from your public library. This is often a good way to help you decide which book you prefer so that you can make a wise purchase.

Food is one category on which you can easily economize but should never skimp. Learn all the gourmet tricks that make inexpensive foods appetizing, but do not cut down on the meat, milk, eggs, and fruits that are more costly but have so much nutritional value. Discover how to buy and cook the cheaper cuts of meat and how to treat them with meat tenderizer. Use powdered milk for cooking, and develop a repertoire of good cheese dishes. They are often money-savers.

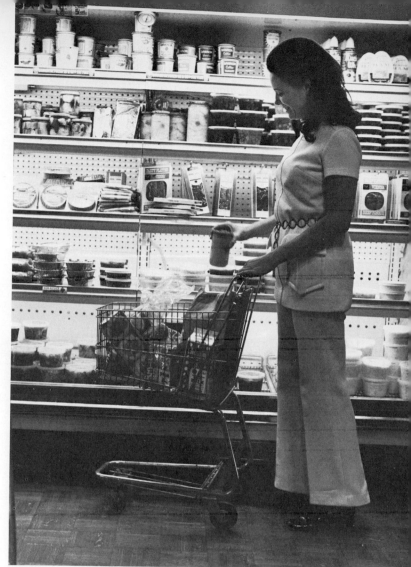

B. D. Unsworth

To stretch your food dollar, plan your meals in advance and either avoid or make use of leftovers. When you shop, read labels and check weights carefully. Don't let the size of the box fool you. Newspaper ads list daily specials and enable you to choose the best buys. Often you can buy extra quantities of durable goods and save.

If you have budgeted a reasonable amount for food but find that you are still running over this figure, don't go on an enforced diet of peanut butter sandwiches toward the end of each week in order to save money. Instead, take a good look to be sure all waste and extravagance have been eliminated, and plan your menus for the week, making sure Friday's dinner will be as satisfying and nutritious as Monday's. Never forget the importance of eating a well-balanced diet for good health.

Lunches can be hard on a budget, and you may spend more than Wilma does if you buy your lunch each day. If your company has an employees' cafeteria or you can bring your own sandwiches, this item can be kept down. Fancy restaurant lunches will probably have to be infrequent until your salary is more substantial.

Before you go to bed, make a sandwich or two for the next day's lunch at work; you'll save a fortune.

Clothing. Back in Chapter 11, you began to figure out your clothing budget for the year. Estimate how much you'll spend, and divide this figure into monthly allotments to see how much you should budget for clothing. This is one variable item where you may be able to cut costs by some shrewd shopping.

Clothing upkeep. Keeping clothing pressed, cleaned, and in good repair will help it last longer. You can help cut cleaning bills by using spot remover, and you can also watch for dry-cleaning specials. Above all, try to wear rubbers and rain gear in wet weather. Soggy, ruined shoes and misshapen clothes can quickly wreck your budget.

B. D. Unsworth

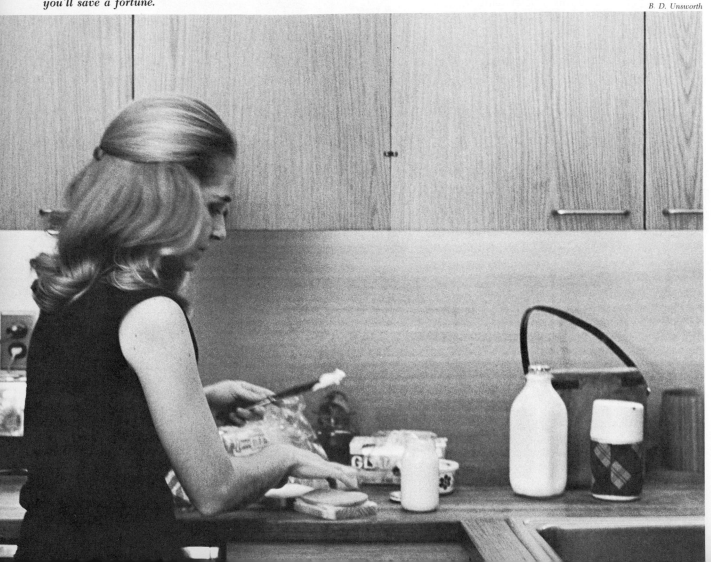

ANNUAL PATTERN OF SALES

Item	Sale Times
Dresses	January, after Easter, late June–July, November
Coats	January, after Easter, August, November
Shoes	January, July
White sales (linens, towels, curtains)	January, May, August
Furniture	February, August
Housewares	January, February, September
Appliances, TV sets, etc.	January–February, June, July
New cars	August
Used cars	July-August
Tires	May–August
Cosmetics	January, July
Storewide clearances	Dec. 26

Personal care. You can save a considerable amount here if you are clever about setting and styling your own hair. A professional cut is usually advisable, but many girls give themselves home permanents and manage the rest of their hair care on their own. If you have difficulty giving yourself a permanent, perhaps you can enlist the aid of a friend—or plan a permanent party in which all the girls help one another.

You may have noticed that the difference between some expensive, nationally advertised cosmetics and the dime store brands is largely in the expensive advertising and more luxurious packaging. This is because one supplier often makes the lipsticks or other cosmetics for several cosmetic houses. Each cosmetic firm purchases and packages the same product, but it is offered to consumers under differing brands—at widely differing prices. If you experiment, you may find the cheaper brands of many items quite satisfactory.

Medical care. This figure will vary considerably depending on your general health, the condition of your teeth, and whether or not you need glasses. It covers medicine, drugs, and medical appliances as well as doctors' fees.

Transportation. Although transportation has been considered as a fixed expense, you may be able to save here if you walk part or all of the way to work. Nevertheless, a little leeway should be allowed in case a sudden downpour or a late start makes a taxi essential. If you think you may want to own and operate a car the *minimum* annual cost will be:

Insurance	$272.00
Taxes, license	26.00
Depreciation	684.00
Gas and oil (10,000 miles)	265.00
Tires	47.00
Repairs, etc.	68.00
Total	$1,362.00 a year or $113.50 a month

These figures are based on averages as reported by AAA. This is the minimum cost you can expect. The actual figure will probably be higher. Nothing has been allotted for tolls, parking, or garage rent—to name a few of the extras you may have to contend with. The tax and insurance rates may differ, of course, depending on where you live.

Recreation and reading. The amount you allot will be influenced by whether you need any sporting equipment, what types of recreation you prefer, what organizations you belong to, what reading you do, whether you plan to continue your education, and so on. This is an individual matter that only you can decide. In this category cuts are always possible, but here they often hurt most. However, by reading the

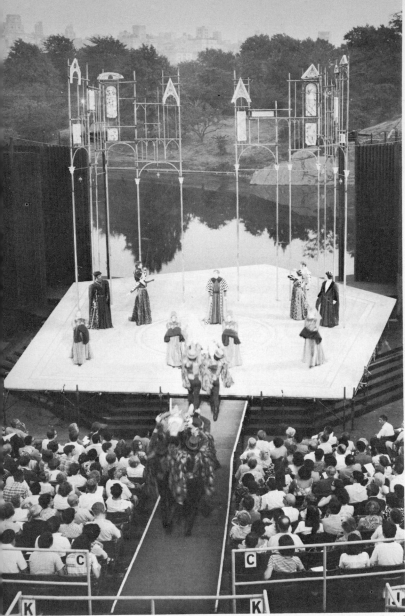

Every summer the New York Shakespeare Festival stages performances in an open-air setting in Central Park. Admission is free, and leading stars often participate, so the plays are quite popular. Many people have picnic suppers on the lawns in the park and then watch Shakespeare under the stars. It is a rewarding and inexpensive way to spend an evening.

newspaper carefully you can get the most out of your entertainment budget. Many cities have free performances of plays and concerts that are announced on the entertainment pages. Usually advertisements for these activities are not large, so you have to look for them. Sometimes you have to write for tickets to free events in advance; at other times all you have to do is show up. Museums often have free exhibitions and some show free movies. You can borrow books from the public library and spend several evenings engrossed in a novel. Sports can also provide inexpensive recreation. Many towns have public tennis courts, skating rinks and swimming pools, which can be used cheaply.

Incidentals. Church and charity contributions, film, film processing and camera supplies, stationery, postage, and your occasional petty indulgences (such as special snacks) are included in this category.

Gifts. You know pretty well what your personal gift-giving schedule is and can guide yourself accordingly. Office collections are not so predictable. Weddings, approaching births, retirements, and other leave-takings are often celebrated by luncheons, parties, or gifts financed by contributions from the staff. A newcomer should not be expected to join in on these unless she knows the person well, and her contributions need not be as much as those of someone with a higher salary.

In some offices the problem has been lessened by collecting a quarter or so from everyone each payday. This money is then put into a general fund to be used for all parties and gifts. In a few organizations the employees have received the permission of management to have candy and soda vending machines installed, and the profits from these machines are used for such celebrations.

Medical insurance. Everyone should have some form of medical insurance. In these days of staggering medical costs, this sort of protection is particularly advisable for the young working girl who has little financial reserve.

334

Many companies have set up group plans for their employees. A group plan has lower rates because of the large number of members in the plan. Some corporations even pay part or all of the cost of medical insurance.

Other insurance. Because life insurance and annuity contracts are forms of enforced saving as well as financial protection for your family in case something happens to you, you may want to make this part of your budget, too. Single women with no dependents and many present needs may prefer to forgo life insurance and keep their savings in a bank, where it is more easily accessible and where interest rates are higher than those offered by insurance companies. However, if you choose some form of annuity plan by which your money is available to you about the time retirement cuts your earning capacity, you're *sure* of having the money at a time when you're likely to need it. Unless you are concerned with death benefits for dependents, the pro and con of insurance boils down to this: intelligent foresight and the determination to maintain a good nest egg can get you a better bargain in savings, but for the average, less strongly fortified person, insurance is a good buy.

Many firms have set up group plans that provide their employees with life insurance at very reasonable rates. Group life insurance plans are usually term insurance. These provide low-cost coverage during your employment, but they terminate when you leave the company, and they do not build up any cash value as straight life insurance does. They are therefore not to be considered a form of savings. You are merely getting insurance. The advantage of a group plan is that you are insured at much lower rates than are otherwise available. Before joining any company insurance plan, you should ask yourself whether you are more interested in life insurance at bargain rates (a group plan)—with savings left to your own initiative—or in an individual straight life insurance policy which, though more expensive, accumulates a monetary value that can be cashed in should you need it.

Don't, however, overload yourself with such a steep policy that you weary of paying it and let it lapse. This happens all too often. One advantage of taking out life insurance when you are young is that the premiums you pay are lower. The rates are higher when you subscribe at an older age.

Savings. The time is sure to come when you will need some ready cash. For this reason, you would be wise to build up as soon as possible a cash reserve of at least four to five hundred dollars for emergencies. A minimum of five percent of your salary should go into savings. Ten percent or more is preferable, at least until you have built up a substantial reserve fund.

The experts advise that your goal should be to maintain a rainy day fund equal to half your yearly salary after taxes. This may seem pretty high, especially from your present financial vantage point, but if you intend to rely strictly on the sweat of your lovely brow, this is none too much to allow for peace of mind regarding future emergencies.

Taxes. Social security (F.I.C.A.) taxes and state and federal income taxes will probably be deducted from your paycheck by your employer. Some states have more taxes than others, so this figure will be determined by where you live.

Any other categories? If you are planning to continue your education, you may also want to set up a category to cover this figure. How about a vacation allotment? And one for Christmas gifts? Many banks have Vacation Clubs and Christmas Clubs to help you save the amount you desire. You agree to pay a certain amount each week, and the bank holds the money for you until the proper time. Club accounts usually pay no interest, and you can't withdraw the money until the end of the time agreed upon. Some girls with a good supply of financial self-discipline prefer to add this money each week to their regular savings account, which does pay interest, but the little nudge a club account offers is very helpful to those with less resoluteness.

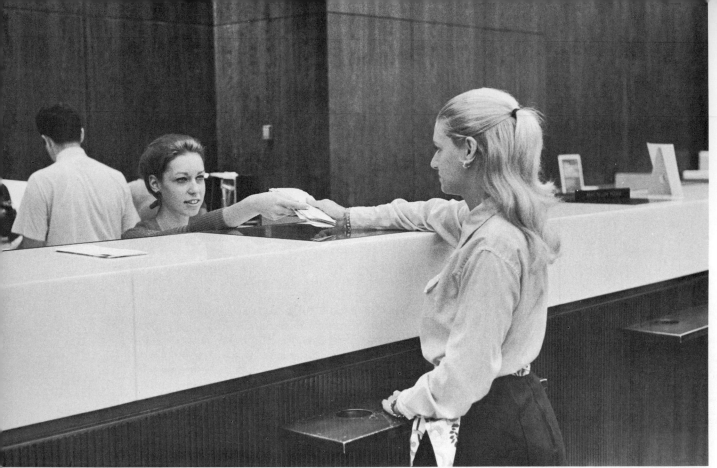

🌷 Banking Your Treasury

Every girl with a paycheck should have a savings account and a checking account to help her take care of her money.

Which bank for savings? When you choose the bank to favor with your savings account, you'll want to select one that pays you the best interest. Investigate the interest rate, but find out also how often this interest is compounded (daily, quarterly, semi-annually), when your money begins to earn interest (from day of deposit, the beginning of the next month, the beginning of the next quarter), and how long your money must remain in the bank to earn higher interest rates (higher rates are often paid if the money is untouched for a certain period of time). In general, savings banks and savings and loan associations pay higher interest than commercial banks. Shop around for the one that offers you what you want.

You needn't select the bank with the most convenient location as your financial storehouse. Most banks offer free bank-by-mail services, so that you can choose a bank in another part of town or even in another state if it pays higher interest. If you do select a distant bank, you may find it helpful to maintain an account in a nearby bank as well. Although you would put most of your money in the account that bears the higher interest, you could keep a small amount in the local bank so that it would be quickly accessible if you needed it.

It's wise to have as little cash as possible around home or in your purse. Too many sad tales of break-ins or purse-snatchings have

336

proved how fragile the unprotected nest egg can be.

Checking accounts. A checking account is a wonderful convenience. It enables you to pay bills conveniently by mail and to conduct most of your larger money transactions by check. It relieves you of the burden of carrying large amounts of cash. Your checkbook also provides a record of expenditures, and your canceled checks serve as proof of payment. Checking accounts do not pay interest, however, so they should be used only for money you use to pay your expenses—not for savings.

Again you will want to shop around to find the right bank, because charges and services vary. Some banks have low service charges if a certain minimum balance is maintained. Others require no minimum balance but instead have a higher service fee. You will find that these service fees also vary. Some charge a certain amount per check and have no service fee; others charge a monthly service fee but allow unlimited checks; still others charge both fees. If you need only a few checks each month, the first type mentioned is better.

🌷 Glad Money

If you've ever watched your last quarter go rolling down a drain as you were waiting for the bus on payday morning, you know the woes of letting yourself get flat broke. To avoid this sort of tragedy, many girls like to carry a small emergency fund—glad money—that they can dip into if necessary but which they always replace so that it is ready for the next emergency. One girl who received a dollar in a gift wallet tries never to spend this last dollar. Another girl who once found a five dollar bill used this for her emergency fund. Carry your glad money with you, but keep it in a separate change purse or envelope—isolated in some way so that you won't spend it by mistake. Probably the time will come when it will save the day for you.

337

🌷 Help Yourself to Save

If, after figuring out your budget, you've come up with the conclusion that there's just nothing left for a vacation or for Christmas gifts or for any other special spending, you probably need a saving scheme to help. Many a girl who's made just such a complaint is now sporting a new fur coat or enjoying an exciting, romantic, adventurous vacation in Mexico.

The first step in any saving plan is to have a goal—something tangible provides the most incentive. You might want to start out with an item that's not too expensive, such as a bowling ball of your own, an overnight bag, or a hair dryer. Once you have a goal, you will probably discover all sorts of ways to catch money that has been slithering through your hands. When you stack up that afternoon piece of cake against your savings goal, it may be easy to pass up the cake. In a month that daily fifteen cents can add up to something like three dollars, saved just from this one item. Every time you

U.S. Virgin Islands Gov't. Photo

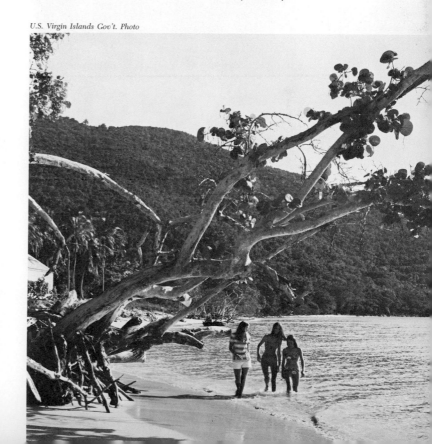

are tempted to spend money on something you really don't need, think of your lovely savings goal and it will be much easier to resist.

Once you've achieved a small goal, you'll have established saving habits and will have the zest to start yourself off on other, perhaps larger, goals.

❦ Saving Devices

Everybody has her own way of making herself save, but here are methods that have helped other girls.

• Keep-the-change method. Each night deposit in your piggy bank all the change you've accumulated during the day.

• Dime collector. Decide to save every coin of a certain denomination for your piggy bank. Instead of dimes you may want to begin with

nickles—or, if you're feeling flush, with 25-cent pieces.

• Splurge box. This is a technique roommates like to use to help save for special splurges. They each agree to deposit a certain amount each week in a special box or bank. It may be only a quarter or fifty cents, but it will soon mount up to enough for dinner in an elegant restaurant or maybe theater or concert tickets.

• Give up some regular expense. Perhaps it's only a candy bar each day, perhaps luncheon dessert (the latter is recommended only for the very determined), or the extra bus you take for the last few blocks. Even a small daily saving, when multiplied by the number of days in a month, becomes a figure to be reckoned with.

• Count your bargains. Every time you get an unusual bargain (a blouse reduced one dollar, hosiery purchased at a semiannual sale) deposit the amount saved in your piggy bank.

• Slice it off. This more drastic method involves deducting a certain amount from your pay as soon as you get it, then trying to do without the extra cash until next payday. Some sturdy souls guard against backsliding by immediately depositing this money in their savings accounts. One girl who did this was forced to withdraw some money one week to carry her through. When she confronted the teller with her withdrawal slip for two dollars, he smiled and asked innocently, "How do you want it?" (P.S. She eventually saved enough for a trip to Europe.)

❦ Earning Extras

The easiest way to have more money is, of course, to earn more money. If an increase in salary is not in the immediate future, you may wish to take on an extra job to add to the exchequer. For a girl with good typing skills, there are many opportunities. Try inserting a classified advertisement in your newspaper, offering to type letters, business reports, manuscripts, class papers, thesis papers, and other typing chores. Many small businessmen often need part-time services of this kind. You could also contact political and charity organizations, which have occasional busy seasons, and your

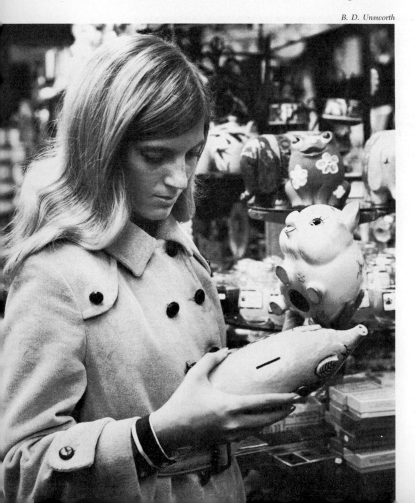

338

local government and school offices, which may sometimes farm out rush jobs.

Some girls prefer a change from their office work and forsake the typewriter for selling jobs. One girl who worked in a department store on Thursday nights and Saturdays said that, although she didn't earn a great deal, the saving she made on clothing purchases, through her employee discount, helped bolster her savings considerably. Another girl who worked in a music store on Saturdays said she loved the job so much that she hardly considered it work and actually looked forward to it. You might find another refreshing change from office work by helping out in the local library evenings or Saturdays. ''That's where I keep up on all my friends,'' explained one library assistant. Baby-sitting is also popular because, even though it is low-paying work, it usually isn't very demanding and your time can be put to good use on your own projects while the children sleep.

Another girl used her car to earn money, changing it from a deficit to an asset. She had driven her car to work but realized that the convenience cost her much more than the bus fare. To turn this into a paying proposition, she advertised for riders, took on four at bus-fare rates, and got herself a free ride plus something for the savings account besides.

If you are still in school, don't overlook the possibility of vacation employment. Many department stores and supermarkets are so short of personnel that they will gladly take on students for such short periods as Christmas or Easter vacations. Many girls look back fondly on jobs spent selling toys or creating elegant gift wrappings at holiday times.

1 *For one month keep an account of your actual expenses (including those expenses that your family now pays but that you will assume when your salary permits). Use a separate notebook page or piece of paper for each category. At the end of the month total up each category of expenses. You may be surprised at how much it costs you to live.*

2 *Plan a budget for yourself based on the information in this chapter. When you have completed your month's accounting of your actual expenses, compare this with your budget to see what changes are necessary to make your dollars do the most for you.*

3 *Do a little investigating about the cost of carrying charges for installment plan purchases. Compare the cost of a TV set purchased for cash with the total cost for the same set purchased on the installment plan.*

4 *Find out what type of work might be available in your area for an office worker with your skills who wishes to earn extra money in her free time.*

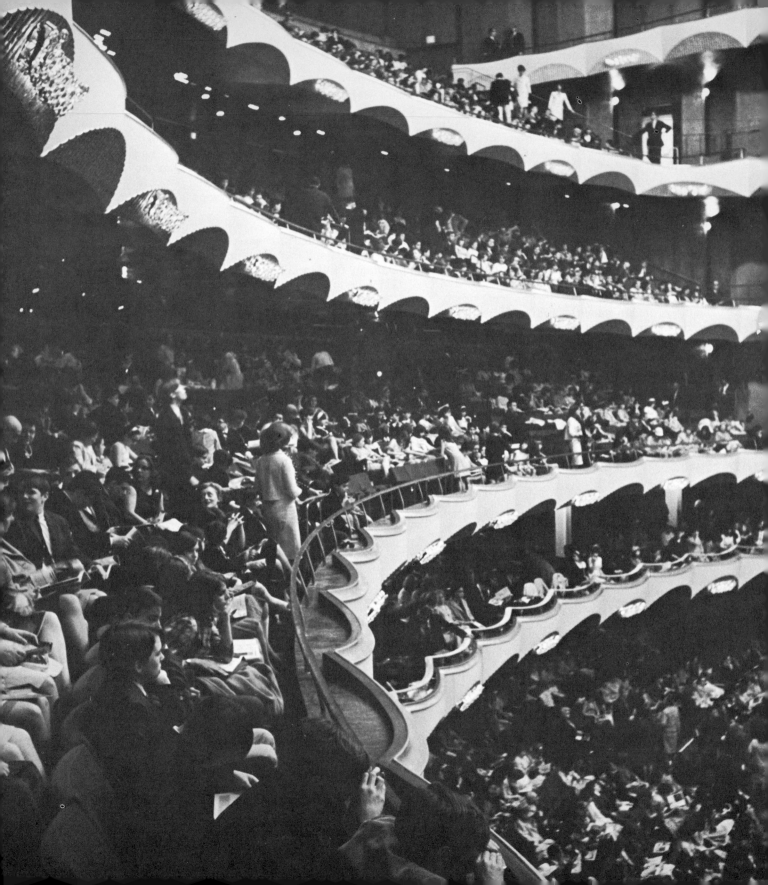

FUN WITH
A FUTURE

During childhood you probably often had more time on your hands than you knew what to do with. "What can I do now?" is an all-too-frequent wail from youngsters. But as you became more occupied with school activities, your spare time dwindled. Now, as a full-time working girl, your free time will be at a premium. It's positively precious. You'll want to use it cleverly so that it can do the most for you. Squander it on the same old routine activities in the same old places, and you add little zest and freshness to your life. Cram it brimful of the best in fun—especially fun that will help you develop greater understanding and knowledge—and your reward will be ever-increasing charm and sophistication.

Sophistication is the highly admired polish that comes from being acquainted with the many things that interest intelligent people. It's being in the know about what's going on and about the important names and happenings, past and present, that affect our society and culture. It's also knowing what to do when.

The sophisticated person is admired because she has learned what to do and how to do it gracefully. You learn sophistication from many sources. Mostly you absorb it bit by bit from what you do and observe. Invest your spare time in activities that will help you learn and grow, and you will add to your sophistication. You will develop a brighter, richer personality. No matter how smart you are or how good your education has been, there is tons more to learn. How much do you really know about art, opera, ballet, or the great writers or philosophers.

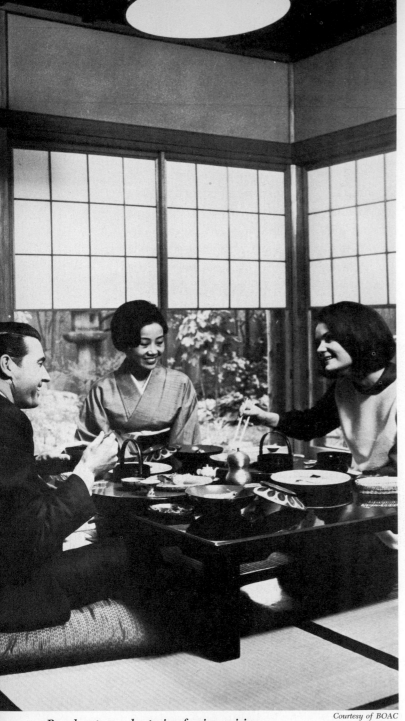

Be adventurous by trying foreign cuisine. If the cooking doesn't suit your palate, you need never have it again, but if it pleases you, you can enjoy it for a lifetime.

Courtesy of BOAC

❦ Fun Well Spent

How do you usually spend your evenings? If it's watching TV programs you don't particularly care about, chatting or playing bridge with the crowd whose every thought you already know, or just puttering around the house, you might give heed to ways in which you could get more value for your time. Is there some subject you don't know about that gives you an uneasy feeling of inferiority whenever it comes up? Would a course in music or art appreciation or would just reading some good books help fill the gaps in your background? Would you like the creative satisfaction of expressing yourself through hobbies such as art, craftwork, playing a musical instrument, or performing in a theater group? Look around for activities that will give you solid satisfaction and inspiration. Some criteria that might be used in planning your free time:

- Will I learn something new and interesting?
- Will I obtain practice in some of the social graces about which I'm a bit shaky?
- Will I be improving my health and physical well-being?
- Will I be doing something worthwhile that will help others?

And, of course, to each of these must be added the further qualification: Will I enjoy it? On this last point, however, don't cross out something you haven't tried until you've given it a fair chance.

One further suggestion: Keep your activities varied. Tennis is an excellent sport—good fun, good for the figure—but the girl who spends every weekend on the tennis court takes care of only one of her needs. Her backhand returns may be great, but her head may rattle emptily when the conversation ball bounces her way.

Susan Sawyer had lived in a suburb of New York all her life but felt that despite her closeness to the metropolis she was provincial and inexperienced in the ways of any but her own immediate set. To develop more smoothness and confidence, Sue enlisted her friends in her project of absorbing the sophistication that could be gleaned from New York. She went to plays, lectures, TV broadcasts, concerts, foreign movies, museums, and art exhibits, and she attended some of the famous churches to listen to their celebrated clergymen. If she was hesitant about something—such as how to act at the Plaza—Sue found out by going there on her own. (Lunch or tea doesn't put as big a dent in your pay as dinner, she advises.) She and her friends also tried foreign restaurants so that they'd have an acquaintance with unusual foreign foods. Wherever she went, Sue watched and learned and evaluated so that she would develop naturally a cosmopolitan air.

❧ Wonderful Weekends

In each year we have 49 free weekends, assuming the others are taken care of by vacation plans. Each is a marvelous opportunity for special fun. When the budget permits, you might take off on a special weekend excursion—perhaps to a ski resort in the winter, a lakeside resort in the summer, a riverboat excursion for spring or fall, or a hiking or biking trip (especially inexpensive for American Youth Hostel members who can stay overnight at one of the A.Y.H. hostels for a dollar or two). Good anytime is a weekend of sightseeing: a visit to some historical area or to one rich in local color, such as the Pennsylvania Dutch country around Lancaster, Pennsylvania, the Indian reservation at Taos, New Mexico, or historic Williamsburg, Virginia. A sports area like Sun Valley, Idaho, Lake Tahoe, California, or the Dells in Wisconsin, can be varied and exciting. With so many wonderful opportunities available to all of us, no girl should let her weekends sink into an uninspiring sameness.

❧ Two Weeks to Play

Vacation time, those precious two weeks of your very own, offer a chance to do something very different. After being attached to a job for nearly a year, you're off the leash to run far and

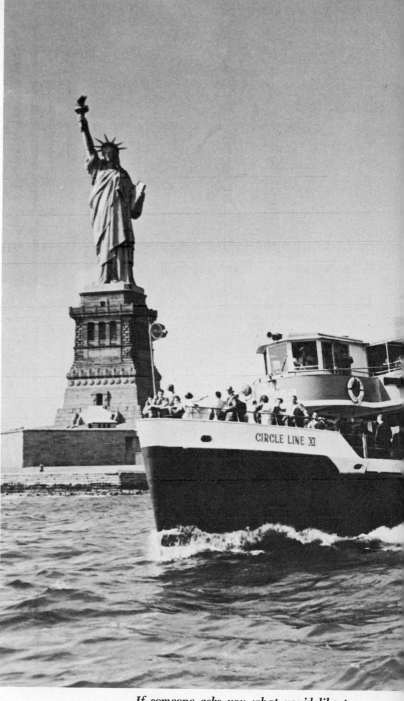

If someone asks you what you'd like to do on a given day, why not suggest something a little different? A boat ride or a trip to a local scenic spot can be interesting and fun.

343

to live it up as you please. Take advantage of this once-a-year opportunity and get an invigorating change of routine. The girl who hangs around the local haunts all vacation, perhaps even joining the office crowd for lunch, misses the marvelously refreshed feeling to be gained from new places and new faces.

Plan early and well. Start your planning in the early spring. If you want to stay at a specific place for several days, you had better make advance reservations—the earlier the better—to be sure space will be available for you when you want it. If you are planning a trip that will mean overnights in certain cities, you might do well to make reservations ahead of time. The joy of a vacation can be ruined if you must spend time searching for lodging and transportation when everything is booked solid because of a convention.

How do you decide where you want to go? The travel sections of the large newspapers offer many suggestions, and if you have decided on a certain locality, you can write to the state or city chamber of commerce for more information. Whenever possible, consult a travel agent. A travel agent is an expert on vacation opportunities, and his services cost you nothing. Tell him what you want, and he can probably suggest the right place for you—and for your budget. He will also save you time by making travel reservations and booking accommodations. You pay nothing for this service because his commission comes from the other end—from the bus line, hotel, or whatever. Consulting an agent can often get you more for your money, because he may know of tour plans that give bargain rates and include features not available otherwise.

Look for a change of pace. If you sit at a desk all day and don't need a rest, there's little to be gained by spending your vacation sitting on a beach or lolling on a hotel lawn. How about a dude ranch, a windjammer cruise, a riverboat tour, or a resort that is noted for lots of scheduled activities? If you want the latter, pass up the glamour hotels and consult a travel agent or study the advertising literature that promises hayrides, masquerades, amateur nights, and the like. If the resort brochure plays up facilities for children, probably you can rate it as more of a quiet, restful family place.

As you make plans, ask yourself if the main feature of this vacation idea is something you enjoy. If you don't like roughing it, a camping trip will hold little charm for you.

Look for congenial company. Check the age group. Does the place seem to cater to young people? If you want a young crowd, study the

Courtesy of Burdine's, Miami

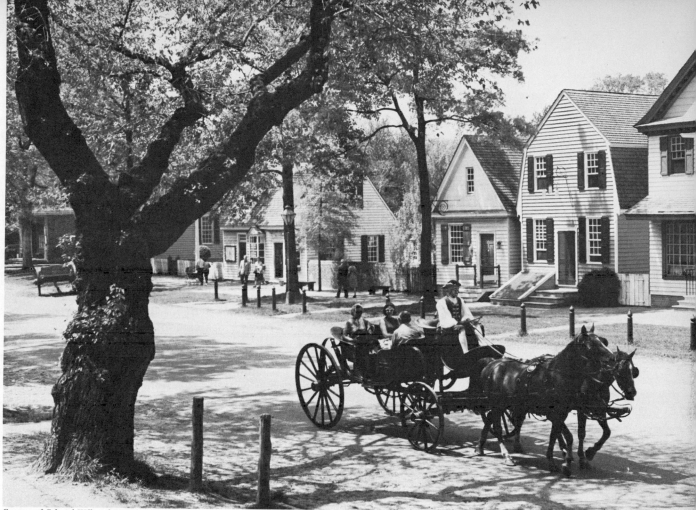

Courtesy of Colonial Williamsburg

pictures and other clues in the advertising matter. Better yet, consult a good travel agent. It's his business to know about the atmosphere as well as the facilities.

Sample new places. Whenever possible, try to get away from the type of people you associate with each day. If you live in Boston, don't follow the rest of the Bostonians to Cape Cod or the Berkshires each year. Go where people think a little differently from you.

When you travel, try to absorb the color and flavor of the area. Talk to the people who live there, read the local newspaper, and eat the regional specialties so that you can get a good picture of the place. Don't act condescending, however. No tourist who has a we-do-it-better-back-home attitude is appreciated. Your trip will also be more enjoyable if you read up on the area before you go. If New Orleans is your goal, for instance, how much more fascinating it will be if you know something about the early French and Spanish settlers, understand the Creole heritage, can tell stories about such pirates as the dashing Lafitte, and have read an article or two about the French Quarter.

In many parts of the country there are special festivals such as the Maine Seafoods Festival at Rockland, Maine, or the Cheyenne Frontier Days in Cheyenne, Wyoming. Perhaps you can make your vacation even more interesting by scheduling it at festival time.

If you live and work in the country, a city vacation may be your ticket for fun. Treat yourself to a glorious week of theatering, dining grandly, sight-seeing, shopping. Perhaps you can pamper yourself with good-for-the-morale beauty treatments at one of the elegant (though expensive) beauty salons. A city vacation is an excellent idea for the girl who entertains thoughts of coming to work in the city at some future date. She has a good opportunity to look it over and examine job opportunities firsthand.

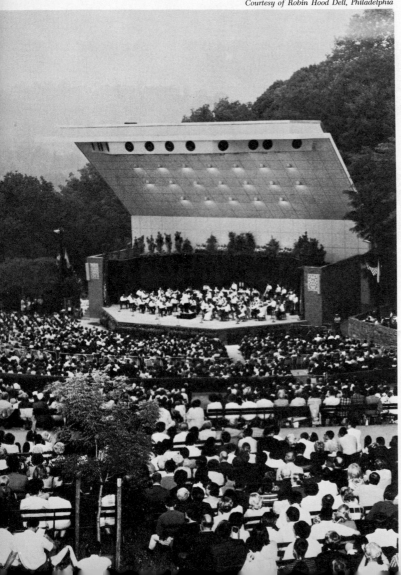

Gather new thoughts. If you want an inspiring vacation, you might consider a place like Aspen, Colorado, which is noted for its plays, concerts, and lectures. Lenox, Massachusetts (in the Berkshires), features the Tanglewood Concerts, and nearby is Jacobs Pillow, noted for its modern dance group, and also the Berkshire Playhouse. At Isomata (Idyllwild School of Music, Idyllwild, California) you can take short courses in music or the arts as well as enjoy being part of the audience.

If you are a Sunday painter or musician, you can investigate the art colonies and music resorts where you can receive expert instruction along with your vacation fun. Consult your newspaper travel section or advertisements in magazines catering to these fields.

Go with good company. If you want a change, don't go with the gang from your neighborhood or with the girls from the office. Vacation time should let you get away from it all. Choose one or two good friends who will keep their good spirits through thick or thin. Or don't be afraid to try it alone. If you're planning a resort vacation, your chances of making new friends will probably be enhanced if you go solo. Conducted tours are often a good choice for lone vacationers because you travel with a group and because the tour director handles all the details of reservations and transportation. Some tours are limited to single people, with further classifications according to age.

What not to look for—a husband. It's sad but true that very seldom do wedding bells chime tidings of a vacation romance that actually ''took.'' As with adult vaccinations the reason few vacation romances take is that many of the men at resorts are already immune—they have the Ideal Girl back home. Men on vacation are looking for fun—for someone to have a good time with. They feel free to ask anyone out, with no strings attached, for they are far from hometown gossip and may want to have a bit of a fling. You, too, have a chance to expand your knowledge of people, to break out of a rut. But be casual about it, be yourself, don't

346

lower your standards just because you're on vacation. If he's really interested, he'll call you again, and then you can judge each other in more prosaic surroundings. If he's just having a fling, you won't get hurt, and you'll have a wonderful memory of fun.

What to wear en route. Although travel ads often show glamorous models descending from trains or planes in slender Sunday-best suits, a good suit is not the most practical attire for travel. That Sunday-best outfit is likely to be subject to more abuse in one train, bus, or plane trip than in six months of Sundays. Under the strain of toting heavy luggage, waiting in dirty terminals, and sitting in cramped seats, clothes get wrinkled, stretched, and soiled. If you eat en route, there's the added danger of food spills. All it takes is a sudden bump or lurch just as coffee is served and that lovely suit may be the victim of an unhappy accident.

The best bet for travel is a dark colored outfit with a comfortable crease-resistant A-line skirt plus a removable knit jacket or cardigan sweater. A sweater is particularly desirable on air trips, where the cabin temperature sometimes fluctuates. Well-cut pants suits are also practical travel wear. Pants are very comfortable, and they conveniently do away with the need for wearing delicate nylons, which are easily snagged by suitcases and other luggage.

❧ Travel Tips for Trains

In addition to regular coach seats, there are several other types of rail accommodations available for long trips. These usually must be reserved in advance. Many trains have special streamlined coaches with reclining seats that make them fairly comfortable for sleeping; these are available for a small additional charge. The least expensive accommodations with beds are Pullman cars, which have upper and lower berths, the lower berths costing more. A roomette, which contains a washbasin and toilet and a bed you can let down yourself, costs a little more than a lower berth. Larger versions

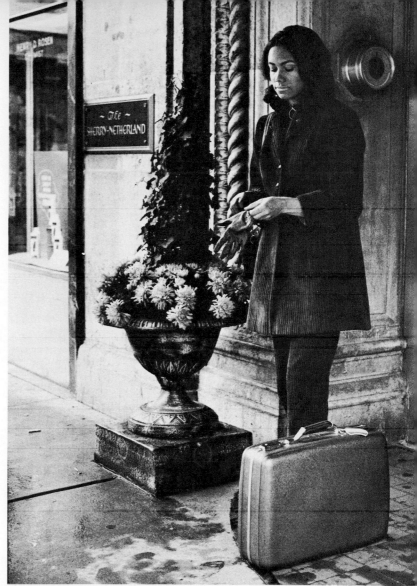

B. D. Unsworth

are bedrooms, compartments, and drawing rooms, which hold up to two, three, or four persons, respectively.

Managing your luggage. The secret of easy travel is to avoid taking too much luggage—never more than you can carry if you don't want to risk being stranded when no porter service is available. A redcap or porter is handy as a guide if you are in a large, unfamiliar station. He will steer you quickly through the labyrinth of tunnels and find you a seat on your train, determining your correct

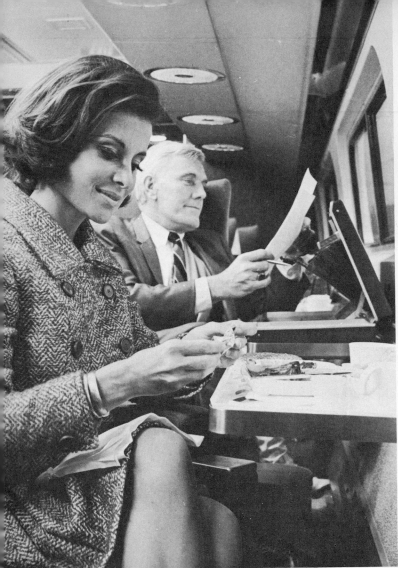

Courtesy of Penn Central Railroad

usually puts large suitcases on shelves in the rear of the car unless they fit under the seat; an overnight bag is kept handy for your nighttime needs. A roomette or compartment has space for hand luggage. Large or heavy pieces (up to 150 pounds) can be shipped free if you check them at the baggage room at the station. Be sure that all luggage bears your name and address—inside as well as outside—to guard against mishaps.

Mealtime manners. You can bring a box lunch or eat in the dining car, where prices will be somewhat higher than usual restaurant prices. Some trains have snack bars, which are less elegant and less expensive. Most have someone who goes from car to car selling sandwiches and beverages. Eating in a dining car is similar to eating in a restaurant except that you write out your order. Also, people are more likely to chat with each other in a dining car than in a restaurant.

Pullman etiquette. Because the lower berth passenger pays a higher fare, he has the privilege of riding forward during the day. The passenger in the upper berth rides backward unless the lower-berth passenger offers to share his seat with him, which a considerate traveler will do.

When the berths are made up, the seats can't be used. At night if your berth hasn't been made up by about ten o'clock, you might ask your seatmate if he would mind if you asked the porter to do so. A passenger who wishes to stay up later can go to the club car or observation car. These are usually at the rear of the train. You ring for the porter, and while you are waiting for your berth to be made up, you can move to an empty seat or to another car, or you can take your toilet articles to the ladies' room and prepare for bed. If you have an upper berth, you must ring for the porter to place the ladder for you. A passenger is not allowed to move a ladder, even if it is right across the aisle.

Once you are in your berth, you close the curtains and undress, using the hangers and net

accommodation if you have a reservation. In most larger cities redcaps receive a standard fee of 35 cents for each piece of luggage, regardless of its size or the distance it is carried. If you'd rather tote your own, you need feel no qualms about politely refusing a redcap's services.

Don't let your luggage become a nuisance—to you or to anyone else. You are entitled to half the overhead luggage rack by your seat. If this is not room enough, ask the conductor where you can put the rest. Don't leave it in the aisle. In a Pullman the porter hammocks provided for your clothes. If you must leave your berth during the night, you will wear a robe (or your coat) and will take your valuables with you. Leave the curtains open and the light on so that you can find the right berth when you return.

In the morning you usually dress first, call the porter for the ladder if you have an upper, and then go to wash. Be sure that all personal articles are removed from your berth before you go to breakfast, because it will probably be folded up by the time you return.

Other services a porter will perform if requested: call you at a specific time, bring a pillow or a table for writing, shine your shoes, send letters or telegrams. When you reach your destination, he will brush your coat, take care of your luggage, and help you off the train. You will tip him 50 cents to $1 for a night berth (more for special service), $1 to $1.50 in a roomette or compartment, slightly less per night for longer trips.

❦ Traveling by Bus

Long-distance travel by bus is popular because it is less expensive and because it often

Courtesy of Union Pacific Railroad

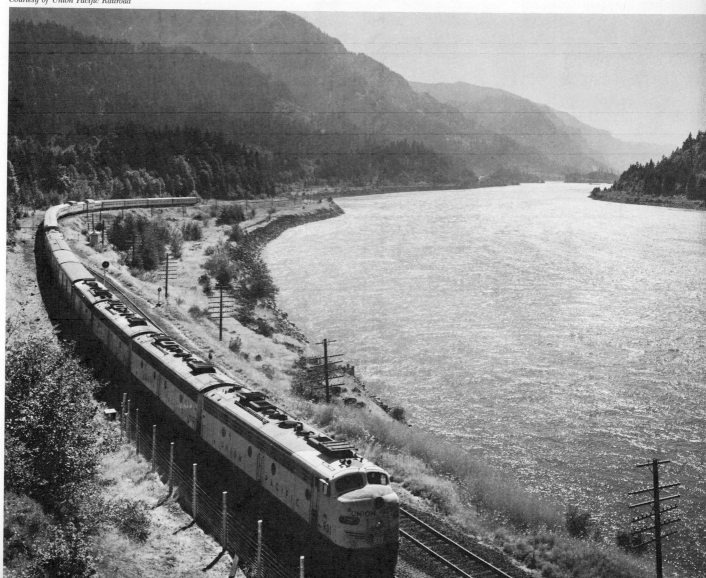

allows you to see more interesting scenery than the freight-yard end of towns. Reservations are made in advance for most long-distance buses, although no reservations are required for most intercity buses that leave regularly every hour or so.

Etiquette for bus travelers boils down pretty much to being considerate of the driver and of other passengers. Don't disturb the driver by talking to him unnecessarily, and do take with you a small bag that contains everything you'll need during the trip. No driver will appreciate the backbreaking job of trying to extricate your suitcase from the luggage compartment because you forgot your makeup kit. Be considerate of other travelers by not taking too much time at wayside stops, by not disturbing sleepers at nighttime, and if you smoke, by being careful that your smoke and ashes do not annoy others.

❦ Airplane Travel Tips

Most air flights require reservations, which can be made through a travel agent or at the airline terminal. At the time you make your reservation, check the amount of baggage allowed on the flight and whether meals will be served. Complimentary meals are served at meal hours on all first-class flights and on many tourist flights. If they are not, bring something to eat or purchase a box lunch at the airport. You will also want to inquire about transportation to the airport. Generally there is a bus or limousine service that leaves from the airline terminal or from some specified central place in the city. The charge for this is usually much less than the cost of a taxi.

Checking in at the airport. First you take your luggage to the desk to be weighed, if necessary. (If a porter carries your luggage, look for a sign specifying a standard porter's fee. If there's no sign to guide you, tip him 25 cents for each bag, more if he's especially pleasant or helpful. No one else at the airport need be tipped—*never* tip a stewardess or other uniformed airline employee.) Three pieces of luggage may be shipped free on any class flight in the continental United States. Weight is no longer considered. The size of the suitcases is the only concern, and these limits are quite generous—the combined length, height, and depth of the largest suitcase may be up to 62 inches, the next largest may be as large as 55 inches,

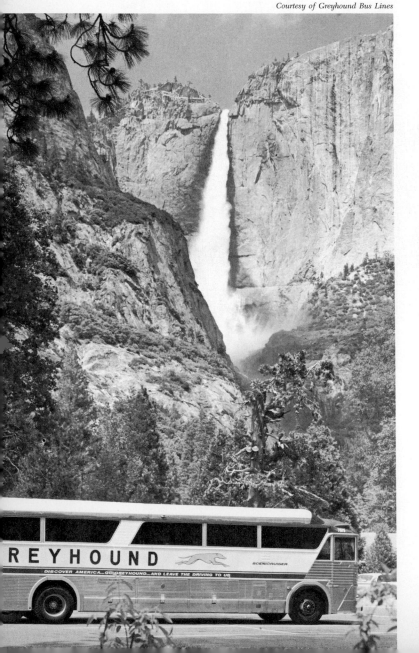

Courtesy of Greyhound Bus Lines

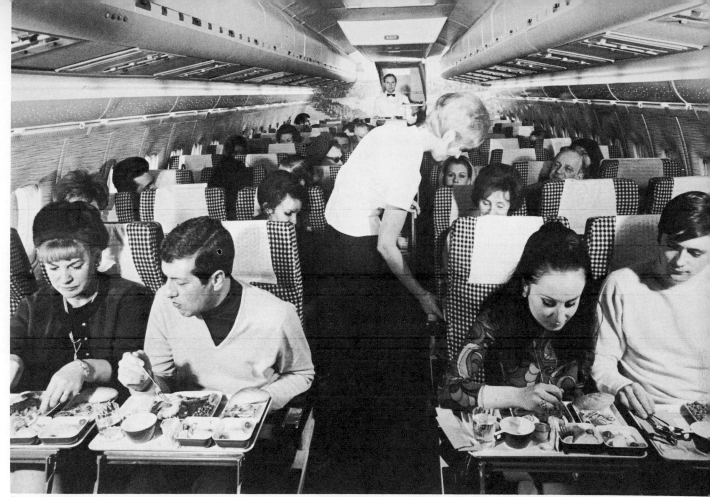

Courtesy of BOAC

and the third can have a 45-inch total for dimensions. An extra charge is made for suitcases that exceed these limits or for more than three suitcases.

Suitcases will be stowed in the plane's baggage compartment, but you are allowed to keep with you your coat, camera, binoculars, and a small bag for personal grooming essentials. Many women prefer to use a large purse for this purpose. The attendant at the desk will verify your ticket and give you checks for your baggage. Then you will wait while your plane is being loaded. Be sure you know your flight number, because this will be announced over the loudspeaker when your plane is ready. Then you will go to the gate specified and board the plane.

Which seat? If reserved seats are available, the attendant who verifies your ticket will ask you to choose your seat and will tag your ticket with your seat number. If seats are not reserved, you will choose your seat when you get on the plane. In either case, you will be wise to arrive early so that you have a better choice. Seats in the rear of the plane have the best view but may be bumpy in bad weather. Seats over the wing offer a smoother ride. If you suffer from motion sickness, you'll be wise to take a preventive pill before you leave. For emergencies special plastic bags are in a pocket on the back of the seat in front of you.

Mealtime manners. Despite cramped facilities, delicious meals are served on planes. If the

351

flight is at all rough, it is considered perfectly proper to tuck your napkin under your chin.

After you land. Your baggage may be claimed at the baggage enclosure, where you surrender your baggage checks. If you are planning a return trip by air, you will be wise to check your return reservation while you are waiting for your luggage.

Experienced travelers often mark each of their suitcases with a small but easily recognized symbol (an initial, a small stripe, a star, or other design) of brightly colored adhesive tape.

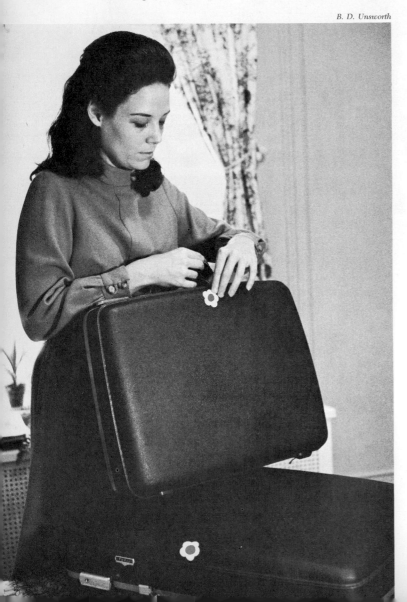

B. D. Unsworth

Anything unique makes it easy to distinguish your blue suitcases from the multitude of similar blue bags and helps avoid confusion and mix-ups. Porters particularly appreciate this sort of identification device.

❦ Shipboard Etiquette

If a sea voyage is in your plans, you should make your reservations months in advance, especially if you plan to go during the peak vacation season. Reservations can be made through your travel agent. He can also arrange for your table and deck-chair assignments. (You will have your choice of early or late sittings for meals and of the location of your deck chair, sunny spots usually being preferred.) As soon as you embark, you should check with the stewards in charge of these services to confirm the reservations. You will sit at the same table throughout the trip, unless you want to change for some reason. The livelier crowd usually prefers second sitting—breakfast is later and the time between dining and dancing is shorter!

On shipboard all the luggage that you will need during the voyage can be kept in your cabin. The ship's advertising material will probably contain information about the type of clothes to be worn, and your travel agent can also advise you about what to take. If you share a cabin, you will want to be careful about usurping too much space.

A resort atmosphere prevails on shipboard. Most people are friendly and congenial, and you will be expected to chat casually with them.

Tipping is usually done at the end of a voyage or weekly if the cruise is a long one. Ten percent of your fare is the usual amount to count on for a transatlantic trip. (Those traveling first class tip proportionately more.)

- Cabin steward—$1 per day
- Night steward—$1 per day (if you utilized his services, such as coffee and sandwiches at 2 a.m.)
- Dining steward—$1 per day
- Deck steward—$2 to $3 (tipping in advance may result in a more desirable position)

352

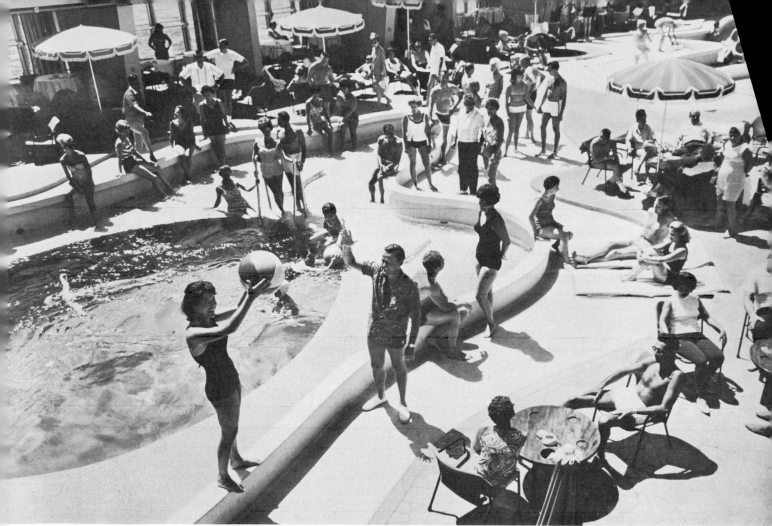

❦ Hotels and Motels

The most luxurious way to travel is by ship. You have the choice of relaxing or participating in a whirl of activities.

In this country most hotels and motels operate on the European plan, which means that rates are quoted without meals. Often resort hotels quote rates on the American plan, which means that three meals (two at some beach resorts) are included. If you are traveling on a limited budget, don't hesitate to ask about a minimum-rate room. In a large metropolitan hotel, you won't ask to see your room before you engage it, but if you find it unsatisfactory, you won't be out of order to ask if something else is available. In small hotels and in motels you will probably want to look at your room before registering. When a woman signs the register,

she includes either "Miss" or "Mrs." before her name. You are expected to tell the clerk how long you will be staying. If you are merely staying overnight at a motel or tourist home, you usually pay when you register, particularly if you plan to leave early the next morning. At a hotel it is more customary to pay when you leave.

A bellhop will usually take your luggage and show you to your room. The standard tip is 25 cents for each bag, but not less than 50 cents. Pay him separately for extra service. Bellhops who deliver telegrams, newspapers, or small items to a room usually receive 25 cents; 50 cents is given for larger deliveries. Any such room service can be obtained by phone by asking the operator.

Hotel manners. When you are staying overnight at a hotel, you should bring some sort of suitcase, even if all your personal needs can fit in your purse. Hotel management is inclined to view with suspicion any young woman without luggage. Similarly, for the sake of your good name, you would not invite a man into your room alone nor go to his alone. Most people, unless they have a suite with a sitting

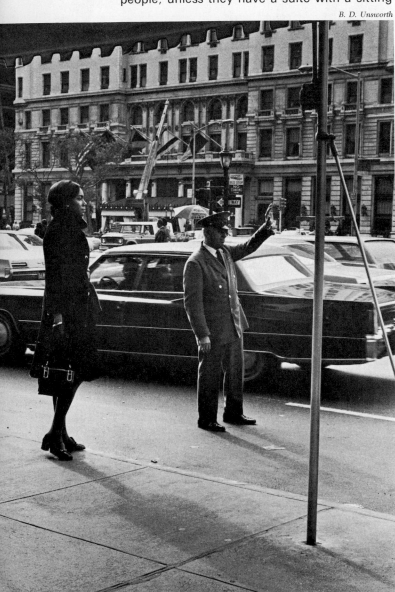

B. D. Unsworth

room, entertain in one of the public lounges or dining rooms.

Incidentally, when a secretary or other female employee is traveling with an executive, reservations are requested for two single rooms for "Mr. John Craig and secretary." This indicates to the hotel staff that the two rooms should be on different floors or at least not next to each other. If work is to be done, the secretary goes to her employer's room. He does not go to hers.

Metropolitan hotels are quite formal, and usually the guests do not chat together or greet each other. Resorts, on the other hand, are much less formal, and guests are expected to introduce themselves and be friendly.

When you leave, please don't collect any of the hotel property as "souvenirs." Although many respectable people consider this good sport, walking off with hotel towels, ashtrays, stationery, or other supplies is stealing just as much as if these items were taken from a store.

Tipping. Other types of tipping that you might run into during your stay at a hotel are the following:

• Room service waiter—15 percent of the check but not less than 25 cents. This can be paid in cash or, if you sign the check indicating that the bill is to be added to your hotel bill, you can note that a certain amount is to be added as a tip for the waiter.

• Chambermaid—no tip for a very short stay, probably $2 for four or five days (leave it on the dresser or under the pillow). At a resort hotel the maid is usually tipped when you leave, at the rate of about 50 cents a day.

• Doorman—25 cents if he finds a taxi for you, more if he lets you leave your car near the entrance for a short time or has it parked for you. If he unloads your luggage and carries it into the lobby, tip 25 cents per bag ($1.00 tops).

❦ Safety First

Travel is always an adventure—full of new experiences and surprises. The knowledgeable traveler takes everything in stride, but she also takes a few simple precautions to prevent unhappy experiences and to make sure that even unpleasant surprises leave her unharried.

Traveler's checks. If you are planning to carry large sums of money while you are traveling, you'll be wise to use Traveler's Checks. These can be purchased from your local bank or American Express office. They are easily converted into money by countersigning at the time you wish to cash one. Since your second signature is proof that the Traveler's Check belongs to you, it should never be countersigned beforehand. Follow the instructions for recording serial numbers in case of loss or theft.

Protection for valuables. If you have any large amount of money or valuables with you, you will be wise to leave them in the office safe if you are staying at a resort or hotel. On shipboard you can leave them with the purser. Most hotels caution you to keep your room locked at all times for the sake of your privacy as well as your valuables. Never leave anything precious in your room when you go out.

Strangers. Mother has surely warned you about strangers, and you'll do well to remember her advice. It's fine to be friendly and pleasant to fellow travelers, to chat with your seatmate in a train or bus if he is in the mood to talk. (You won't, of course, be forward or force conversation on someone who'd rather keep to himself.) To avoid embarrassing situations, keep the conversation impersonal and don't obligate yourself in any way by accepting favors. If a stranger offers to pay for your meal or to give you a lift in his car, it's better to thank him but refuse politely. Most strangers mean well, but every Little Red Riding Hood may not have a handy hunter to come to her rescue if the stranger turns out to be a wicked wolf.

Need help? If you have lost your wallet or run up against some other difficult problem while you are traveling, you can consult a policeman or the Travelers Aid Society, which usually has

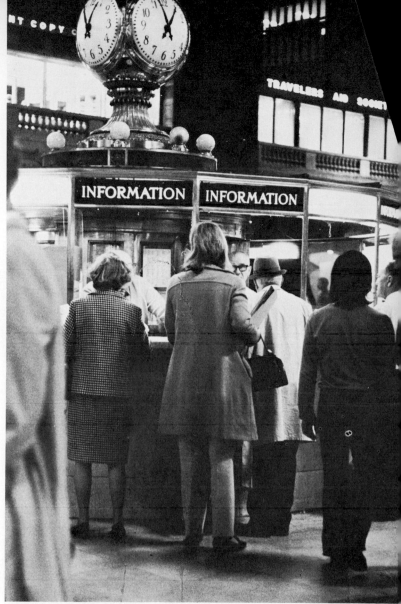

B. D. Unsworth

a desk in large stations and terminals. If you are on a train or plane, the conductor or stewardess will help you. It's always best to seek help only from an authorized person.

❦ Guest Etiquette

You'll be a welcome guest in someone else's home if you can show the consideration and thoughtfulness you'd like a guest to show in

355

your own home. This means being careful about the furniture—no suitcases on beds (the floor is always safe), no wet glasses on wooden tables, no wet bathing suits on chairs. When there are dishes to be done or other work in the offing, the thoughtful guest pitches in. She also praises the cooking, even dutifully downing the turnips she abhors. She wouldn't think of raiding the refrigerator and accepts her hostess's preference in records, television, or radio programs.

If you're visiting at the family home of a friend, you'll win her parents' appreciation by relating complimentary stories about her. (You can discreetly skip any stories that might embarrass her, no matter how hilarious they seem.) Enter enthusiastically into her plans, and show your appreciation of her friends. You shouldn't accept a date, however, unless you're sure your hostess has one, too.

Find out when you're expected to rise in the morning and make an effort to get up on time, taking your turn in the bathroom as quickly as possible so that you won't interfere with others. A hostess appreciates guests who stick to family timetables, particularly regarding meal hours.

You should also abide by family bedtimes. If the hour grows late, you should gracefully let the conversation ease off at intervals in case your hostess wants to suggest retiring. Resist the urge for a midnight swim, a wee-hours walk in the rain, or any other unorthodox whim, because you would not want to upset family routine any more than necessary.

When the time comes to leave, do so on schedule. Don't be tempted to linger. The menus and weekly routine were planned around a certain length visit. Though your hostess may say with sincere sorrow, ''Oh, I wish you didn't have to leave,'' exit smiling.

A thank-you note for any visit of overnight or longer should be sent within a day or two after you return. If you didn't take a hostess gift with you, it would be thoughtful to send something at that time—a record or book you had discussed or something else pertaining to your hostess's home or interests.

❦ Packing Tips

The experienced traveler knows the wisdom of traveling light. One woman who is noted for her attractive appearance spent two months in Europe with a total wardrobe of three basic dresses and a limited assortment of carefully selected accessories. When you are choosing clothes for travel, be guided by their versatility, soil resistance, and wrinkle resistance. Next time you take a trip, try the following suggestions for organizing your suitcase efficiently.

• Put jewelry in pockets of a sectional silverware bag to prevent scratching and scattering. When the bag is rolled up, it fits compactly in a corner.

• Use plastic jars for cosmetics. Store spillables in plastic bags for extra insurance.

• Use a plastic bag (or shower cap) for washcloth and toothbrush in case they are still damp at packing time. Carry an extra plastic bag in case things you have washed out don't dry in time.

• To save stockings, tuck them in gloves and socks, put gloves and socks in shoes; put shoes in plastic bags.

• Arrange your clothes in this order: shoes and heavy items on the bottom, then lingerie, accessories and blouses, suit, and dresses on top.

• If you are making several overnight stops, keep your nighttime articles together where they are easy to get at. Grooming items can all be kept in one plastic bag so that they can be carried to the bathroom easily.

• Prevent creases by padding shoulders and folds with plenty of tissue paper or, better yet, use plastic bags. The large dry cleaners' bags are especially good for layering between outfits. Plastic won't become flimsy the way tissue paper will, and a large-sized bag allows you to lift out top layers undisturbed when you must dig for something in the bottom of the bag.

• To pack a suit, fold the skirt lengthwise with the hem end hanging out over the side of the suitcase. Place the upper half of the jacket in the suitcase on top of the skirt at the waistband end and fold the sleeves across. Now fold the hem end of the skirt over the jacket top; then the bottom of the jacket up over the skirt. The resulting layers of skirt top, jacket top, skirt hem, jacket bottom act to cushion each other and to prevent creases.

This same principle works with dresses, blouse sleeves, and slacks—wrap one garment around and over another for added cushioning and no sharp creases will form.

• Include several clip clothespins. When clipped over wire hangers, they make excellent skirt hangers or dryers for hosiery and other wash. Take some sturdy cord, and you can easily rig up a bathtub washline when necessary.

• Nice to have—travel iron, travel alarm clock.

• Extras for emergencies: your own version of a first-aid kit with aspirin and indigestion remedy, spoon and bottle opener, sewing kit (plus a roll of cellophane tape for loose hems), also scissors, a small flashlight, a miniature clothes brush, shoe polish, razor.

Before you begin your packing, make a list of all the things you will take. This makes the job of assembling all the items much easier and, if you carry the list in your suitcase, provides you with a ready reference at homecoming time to make sure nothing has been left behind.

How could you make your life more interesting? What new activities could you try? What different places could you visit? Plan to spend your next free weekend doing something special. Perhaps it can be a sight-seeing trip, maybe a lunch at an interesting restaurant, an evening at the theater, or possibly just a try at a different sport. Any worthwhile change of place or pace will put more zest in your life.

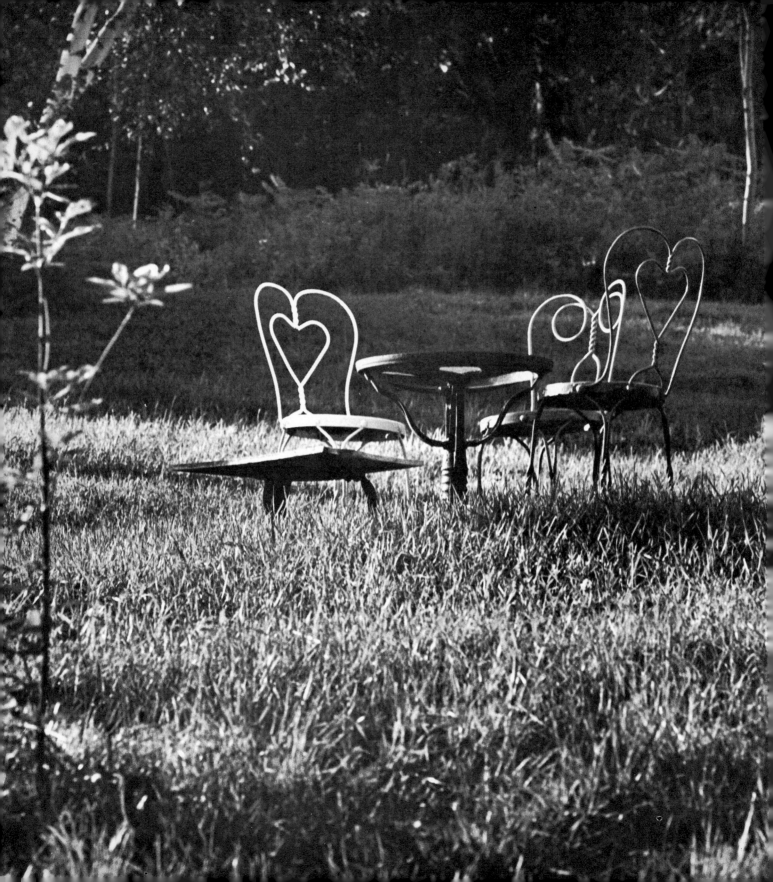

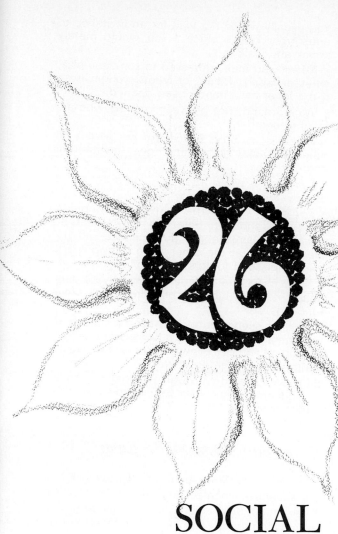

26

SOCIAL GRACES

A thorough grounding in the basic rules of etiquette is just as vital to the success of a business girl as knowing which key is which is to a typist. If you are to appear poised and socially mature, manners must be something you just do, something so second nature that you don't have to think about them. Being constantly aware of the situations that call for special actions and taking the trouble to follow correct procedures will result in a smoothness that sets you off as a cultivated, well-bred young lady—a high reputation that cannot be over-estimated. Another important consideration is that good manners make a person vastly easier to get along with, whether at work or at play. They are also often taken as an important gauge of personality, for good manners are an indication of other virtues, and lack of them is often considered an indication of other lacks.

There are many small courtesies that rate high when it comes to making a good impression. They are rules that everybody knows but which, sadly enough, are not always observed. In many ways the little courtesies are far more important than the fancier rules of etiquette. It's nice to know how to eat an artichoke or what to wear on what occasion, but these are bits of information friends are always flattered to share with you if you are at a loss. Far from being critical of you in such a situation, they'll simply realize you're doing something you haven't done before, and they'll admire your sense in asking for help. But let a girl be lacking in the respect and consideration for others that those little courtesies demonstrate so clearly and she's likely to find her friends rapidly cooling toward her. The simple truth is that anyone who genuinely respects and considers others will observe the little rules as a matter of course. For most people such respect is far more important than being able to display the most elegant of manners. And such respect is the only guide you'll have in situations for which there are no rules.

Here, then are some of the little courtesies you should always observe.

• Do not interrupt someone who is speaking.
• Respect the privacy of others. Knock on a closed door and wait for a response before entering. (Business is an exception, however.

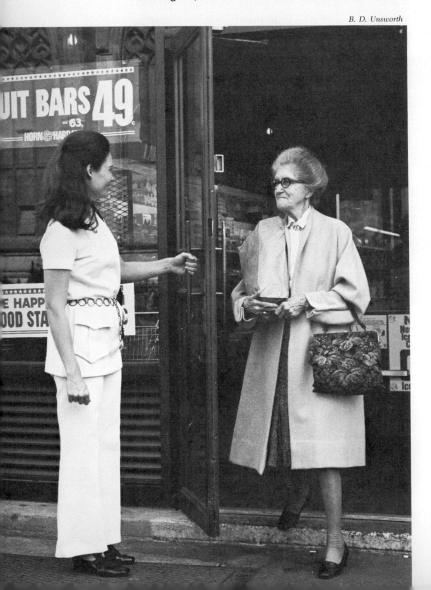

B. D. Unsworth

You usually would not wait for an invitation to enter your boss's office. You would merely knock and walk in.)

• Never read mail addressed to someone else, whether family, friend, or fellow worker, even if the letter has already been opened.
• Walk around, not between, people who are talking together.
• When in a hurry, be careful not to cut off others who may be strolling down the street or corridor.
• Don't push when attempting to enter a bus or elevator.
• Avoid making a scene of any sort in a public place—no shouts to friends in a restaurant, no noisy complaints about poor service, no unpleasant digs at the other team during sports events, no loud to-do's in the office.
• Don't chew gum except at extremely informal affairs, *never* at business or more formal social functions.
• Observe silence during a meeting, speech, or performance. Jokes and other side remarks or rattling of papers disturbs others and is discourteous to those on stage.
• Cover a sneeze or cough with your hand or a handkerchief and turn your head away from others near you.

❧ Introductions Made Easy

The important thing about introductions is that we should not neglect to make them. While there are many technicalities regarding the exact wording, few are vital. The fact that you make an introduction is often more important than the precise words you choose. Introductions should always be made whenever you talk with someone who does not know the others with you. If you are with some friends and another acquaintance joins you, you should introduce her to the others. If you are walking with someone and pass an acquaintance on the street, you need not bother to make introductions unless you stop and chat. If you are hostess at a large gathering, introduce a guest to a few people to make him feel at ease. Don't attempt to have him meet everyone at once.

360

Wording the introduction. The basic rule to remember is that *the person you mention* First *is the one you are honoring.*

• A man is presented to a woman: "Mrs. Hendricks, this is Mr. Briggs" or "Debby Campbell, I'd like you to meet Jerry Jackson." In each case the woman's name is mentioned first. (An exception to this rule is usually made in business when a woman employee is presented to an important executive of the firm. In such situations respect is shown to the executive by mentioning him first: "Mr. Gilbert, this is our new receptionist, Ann Bartlett.")

When you are introducing members of the *same sex,* the guiding factors are age, rank, or degree of distinction. Again, the person to be honored is mentioned first.

• Present the younger to the older person: "Mr. Elder, may I introduce Mr. Young."
• Present the lower in rank to the higher: "Mr. Aldridge (vice-president of your firm or another firm), this is Mr. Adams" (a junior executive of either your firm or of another firm).
• Present a less distinguished person to a more celebrated person: "Miss Celebrity, may I present Miss Smith?"
• Present a layman to a clergyman: "Father Higgins, Mr. Hudson." Catholic priests are called "Father." Protestant clergymen should be addressed as "Mister" or if they have a degree, as "Doctor." A few Episcopalian clergymen are called "Father." For Jewish rabbis, "Rabbi Stein, this is Mr. Hudson," is the correct form.

Usually you would honor your mother and father by presenting others to them—your employer and instructors and professors, as well as your other acquaintances. "Dad, this is my friend Carol Welles." "Mother and Dad, I'd like to introduce Professor Carlson." The only exception would be some very distinguished person.

When two people of the same sex are approximately the same in age, rank, and prominence, it doesn't really matter which name is mentioned first.

The following forms of introduction are all acceptable.

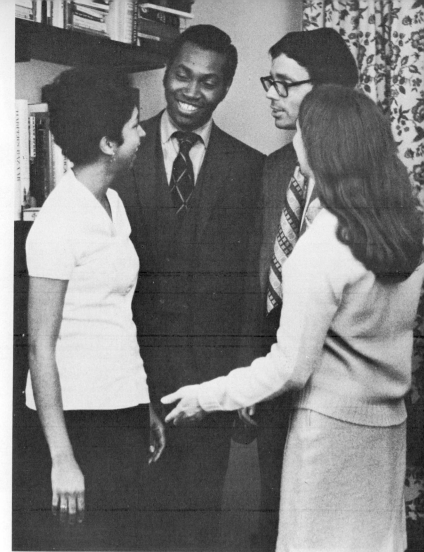

B. D. Unsworth

• "Sally Green, Herb Thompson."
• "Sally Green, this is Herb Thompson."
• "Sally, this is Herb Thompson. Herb, Sally Green."

More formal but equally correct are:

• "May I present . . . ?"
• "May I introduce . . . ?"
• "I should like to introduce . . ."

If you are not sure whether they are acquainted, you can forestall any embarrassment by saying:

• "Sally, do you know Herb Thompson?"
• "Sally, have you met Herb Thompson?"

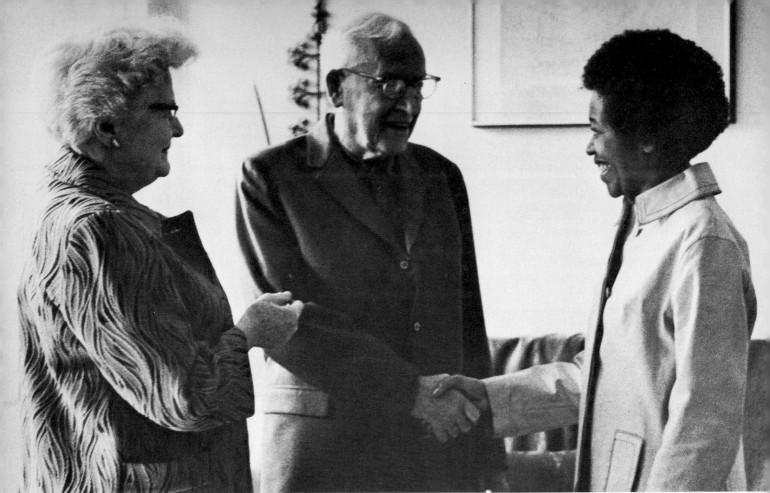

Mention both names because even though they may have been introduced before, one of them may have forgotten the other's name. Thanks to your tact, the lapse of memory won't have to be confessed.

Acknowledging an introduction. The best acknowledgment to an introduction is "How do you do." Mentioning the person's name in your reply helps fix it in your mind. With people your own age, you might reply informally, "Hello, Karen" or even "Hi."

If you have heard a great deal about someone and are especially glad to meet him, you might add sincerely, "It's a pleasure to meet you," or "I'm very glad to have the opportunity to meet you." You'll want to avoid such crass

phrases as "Pleased to meet you" or "Charmed, I'm sure."

In the rush-rush of business, your employer is not likely to introduce you to many visitors, even if you are his private secretary. If he does, you should merely smile and say, "How do you do, Mr. Jones" (even if he was introduced to you as Dick Jones), and you should quickly return to your work unless the men have something further to say to you.

Shaking hands. Shaking hands when introduced is not quite as customary for women as it once was. Although a man always shakes hands when introduced to another man, he may merely nod to a woman, and he will shake hands only if she offers hers. Usually you do not offer your hand to someone your own age or to another woman unless she is considerably older. You should, however, be alert to the possibility and be ready to shake hands if the other person offers. If you are introduced to an older man or woman, you will want to extend your hand. Let your handshake be brief, firm, and friendly, neither a painful grasp nor a limp, unresponsive one.

If you are wearing gloves at the time of an introduction, it is much better to shake hands with your gloves on than to delay the proceedings by hurriedly fumbling to pull off your glove. When possible, it is preferable to remove the right glove as a mark of sincerity and respect for the other person.

When do you rise? While it is proper for a man to rise whenever he is introduced to someone, a girl is not expected to rise unless she is introduced to an older woman, an elderly man, or to someone of great distinction whom she wishes to honor. However, whenever you are a hostess or are in a hostess situation (such as when you greet your boss's visitors), you will probably want to stand up to welcome callers. When in doubt, you can't go wrong by getting to your feet.

The same rule about rising for introductions can be applied in social situations to persons entering a room in which you are seated. Again, a young woman need not rise except for an older woman (especially if she is a housemother or instructor or the mother of one of your friends), a much older man, or a very distinguished person. In the office you would not be likely to rise unless someone very important came to your desk specifically to talk with you. Neither should you expect men to stand up when you enter an office. Convenience overrules chivalry in the business world.

❦ Watch Your Smoke

Medical tests show that there is a definite connection between smoking and certain lung diseases. Smoking is so harmful to the human body that federal law requires that a warning be printed on every package of cigarettes.

Still, many people enjoy smoking enough to ignore its hazards. If you do smoke, remember that where there's smoke, there's often ire—unless the smoker takes care. Those who smoke are seldom aware of the annoyance that this habit can cause.

Smoking often evokes frowns, not because it is harmful but because of the nuisance it creates. Tobacco odor can be very annoying to nonsmokers, and the danger of accidents is ever present. A smoker is literally playing with fire. If you smoke, you should be very careful and very considerate of the feelings of those around you.

B. D. Unsworth

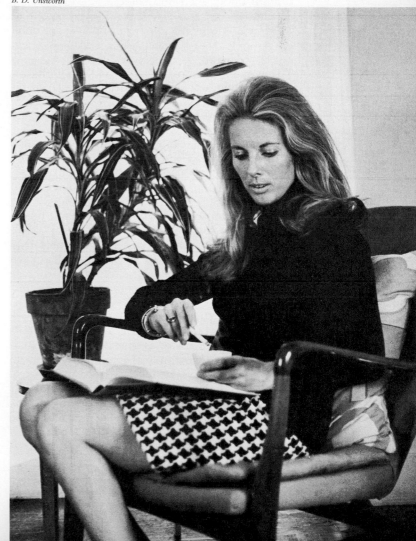

Careless handling of cigarettes is the Number One cause of fires. The office smoker who hasn't a good ash tray with secure resting places for her cigarette should hie herself to the nearest dime store and buy one. A rolling cigarette gathers no friends—especially if it happens to scorch an important report, a desk, or a brand-new suit.

A few good rules to follow:

• At the office never smoke in the presence of customers or visitors, even if smoking is allowed at your desk.

• Put out your cigarette before going into your boss's office to take dictation or to discuss work.

• Between puffs remove a cigarette from between your lips. A cigarette drooper or the person who talks with a cigarette in her mouth looks undignified and cheap.

• Always snuff out your cigarette carefully. Smoldering butts give off an unpleasant odor.

• Empty your ash tray often. A heap of lipstick-smeared butts is a definite eyesore. However, be sure matches and old butts are completely out before putting them in the wastebasket.

• When you smoke, air the room out occasionally to counteract stale tobacco odor.

• Never, never smoke in an elevator or other small area. The smoke from your cigarette will become obnoxious even to other smokers.

• Avoid blowing smoke in other people's faces, and take the prevailing winds—or drafts—into consideration so that your smoke won't trail in someone's direction.

• Watch your ashes. Don't keep others hypnotized as the ash on your cigarette grows longer and longer.

• Don't gesture with a cigarette. That is a sure way to flick ashes where they may do damage.

• Avoid playing with your cigarette. Affected mannerisms and excessive hand movements give a smoker away as unsophisticated.

• Tote your own supply of cigarettes and smoke them. A cigarette moocher is no joy to have around.

• Guard against cigarette stains by holding the lighted end up so that smoke does not trail through your fingers. (Tobacco stains usually can be bleached out with lemon juice.)

❦ Times of Good Cheer

Office parties. Christmas, a wedding, a lamented resignation—throughout the year there are a goodly number of office parties. Some may be merely department cocktail parties at the close of the day. Others may be elaborate dinner-dance affairs. Good spirits soar freely, and so do the alcoholic ones. This is a time when all is good cheer, yet it's also a time when each employee is on display—an occasion that influences management's opinion of staff members and provides grist for office gossip for weeks to come. Your most charming, ladylike manner is called for.

WHAT DO YOU WEAR? For a normal after-work party you would wear your usual business clothes. If you are the honored guest, you might wear your prettiest outfit, but certainly nothing more dressy. Even a company dinner-dance would not be the occasion for a low-cut dressy cocktail dress. A better choice would be a simple dressy style with a discreet neckline. Let the festive touch come more from elegant fabric or jewelry than from cut.

HOW DO YOU ACT? Act basically the same as you do when you're in the office. Of course, the talk is gay and business is forgotten, but you will show the same deference to those above you and the same dignity and poise that is expected of you on the job.

Management is more likely to mingle with lesser employees at these times. If the man in the formidable office guarded by a gauntlet of secretaries should happen to chat with you, don't let yourself become shy or embarrassed. The great man must talk to someone, and perhaps he feels a little uncomfortable out of his usual office element. Be cordial and friendly and *interested.* Usually part of the reason he has become so successful is that he is a charming person. This is a good opportunity to make a favorable impression, but don't overdo it.

Occasionally some executive may, under the mellowing effects of the occasion, become quite chummy. He may even suggest that those he is with call him by his first name. Although they may do so for that evening, the status shifts back to normal on the next working day, and the "Mister" and other usual formalities apply once more. Just remember: keep the party apart from the job.

TO DRINK OR NOT TO DRINK? A company party may have all the earmarks of a social occasion, but you're still under the scrutiny of those who control your business future. You can't be sure how severely they may judge your behavior if you get high. They may very well laugh at your antics yet mentally cross you off for any job that calls for business drinking while you are representing the company. Play it safe. If a drink or two means you might say or do anything your sober business judgment would censor, better abstain. If you're sure of your capacity, join the crowd, but safeguard your better judgment by setting yourself a quota, particularly if the drinks are unlimited.

If you don't want to drink, ask for a ginger ale or a Seven-Up—both resemble cocktails—or nurse one cocktail all evening so that when Fill-Em-Up Freddy comes your way, you can reply, "Still have some, thanks."

WHEN DO YOU GO HOME? Office parties have a way of becoming more sticky and more difficult as the hour grows later. Those who come off best usually leave fairly early in the evening.

Office luncheons. If a large group from the office holds a luncheon to celebrate some auspicious occasion, they will need to make a reservation. In some restaurants it's possible to obtain a menu in advance so that each person can sign up for her luncheon selection and can pay her money beforehand. If not, one girl usually takes care of the bill and collects from the others later.

A luncheon cocktail? The boss may have no objection, but he'll expect work as usual when you return. Before you indulge, consider whether you'll suffer aftereffects—drowsiness, carelessness, a loosened tongue, or emotional eruptions. If you're not sure of your immunity or if you have a busy afternoon ahead, you'd

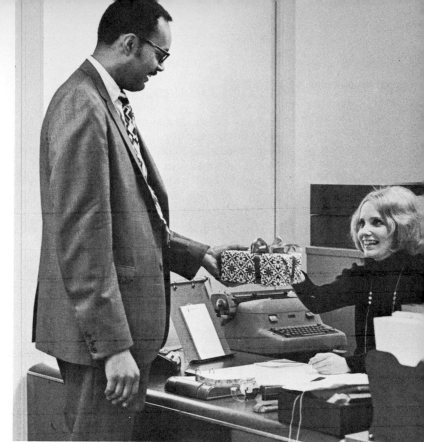

B. D. Unsworth

be wise to abstain. In addition, you won't want liquor on your breath if you have to meet the public.

Christmas etiquette at the office. Many companies give bonuses at Christmas. Some executives give presents to their secretaries. Whatever gift-giving occurs is done down the scale, not up. Employers are never given presents by staff members. You would, of course, probably want to send your boss a Christmas card. If he is married, it should be addressed to "Mr. and Mrs."

In many offices a list of employee addresses is prepared for those who wish to send Christmas cards. It is the custom some places for *everybody* to send cards to *everybody*; other places cards are sent only to those people you feel close to. Generally it would seem presumptuous for a secretary or clerk to send a card to the president of the company unless she really knows him.

❀ Social Drinking

Alcohol is customary at many social gatherings because it breaks down stiffness, relaxes inhibitions, boosts self-confidence, and stimulates friendly feelings. In this sense, drinks act as a social catalyst. But the drawbacks are many too, and it takes intelligence to prevent them from outweighing the advantages.

Tips for drinkers. Be an intelligent drinker and you'll get fun out of your drinks without the drawbacks. The first step is to know your limit—the amount you can consume without getting sick, suffering a hangover, or behaving in a way you would disapprove of afterwards. The second step is simply never to exceed your limit.

Another precaution is to avoid regular drinking, especially if you gain weight easily—alcohol is full of nutritionless, fat-building calories. Regular drinking can also result in dependence on alcohol. If your social life calls for frequent drinking, reduce the limit you allow yourself and occasionally refuse to drink just to exercise your willpower. Remember that the first sign of alcoholism isn't the quantity or regularity of your consumption but the feeling that you *must* have a drink.

The most important rule is never to mix drinking with driving. Take a bus or a cab, ask a friend to drive you home, or arrange to stay where you are—but don't drive, and don't ride with anyone else who has been drinking. Although a drinker may not sense the change, just one drink slows down reactions and can make the split-second difference between a fatal accident and a near miss. Don't let anyone persuade you otherwise. Statistics show that 50 percent of all fatal motor accidents involve drivers who have been drinking.[1] If you ignore this fact, you risk your life.

Tips for nondrinkers. If you don't want to drink, don't. You won't be breaking any rules of etiquette or endangering any friendships. The reason your host or friends urge you to drink is that they think you're missing something—not that they intend to disown you if you don't turn into an alcohol burner.

If your host insists on brewing a special concoction he's convinced you'll like, accept the drink graciously. To reject his special efforts to please you would be rude. Of course, you've already warned him that the drink may go to waste, so you're not obligated to try more than a sip or two.

Occasionally you'll run into the person who persists in urging you to have a drink. Although he's being rude, he probably honestly thinks drinking is essential to a good time.

[1] Accident Facts, *National Safety Council, 1968.*

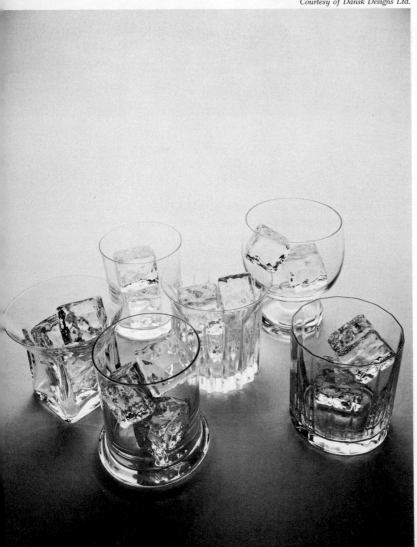

Courtesy of Dansk Designs Ltd.

Escape by excusing yourself and visiting the ladies' room; then insulate yourself by joining a group of people. Never let yourself be bludgeoned into drinking something you don't want. If worse comes to worst, you can always accept the drink, then nurse it along all evening so he'll have no excuse to bother you further.

🌱 Drugs

Undoubtedly you've heard plenty about drugs, but how much is truth and how much rumor? Scare stories abound, while friends who use drugs may minimize the risks because they want you to experiment also. Don't underestimate the temptation—it's not easy to be the will-powered loner while everyone else is part of the group. And it's even more difficult if you're not sure of the facts.

What, then, are the risks? Friends may tell you that marijuana (*pot*, or *grass*) is innocuous. But possession and use of this drug are illegal, and young people *are* being booked on these charges every day. And there may be nothing innocuous about the impurities (rat poison, in a recent case) added to this drug or to others when a crime syndicate wants to stretch a dwindling supply.

The ultimate risk of using drugs for kicks is addiction. Nearly everyone knows that heroin is addictive, but not all people realize that barbiturates also are habit-forming. Although amphetamines (*pep pills, diet pills, bennies, ups,* or *speed*), hashish, and marijuana are not themselves addictive, they can be a first step towards addiction to stronger drugs. Nearly all heroin addicts begin with marijuana. The drug initiate who gets bored with pot and seeks different, stronger kicks is very likely to go on to heroin.

LSD and similar drugs are not addictive, but their results are unpredictable. The hallucinations induced by these drugs can be terrifying; like any other bad experience, they can leave a scar. Cases of violence and even suicide during such hallucinations have been reported. Such effects can't be predicted, nor

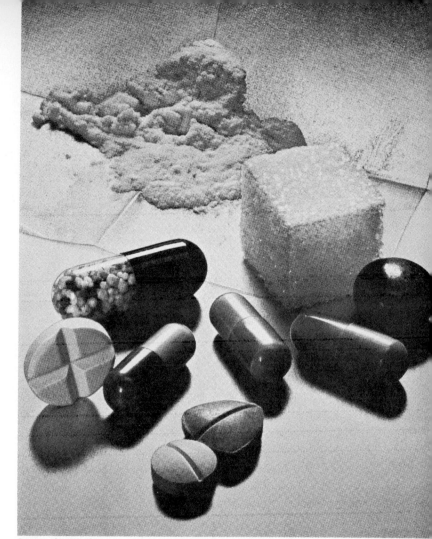

Courtesy of WGN, Chicago

can a person who's had one exhilarating "trip" be assured that his next one won't be a horror.

Even drugs that legally may be prescribed have dangers; that is why the law requires prescriptions. Overdoses of barbiturates are one of the leading causes of accidental death in this country. Amphetamines step up the metabolism but leave the user extremely nervous and fatigued when they wear off.

All drugs, including marijuana, are taboo for drivers for the same reasons that alcohol and driving don't mix. Coordination, sense perceptions, and judgment are all affected. Doctors usually warn patients not to drive when they are taking prescribed drugs, but no warning is issued with drugs that are obtained illegally. Public-interest campaigns have spread the word about drinking and driving, but not so with drugs. It's up to you to remember that riding with a driver who's ''high'' is as dangerous as riding with one who is drunk.

✿ *Manners and Men*

There are many rules of etiquette governing the behavior of men and women. Some are delightful gestures of gallantry that make a girl feel

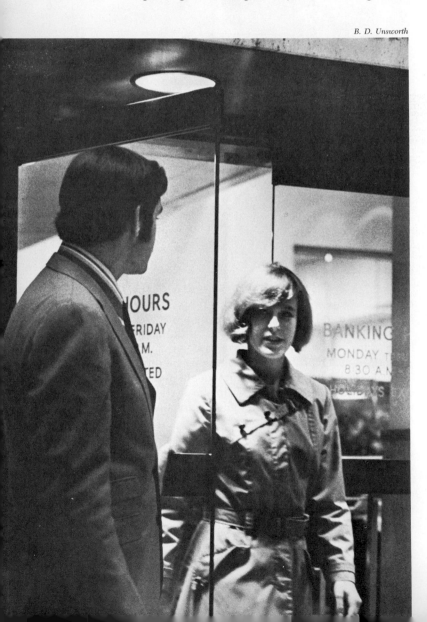

B. D. Unsworth

special and appreciated, such as when your date opens a door or pulls out a chair for you. Some are, however, a bit inconvenient at certain times. Maybe he's digging for change at the precise moment he should be helping you on with your coat. Maybe in your rush to make curtain time he didn't stop to run around to open the car door for you. Don't make him conscious of his lapse. Manners in the social world, as well as in business, often succumb to convenience. By all means, give a man a chance to show off his gallantry. No man appreciates the brusque I-can-do-it-myself attitude of the girl who beats him to the doorknob. Even in the office, nine times out of ten, a male associate will be pleased to hold a door for a girl if she gives him half a chance. But no charming lady will stand there waiting in an obviously expectant pose so that he feels like an oaf if he's preoccupied or his timing isn't fast enough for these little things.

Good manners are born of consideration and thoughtfulness. They are not something artificial we hold up on display merely so that we can say, ''See what lovely manners I have.'' Make sure you know what to do, be ready to let him do his part, but don't embarrass him if he slips up in some way.

When a date is not a date. In offices where a young crowd works together, the boys may treat some of the girls as part of the gang. ''Say, Beth, we're all going over to try that new Chinese place for lunch. Want to come along?'' Or some night when she's working overtime, one of the fellows may suggest taking time out to get something to eat. Such casual invitations, a girl should realize, aren't dates. She's lucky enough to be considered one of the gang, and she should pay her way accordingly. If one check is presented for a mixed group, the girls as well as the men will each put enough money to cover the meal and tip in the center of the table for whoever is going to pay the check. If she's dining alone with one of the fellows and a single check is presented, she should offer to pay her share. Some men are embarassed about having a woman in their company plunk down cash in public, and if she realizes he will be annoyed, she shouldn't insist. Instead, she might tell him she'll settle with him later, which she'll be sure to do promptly—and inconspicuously. A good way to avoid any misunderstanding is to qualify your acceptance of such an invitation by saying, "Sure, if we can go Dutch."

Who goes first? The business of who goes first and who stands where shouldn't be bothersome. Usually it boils down to this: The lady goes first except in those cases where the man precedes so that he can offer some sort of help or protection, theoretical though it may be.

- Entering bus or taxi—girl goes first.
- Exiting from bus or taxi—man goes first and helps her out.
- Walking on sidewalk—man is on the outside (a protective shield from splashes or other street or sidewalk conditions).
- Theater or movie—while her escort is purchasing tickets, the girl waits inside in the lobby. If there is an usher, she follows him down the aisle. Otherwise, the man goes first or they may walk together to find seats. The man then steps aside so that she can enter first. When they leave, he waits in the aisle while she steps in front of him and precedes him up the aisle.

❧ Parties Are for Fun

No matter what kind of affair is planned, from a hayride to a formal dance, you can relax and enjoy yourself if you have that little extra security of knowing that you have answered the invitation properly and understand what kind of behavior is called for. You won't be thrown for a loop by the receiving line at a graduation, tea, or wedding if you expect it to be there and know what to do. And you won't be the only girl without gloves at the President's afternoon reception.

Answering invitations. An invitation to a party should be answered, whether or not R.S.V.P. (short for "répondez s'il vous plait," the French

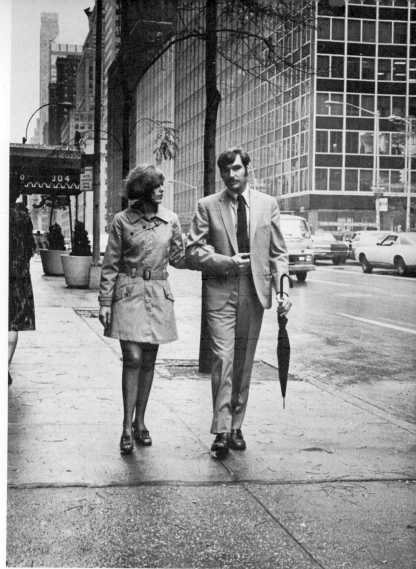

B. D. Unsworth

It is customary, and almost no trouble, for a man to walk on the street side of the sidewalk.

equivalent of "please respond") or a similar request for a reply is indicated. An informal invitation can be answered by a phone call or brief note on plain white paper.

Formal invitations use very formal wording and are usually engraved, although they may be completely or partly handwritten. Formal invitations are used mainly for weddings, dinners, luncheons, and dances.

In regard to wedding invitations, an invitation to the church ceremony doesn't require an answer, but you are expected to acknowledge an invitation to the wedding reception. A reply to a formal invitation must always be handwritten. Use plain white notepaper, and follow the same phrasing and setup of the invitation. Other formal invitations, and your response to them, follow the same pattern.

If you are unable to attend an affair, your reply will state very simply that you regret that you cannot accept the kind invitation.

Party manners. If you have been invited for a meal or if planned activities have been indicated, you should be sure to arrive on time. After greeting the hostess, you will join the other guests. Remember that you were invited because you were expected to contribute to the fun. If you can play the piano, sing, read palms, or perform in some other way, comply without too much coaxing. (Don't begin on your own, however, unless you're sure your hostess wants you to.) When the hostess has planned games or other activities, enter enthusiastically and lend support wherever you can. The surest way to have a good time at a party is to get your mind off yourself and to concentrate on seeing that others have a good time.

Weddings. Although a wedding is a formal affair with a special set of rules and traditions, you can be poised and ready to enjoy yourself when you know what to expect.

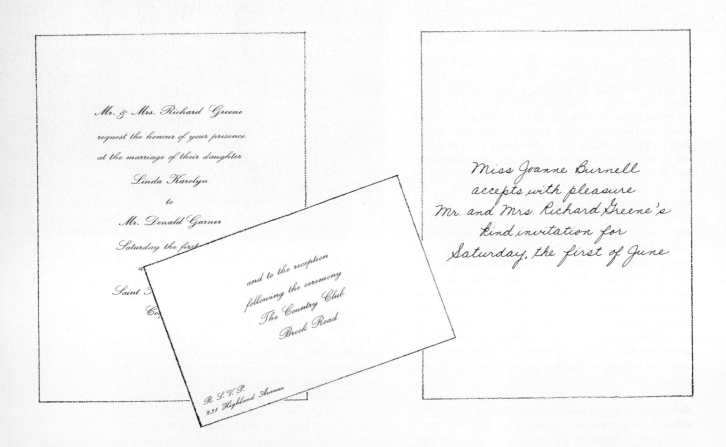

Mr. & Mrs. Richard Greene
request the honour of your presence
at the marriage of their daughter
Linda Karolyn
to
Mr. Donald Garner
Saturday the first

Saint

Co

and to the reception
following the ceremony
The Country Club
Brook Road

R. S. V. P.
231 Highland Avenue

Miss Joanne Burnell
accepts with pleasure
Mr. and Mrs. Richard Greene's
kind invitation for
Saturday, the first of June

What to wear? A morning or an afternoon wedding calls for a simple dress or suit in an elegant fabric, a hat, and gloves. An evening wedding is more formal—wear your dressiest dress, but not necessarily the one with the plunging neckline.

Arrive for the ceremony in good time—at least five minutes before it is scheduled to begin. You don't want to delay the bride, and you want to be present for the whole ceremony. One of the ushers will come up to you and ask, "Bride or groom?" He wants to know which side of the aisle you will sit on—a friend of the groom sits on the right, a friend of the bride, on the left. (If you are friendly with both of them and the groom is from out of town, you might sit on his side because it is less crowded.) The usher will offer his arm. You put your hand inside the crook of his elbow and rest it lightly on his arm. He will escort you to a seat.

When the ceremony is over, it is customary to wait until the families of the bride and groom have been escorted from their seats. Usually you will find your own way out, but if those in front of you wait for an usher, you wait too.

At the reception the first thing you do is greet those on the receiving line. You will give your name to the first person in line, and she will pass your name to the person on her right by introducing you to her. All you have to say is, "Hello, isn't Mary beautiful?" or some similar comment. No conversation is necessary—there may be a hundred people behind you. What you say to the bridal couple depends on how well you know them. Shake hands with the groom and say "Congratulations." Shake hands with the bride, or kiss her if you know her very well, and wish her happiness (*never* congratulate her on securing a husband!). Then move on.

The reception lasts anywhere from an hour to several hours, depending on the time of day, the number of people, and whether or not there is dancing. If you don't know many people, simply go over and begin talking to someone about the bride or the groom—this is what you have in common, after all! You do not have

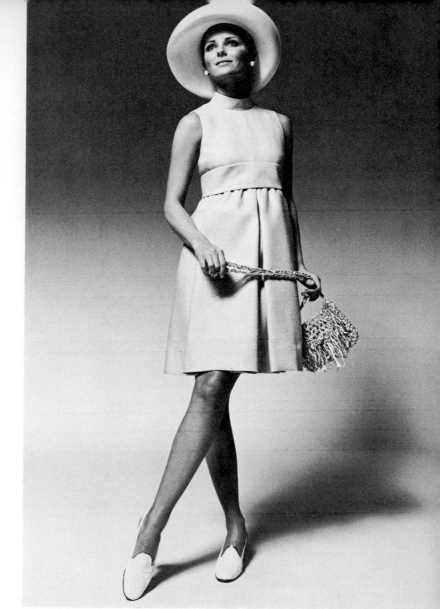

Courtesy of Saks Fifth Avenue

Though simply styled, this dress could do for a daytime wedding if teamed with dressy shoes and bag and white gloves.

to stay until the end, but usually you should wait until the bride throws her bouquet.

Teas and receptions. Teas and receptions are usually given to honor some person or event or, in business, to introduce some new product or development. They are usually held for a specified time period, such as from three to five in the afternoon, and you may arrive any time during these hours. You will probably stay about a half hour unless some form of entertainment or presentation is to take place.

Correct attire would be an afternoon dress or dressy suit, gloves, and in some sections of the country, a hat. If hats are worn, they are kept on, but gloves should be removed when refreshments are served. You will greet your

host or hostess when you arrive. When there is a receiving line, your hostess will be first and will present you to the guest of honor on her right, who will, in turn, present you to the person on *her* right, and so on. You will shake hands and say, "How do you do?" A longer conversation would hold up the line and can be saved until later. If there is no one to present your name, you will introduce yourself.

When you want refreshments, you will go to the table. The person who is pouring may ask, "How do you like your tea?" In a cup, obviously, but she wants to know whether you prefer lemon or cream. (An inexperienced young tea drinker once tried both together much to her chagrin. The curdled mess that resulted is not recommended fare.) You will help yourself to a couple of cookies or fancy sandwiches and can either stand or find yourself a seat while you eat. You'll be likely to mingle with more people if you stand. At a business reception the fare is more likely to be cocktails and canapés. Waiters often circulate with trays of refreshments. If this is a self-service affair and no gentleman is available to get your refreshments, you need not hesitate to go to the serving table yourself.

Dance etiquette. If the affair is formal, there are a few taboos you will want to abide by. Your entire outfit must be keyed to the occasion. Sporty or fraternity jewelry of any kind is out, and wristwatches are not worn unless they are very dressy or jeweled. If you are given a corsage, remember that the flowers are worn blossoms up, as they grow.

At the dance, if you and your escort use the same cloakroom, he takes care of the stubs. If separate checking facilities are provided, you take care of your own stub. After a quick checkup on your appearance, you will meet your date and will then greet the hostess or chaperones. If there is a receiving line, you will go down it together, the girl preceding her escort.

The first and last dance and the one following the intermission belong to your escort. You will usually share refreshments with your last

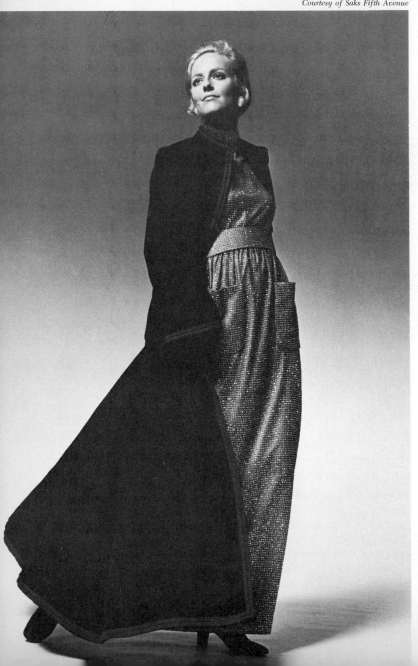

Courtesy of Saks Fifth Avenue

372

partner before intermission. If there is a mixer, be a good sport and join in. In like manner, you and your date should not refuse cut-ins. If you are on the sidelines and someone with whom you do not wish to dance asks for a dance, you had better have a very good excuse before you refuse—and then do so as kindly as possible. During a dance, keep the conversation light; controversial subjects and long, involved stories are out of place. At the end of a dance, your partner will thank you, and you can reply with a compliment on his dancing technique or with a light pleasant remark along the lines of "It was fun."

If you must cross the ballroom for any reason, you will go around the side. No one should ever walk across the floor when a dance is in progress. At the end of the evening you and your date should be sure to thank your hostess, or the chaperones if it is a school dance, before leaving.

WALLFLOWER PROBLEMS? If you've been applying what you have learned so far in this course, the fault can't be your grooming or posture. If you have any doubt about your footwork, try to get in a little extra practice or take a course. A good dancer seldom sits one out. But remember that despite all sorts of allure, even the greatest charmers have occasionally adorned the sidelines for uncomfortable periods. If this happens, don't slink behind a potted palm or hightail it to the powder room for a lengthy stay. Courageously sit out where you can be seen, preferably not huddled with a lot of other girls (or even with only one other). It often requires quite a lot of courage for a boy to ask a girl for a dance. He's much more likely to choose the girl who's sitting alone than the one who is flanked by a group of other girls who are all hopefully wondering if he's going to ask them.

❧ Table Manners

Table manners are basically a matter of courtesy. They developed from a desire to make mealtime a pleasant social occasion, not just a refueling stop. Eat neatly and quietly and you

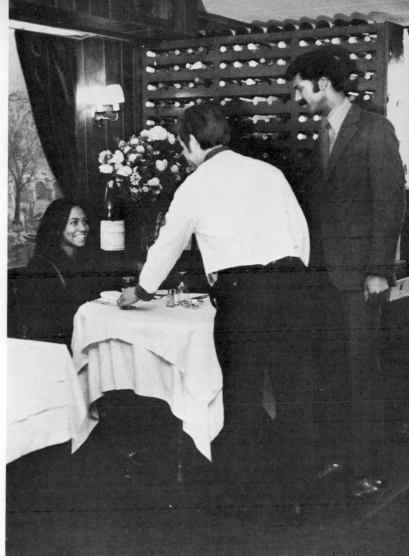

B. D. Unsworth

It is customary in a restaurant for the girl to sit with her back to the wall.

will not have to worry about your manners. The bothersome questions of etiquette at the table are covered generally here, but if you are eating out and are in doubt, just watch your hostess or an older woman and do what she does.

Much of this information you may already know, but it is included to give you a quick checkup on any points that may have been puzzling you or may have been forgotten.

When you are a guest for dinner, you wait behind your chair until the host or hostess invites everyone to be seated. In many homes

373

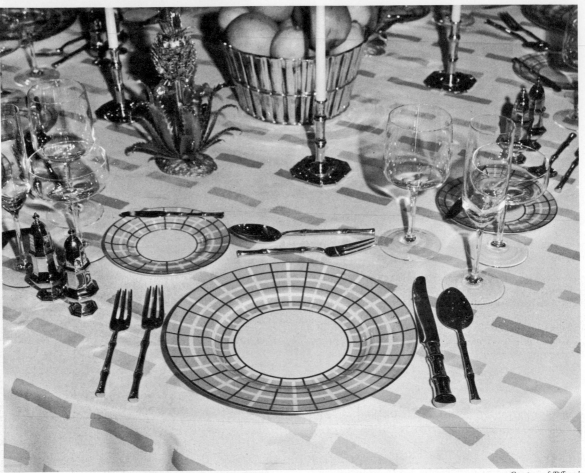

grace is said before the meal is begun. You will be saved possible embarrassment if you watch your hostess for a cue. If no grace is said, guests may begin eating when the hostess starts. If there are many people, such as at an office luncheon or company banquet, you would not begin eating until those around you have been served. It wouldn't be necessary to wait until the entire group had been served, however, because your food would become cold.

Proper eating techniques. Silver is usually set beside your plate in the order in which it is to be used, the outer pieces being those you will need first. If there is any doubt about which

to use, take your cue from your hostess. If you make a mistake, just continue eating nonchalantly. Don't put the silver back on the table.

Soup is spooned away from you and sipped noiselessly from the side of the spoon. If soup is served in a cup, it is also correct to drink the soup directly from the cup. Your soup plate or cup can be tipped slightly away from you (never toward you) when the contents become shallow, but it is politer to leave a little soup and *not* try to get every drop. If there is no serving plate beneath your soup dish, your spoon should be left in the soup dish when you are finished.

There are two knife-and-fork eating styles that are correct: the American, in which you eat with the fork in the right hand and change over to cut, and the Continental, in which cut-off bites of meat can be speared with the fork, tines down, in the left hand and transferred to the mouth with the left hand. Although the latter style is considered the preferred method of eating in certain cosmopolitan circles, it has not been widely accepted in our country.

When you have finished with any course, center the utensils on the plate so that they won't fall off, keeping the handles on the right and the knife blade furned in toward the fork. No piece of silver that has been used should ever be put back on the tablecloth, nor should it touch any dish that other people eat from. A spoon is always left in the saucer beneath your bowl, cup or glass. If no saucer is served with your iced tea, the iced-tea spoon can be placed on your salad or dessert plate or on the edge of your dinner plate.

At the start of a meal, unfold the napkin halfway and spread it across your lap. Do not tuck it in a belt or skirt. After a meal your napkin should be kept on your lap until everyone is ready to leave the table. Then it is placed in a semifolded condition (neither completely refolded nor crumpled in a tight ball) at the left of your place.

When a maid or waiter serves, you wait until he is at your left; then you take the food from the serving dishes yourself. With the serving spoon in your right hand and the fork in your left, you take the nearest (not necessarily the choicest) portion. When a maid passes food, you needn't thank her each time you are served. A few additional pointers: nothing from a serving dish should ever be placed directly in your mouth. Even something small, such as a cookie, should be put on your plate first.

• When you pass a pitcher, cup, or piece of silver, turn the handle toward the person who is to receive it.

• A goblet should be held by the stem and the *lower* part of the bowl, whether you are drinking from it or just passing it.

• It is perfectly proper to reach for dishes directly in front of you, but ask your neighbor to pass you the salt if it is in front of him.

375

• Salad greens may be cut with a knife, but using a fork is preferable.

• Only one or two bites of meat should be cut at a time. You are not running an assembly line.

• Take a portion of butter and place it on your bread and butter plate, if there is one, or on the side of your dinner plate. If you wish to add butter to vegetables or potatoes, take it from the bread and butter plate with your fork.

• Bread should not be cut with a knife. Break off a small piece of bread or roll with your fingers and butter it, on the plate, with your butter knife. Take only one piece at a time.

B. D. Unsworth

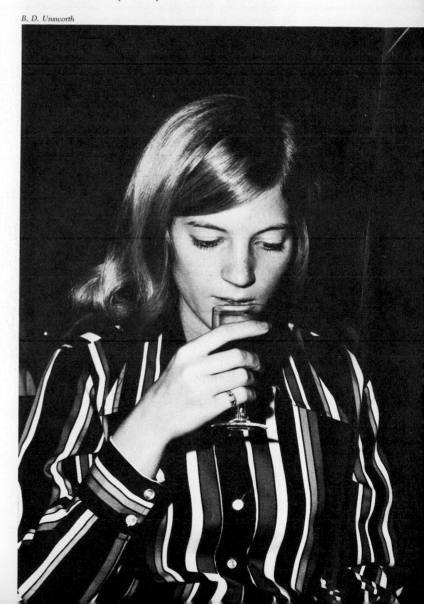

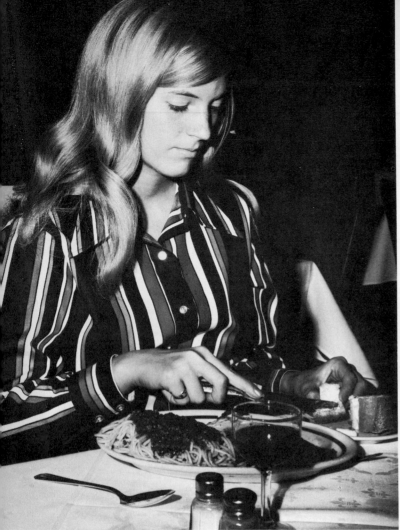

B. D. Unsworth

• At no time should silver dangle off a plate.

• Since it is very impolite to talk with your mouth full, ease the problem of being caught by a question in mid-chew by taking only small bites. In any event, you would finish chewing before you replied.

• If some food needs to be removed from your mouth, don't hesitate to do so. Clean things, such as fish bones, olive pits, and fresh fruit pits, can be removed with the fingers. Other items, such as a bit of gristle or sticky pits from stewed fruit, should be removed the way they went in—with the fork or spoon you are using—and should be placed on the edge of your plate.

• No well-bred girl ever chews with her mouth open or smacks her lips as she eats.

• Whenever you take a mouthful, lean slightly toward your plate. Then if anything drops, it lands on your plate, not on your lap or on your hostess's tablecloth.

• Don't gesture with silver in your hand—you'll stir up nothing but trouble.

• In a restaurant the vegetables that accompany the main course are often served in side dishes and should be eaten directly from these dishes. Sometimes a main course, such as a stew or a chicken pie or a chef's salad, may be served in a side dish. In this case you would spoon a serving onto your dinner plate.

• Elbows should never be a hazard to table partners. Keep them close to your sides, especially when cutting food.

• If finger bowls are used, they are served on the dessert plate, although they are not used until after dessert is finished. Remove the finger bowl, with its doily, and place it on the table at the upper left of your plate until dessert is finished. Then dip the tips of your fingers in the water and wipe them on your napkin.

❦ *How Do You Eat It?*

ARTICHOKES. Use your fingers. Take off one or two leaves at a time, dip the soft end into the sauce, and scrape off about a third of the leaf by drawing it through your teeth. Don't try to swallow the whole leaf; it won't digest well. Pile the used leaves on the side of your plate. When all the leaves are removed, cut away the prickly part with your knife and fork and eat the heart with your fork.

ASPARAGUS. Break off the tender part with your fork, eating it in several sections. Eat only what can be cut with your fork. At home you might pick up the end in your fingers and nibble a bit more.

AVOCADOS. No problem if they are served cut up in a salad. When they are split in half and the seed cavity filled, you scoop the fruit out of the shell with your spoon, as with a melon.

BACON. If it is crisp, eat it with your fingers; otherwise, use a knife and fork.

376

CAKE. Dry cake may be eaten with the fingers. A layer cake or gooey cake should be eaten with a fork. Cake or pie á la mode is eaten with a fork rather than a spoon, although a spoon may be used if the ice cream is very runny.

CANDY. When a box is offered to you, take the frilled paper cup as well as the candy.

CHICKEN. Use a knife and fork in public. At home or at a picnic you might pick up the bones, but you should always get off as much meat as possible first.

CLAMS. When you eat clams on the half shell, lift the clam from the shell with your oyster fork and dip the clam in the sauce. Put it whole into your mouth. Steamed clams may be eaten with the fingers.

CORN ON THE COB. Eat it with your fingers. Butter only a few rows at a time.

CRABS. *Hard-Shelled:* Pull off the small claws, and suck or chew the meat out of the open end. Then lift out the body meat, cut it with a knife and fork, and eat it, dipping each piece into the sauce. The coral and green part is also good. If a nutcracker is served with the crab, you may want to crack the claws more. Break the claws with your fingers, take out the meat with your oyster fork or a pick, dip it into the sauce, and eat it. *Soft-Shelled:* Everything is edible.

LOBSTERS. Same technique as for crabs.

MUSSELS. Use a fork to take them out of the shells, or pick up the shell and suck the edible part out of it. Shells go on a side plate so that you can spoon up the sauce afterwards.

OLIVES. Eat with the fingers. Pits go into your hand and then onto your plate.

OYSTERS. *On the Half Shell, Raw:* Eat like clams. *Cooked:* Use knife and fork. Dip in sauce, if any.

POTATO CHIPS OR STICKS. If no spoon is served with them, help yourself with your fingers. Eat with your fingers.

PICKLES. Whole pickles and pickles served with sandwiches are eaten with the fingers. Sliced pickles served with meat are eaten with a fork.

PINEAPPLE RINGS. *Fresh:* Use a knife and fork. *Stewed:* Use a spoon.

RELISHES. Put them on the dinner plate beside the food they go with, and eat them with your fork along with the bite of food.

SHRIMP COCKTAIL. Eat with an oyster fork. Sauce may be served on the shrimp or in a separate small cup. If the lettuce on which the shrimp is served is hard to manage with a fork, skip it. Although on other occasions you might cut lettuce with a knife, it looks rather awkward to attack a cocktail glass with a big dinner knife. If the shrimp is too big to eat in one bite, bite a piece off and then redip the remaining portion in the sauce and eat that.

FRIED FANTAIL SHRIMP. Using your fingers, pick it up by the tail, dip in the sauce and eat, leaving the tail.

UNSHELLED SHRIMP. Shell with your fingers and eat.

SPAGHETTI. If you've acquired the knack of rolling your own, good. To do this, hold the spoon in your left hand, take a few strands with the fork in your right hand, and wind the fork, keeping the prongs against the spoon. The result should be a neatly wound mouthful. Only a few strands should be used, or you'll end up with much too much. If you can't do this expertly, it's better to cut up the spaghetti with a fork.

❦ Dining Out

Most fashionable restaurants have checkrooms, where a man will check his hat and coat. A woman usually keeps hers and slips the coat over the back of her chair. She might, however, check packages or an umbrella or raincoat.

If there is a headwaiter or a hostess, the girl precedes her escort and follows the headwaiter to the table he indicates, taking the seat he offers and allowing him to help her with her

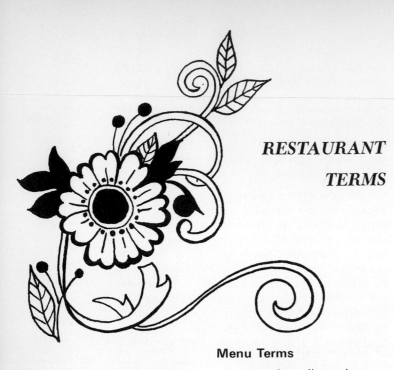

RESTAURANT TERMS

French Terms

Bisque	– a thick cream soup
Consommé	–clear, thin broth of vegetables and meat or chicken
Potage	–a thick, rich soup
Vichyssoise	–creamy potato (and leek or onion) soup, usually served cold
Bouillabaisse	–a dish ranging between soup and stew consistency, made with various fish, saffron, and wine
Poulet	–chicken
Veau	–veal
Boeuf	–beef
Ragout	–stew
Haricots verts	–green beans
Petit pois	–small green peas
Fromage	–cheese
Crêpes suzette	–dessert pancakes usually served with grated orange rind and flaming liqueur

Menu Terms

Table d'hôte	–complete dinner is served for the price indicated
À la carte	–each item is priced separately
Entrée	–the main dinner course
Smorgasbord	–a buffet-type meal in which you help yourself to a variety of hot and cold dishes, taking as much as you like and returning as often as you wish
Demitasse	–a small cup of coffee that is usually drunk black
Paté de foie gras	–a finely ground goose liver canapé
Julienne	–cut in long, thin matchlike strips
Au jus	–in its own juice
Au crème	–with cream
Au vin	–in wine
En brochette	–cooked on a skewer

Oriental Terms

Chop suey	–mixture of cooked bamboo shoots, bean sprouts and other vegetables with some form of cut-up meat, usually pork, chicken, beef, or shrimp
Chow mein	–similar to chop suey but served on fried noodles
Sukiyaki	–mixture of cooked vegetables with some form of meat or fish
Foo yung	–eggs and vegetables cooked together (similar to omelets); also obtainable in meat varieties

378

Italian Terms

Zuppa	–soup
Minestrone	–thick vegetable soup
Antipasto	–plate of mixed appetizers
Pollo	–chicken
Manzo	–beef
Bistecca	–steak
Vitella	–veal
Agnello	–lamb
Prosciutto	–smoked ham, sliced very thin
Scampi	–shrimp (large)
Chicken cacciatore	–chicken cooked in oil with tomatoes and wine
Chicken tetrazzini	–creamed chicken on spaghetti
Lasagne	–broad noodles baked in layers with sauce and cheese
Manicotti	–noodles stuffed with cheese and served with sauce
Risotto	–rice dish
Fagiolini	–green beans
Patate	–potatoes
Piselli	–peas
Spumoni	–sliced frozen dessert similar to ice cream, with fruits and nuts
Gelato	–any ice cream dessert

German Terms

Wienerschnitzel	–veal cutlet
Schinken	–ham
Kalbfleisch	–veal
Wurst	–sausage
Geflügel	–general term for poultry
Sauerbraten	–pickled beef stewed in sweet-sour gravy
Hasenpfeffer	–rabbit stew
Grüne Bohnen	–green beans
Kartoffelklösse	–potato dumplings
Erbsen	–peas
Kuchen	–cake

Spanish and Mexican Terms

Sopa	–soup
Gazpacho	–cold soup dish of raw vegetables
Pollo	–chicken
Cerdo	–pork
Ternera	–veal
Vaca	–beef
Cordero	–lamb
Tamales	–highly seasoned corn mixture, stuffed with ground meat
Tortillas (Mexican)	–thin flat cornmeal cakes
Tortillas Spanish)	–Omelets
Enchiladas	–Mexican tortillas stuffed with meat, other ingredients
Paella	–rice dish with chicken, pork, shrimp or other seafood, tomatoes, pimento, and so on
Chili	–kidney beans and meat in spicy sauce
Frijoles	–beans
Guisantes	–green peas
Arroz	–rice
Empanada	–small filled pastry
Flan	–egg custard with caramel sauce

Eastern Terms

Borsch	–soup of beets and other vegetables, served with sour cream
Shashlick or shish kebab	–meat and vegetables cooked on skewers
Beef stroganoff	–slivered beef in sour cream sauce
Pilaf	–rice dish, with meat and seasonings
Blini	–pancakes served with sour cream and caviar or smoked salmon

chair. If there is no one to direct you to a table, your escort will choose the table. You will keep your purse and belongings in your lap, or if there is an empty chair at your table, you could put them there. They should not be put on the table itself.

If you are dining with a man, you will give him your order and let him relay it to the waiter. A girl on a date should be considerate of her escort's financial state. If you don't understand the menu, don't be ashamed to consult the waiter for help.

Courtesy of Kraft Foods

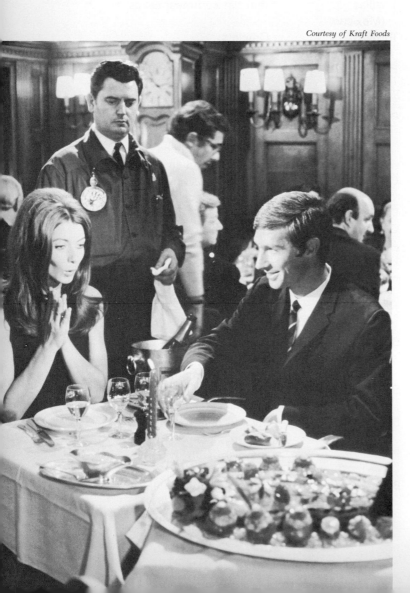

Unless the check advises patrons to pay the cashier, the waiter is paid. Usually, when the waiter is to handle payment, the check is presented on a small tray. This tray will be returned with the change, and the tip (usually 15 per cent, see page 381 for details) can be left on the tray. When checks are taken to the cashier, a tip should first be left on the table. If you haven't the right change for the tip, you can obtain it from the cashier and then go back to put it at your place. If you are with a date, wait by the door while he does this. When a couple leaves a restaurant, the girl precedes her date.

On a date a good time to repair makeup damage is while your escort is waiting for the check. Any face or hair fixing should, of course, *always* be done in the powder room, as the name implies. The sight of a woman applying makeup in public is distasteful to most people.

❁ Tipping Guide

How you tip is almost as important as how much you tip. Let your manner as well as your money express your thanks for the service that has been given to you.

Whom should you tip? You tip only employees who have served you personally. The owner or manager should not be tipped even if, as in a beauty parlor, he does the same work as his employees.

As an average, you would tip about 15 percent of the bill, more for special services. The amounts suggested below are approximate standards.

• Taxi—15 percent or more, never less than 15 cents for a minimum fare.

• Doorman—25 cents for putting you into a convenient cab, more if he goes out into bad weather to find one for you. Apartment dwellers often give a dollar or more every so often instead of giving a small tip for each service.

• Lunch counter—10 percent to 15 percent, but no less than 10 cents. No tip necessary for just coffee, sundae, or soda.

- Waiter—generally 15 percent, but at least 15 to 20 cents per person.
- Headwaiter—no tip for seating you. If he performs special services such as making advance arrangements, $1 to $5 (always paper money) or about 10 percent of the bill. If the location of the table is important, tip before dinner. Otherwise a tip for special services is given after dinner.
- Hatcheck girl—15 to 25 cents per person.
- Rest room matron—for towel and soap, 10 to 25 cents. More for special service.
- Beauty parlor—for a permanent, 15 percent, for a set, 15 percent but not less than 25 cents; a shampoo, 25 cents; a manicure, 25 cents; for hair coloring, facial, massage, or other involved treatment, 15 per cent but not less than 50 cents.
- Shoeshine boy—25 cents.

- Parking lot attendant—if he parks or retrieves your car, 25 cents.
- Telegraph boys, messengers, store delivery boys—25 cents.
- Moving men—for a large load such as all the furniture in an apartment or a house, $5 to $10 to be divided among the men. (Figure about $2 per man.) Less for a single item.
- Tennis—locker-room attendant, 25 to 50 cents at a public court; at a country club, $1–$2 a month for members, $1 per visit for guests.
- Golf—If a set caddy fee is charged, tip an additional $1 for 18 holes, 50 cents for 9. If there is no fixed rate, tip $5 for 18 holes, $2.50 for 9. Many people prefer to tote their own clubs in golf carts. Carts can usually be rented at the clubhouse for a small fee.
- Riding—groom at public stable, 50 cents after you ride.

1 *For the next week or so, look for opportunities to make introductions. The more practice you obtain, the smoother and easier introductions will become.*

2 *Are there any problems regarding introductions, dining etiquette, party or dance etiquette or any other subjects not covered in this chapter that you have some doubts about? If so, go to your library and look up the correct procedure in a complete etiquette book. Don't let any etiquette problems threaten your poise when they can be settled so simply.*

3 *Practice using your very best table manners at all times. If you have been making exceptions at home, try to avoid this as much as possible.*

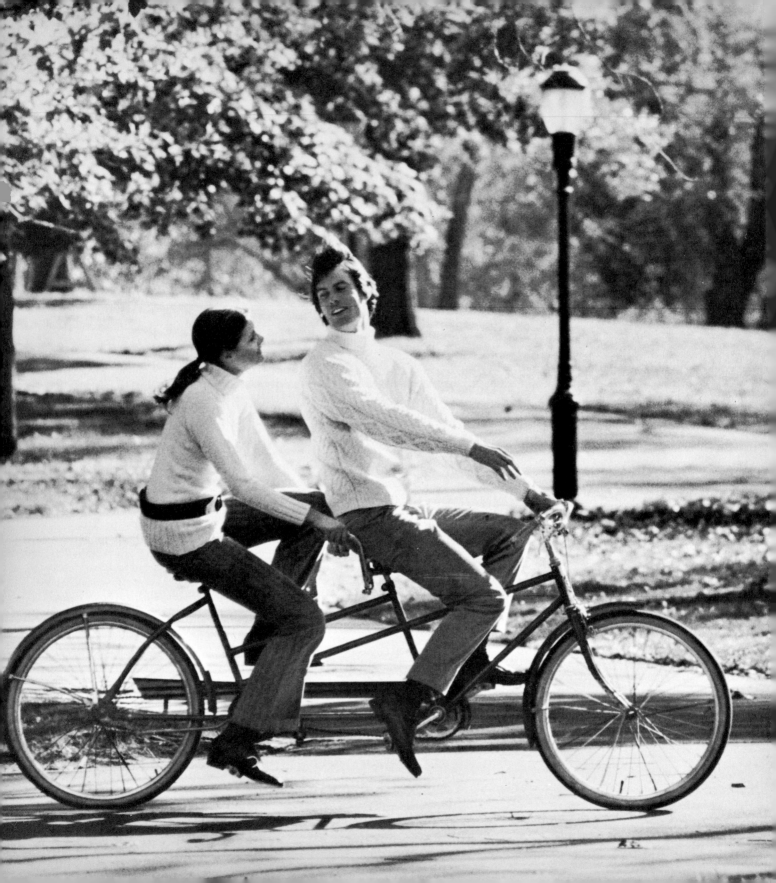

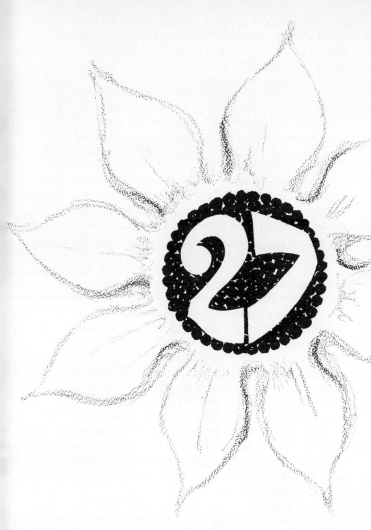

DATING

Charm has its rewards, and dates and romance are usually high on the list. As a working girl you have a distinct advantage. A business office offers a girl numerous opportunities for meeting men, and many a future husband has been found within its gold-lettered portals. Past your desk will go a procession of dynamic executives, genial salesmen, dapper idea men, and suave personality guys, as well as a substantial sprinkling of elite, balding dignitaries and lesser clerical drones. You'll learn to know men of all types from a variety of backgrounds. Not all the men you meet will be eligible for matrimony and not all of them will be desirable marriage material, but most will be well worth studying. In an office you have a golden opportunity to study impersonally the workings of the male mind. Through your day-in-day-out contact with a variety of men, you'll absorb a deeper understanding of what concerns them, what pleases them, and what problems confront them. Because of your understanding and the efficient and kindly way you respond to the needs of others, you just might come upon a man who will want you to help him solve his problems on a full-time basis for the rest of his life.

Business frowns upon any outward manifestation of attraction between the sexes. Flirting, coyness, and other feminine wiles are embarrassingly inappropriate. The work must be done; the profits must be accrued to keep employees on the payroll. Though there may be subsurface ripplings, men and women must work together almost as if unconscious of each other's sex.

❦ Impressive Impressions

Just as the career girl has an opportunity to meet a wide variety of male types, so the man in the office is exposed to a variety of female types. He, too, observes carefully, compares what he sees, and checks the office grapevine to hear what others think of you. He'll be attracted by your smart appearance and friendly smile, yes, and he'll be able to find out how capable you are and how considerate you are of others. He'll notice how you get along with the other girls. Before he makes a move in

your direction, he has a chance to do quite a bit of subtle research. In the office the surest way to catch the heart of a man is to build yourself a reputation for being a mighty wonderful girl. The old-fashioned virtues of kindness, consideration, efficiency, and dependability—in short, character—carry the weight here.

A happy beginning is usually the result of your being observed by someone who liked what he saw well enough to wangle an introduction. Somehow the odds seem to be against the fellow at the desk next to yours. This only serves to point up the fact that you should always be on your most charming behavior; you never know who's watching, and it may be that most important man in your future. Ironically, romance slips away if a girl tries too hard, and it usually sneaks up on her when she least expects it.

Conducting an intraoffice romance requires great skill and delicacy. Mere proximity can be a serious problem. It's hard enough to keep your mind on your work when you're in love, but when the object of your affection is sitting there in full heavenly view, any sort of concentration requires superhuman effort. Your boss —and your beau's boss—are aware that love and efficiency don't mix, and any little slipup is likely to be attributed resentfully to your romance. When the staff knows of the interest you and another employee have in each other, you must both be extra careful that your work is above reproach.

As sometimes happens, even the most torrid romance may fizzle out. The end of an office romance is especially painful. Not only is there the necessity for daily contact with the lad who once played such beautiful music on your heart strings, but there is the added torture of watching from the sidelines when he takes up a new romance with someone else.

All the world loves a lover, and office staffs are no exception. You and your heart throb will be a major source of interest and entertainment to the entire staff unless you are extremely cautious. Any courtship is more difficult when it is being scrutinized by too many interested observers. Some couples have man-

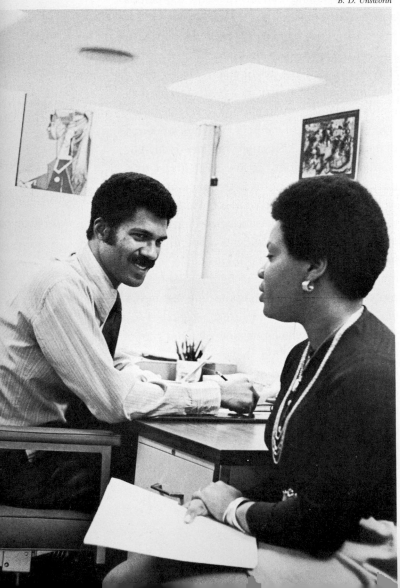

B. D. Unsworth

aged to conduct a flourishing romance by keeping it entirely secret until they could flash the news via an engagement ring. Though this requires great restraint, it assures privacy and avoids criticism. It means, however, that the young man can't hover around her desk, can't phone her at the office, and can't be conspicuous about meeting her after work. Couples who have managed this sort of discreet romance are usually highly respected.

Although the boss-loves-secretary theme is a popular one for movies and magazine fiction, actual cases are extremely rare. Probably this is due partly to the fact that the rising executive is sometimes lowered in the eyes of his peers if he marries one of the girls from the office. In view of this, should one of the young bachelor executives take an interest in a lesser employee, she would most definitely want to keep the romance private so that nothing could spoil her chances before his feelings had become strong enough to counteract any possible criticism.

❦ The Office Wolf

There are several varieties of office wolves. They range from young nobodies to dapper dignitaries. Some are basically nice guys, actually quite harmless, who, because of some inner insecurity, have to keep testing their batting average on every girl within sight. Just don't let yourself become their favorite testing ground. Although they may mean nothing by such action, it demeans a girl if she lets someone take advantage of her. In an office in this day and age a girl can't go Victorian and declare her virtue slandered by the cad who tells her a slightly off-color joke or puts his arm around her shoulders. But expressing displeasure at this stage (either by a feigned look of alarm or by coolly and quietly moving away) will probably discourage further advances. Act naturally, change the subject, and ignore it. The circumstances and the person have a lot to do with how you react, but the wisest course for a girl who's new to the office game is

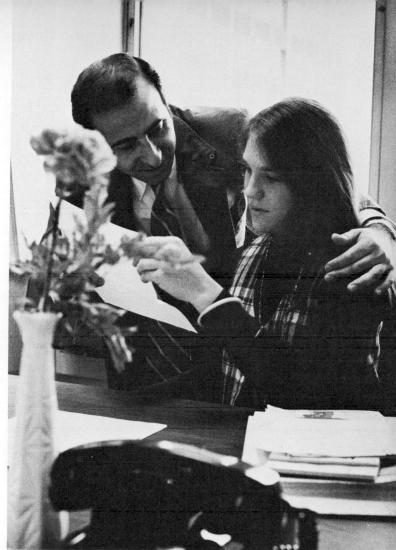

B. D. Unsworth

usually to head off any trouble before it has a chance to start.

Serious nuisances can usually be discouraged if you become desperately busy whenever they hover on the horizon. They, too, realize that work must be done and will usually head for less hectic pastures.

Suppose some night when you are working overtime, Mr. Already-Married suggests you have supper with him. It seems a very natural thing to do, so you agree. About dessert time, all thoughts of finishing that important rush job somehow vanish from his mind and he suggests that instead of returning to the office you go on

385

to another spot for some dancing. Such extra-curricular activity is dynamite when a married man is concerned. You needn't act outraged or prissy about it, however. Simply state that you already have plans for the evening and are counting on getting home soon. He'll get the point. And he'll respect your discretion. A married man looking for a little outside amusement usually is quite easy to discourage, just because he *is* married. No matter how high his rank in the office, you hold the upper hand in such situations and should use it. Even though you might be quite infatuated with him,

don't let anything start. There's nothing in it for you—except trouble. When the affair cools and the executive tires, it becomes inconvenient to have the girl around. She's the one who'll be out of a job, not the boss.

If some roving-eyed menace who is too important to squelch becomes a serious problem, you might as well start looking for a new job. Actually, very few bosses have dishonorable intentions. They realize that they are in the limelight, and they value their prestige and position too highly to risk providing opportunities for unsavory gossip. Usually the girl who takes everyone at face value and assumes he has no dark, underlying motives will find that she is quite right. Even if she isn't, a naive, see-no-evil attitude will usually discourage anyone who might be comtemplating unwholesome advances.

❦ Filling Your Date Book

If you're new in town or feel your date list needs a little rejuvenation, make a special effort to get out and meet men. Sitting back and waiting for Cupid's arrow to strike isn't enough. Skiing (especially ski tours), skating, bowling, and other co-ed sports usually offer natural opportunities for meeting new men. Many towns have social centers that sponsor dances and other get-acquainted activities. In cities the gathering spots for the young crowd may be discotheques. If none of these is available, you might try throwing your own party. This provides an opportunity to invite the man who hasn't quite got around to asking for a date but whose interest you'd like to encourage. But don't let him be the only unattached man present. Perhaps you can ask some of the more popular girls to bring an extra boy or two. Include single friends as well as couples to keep the party moving.

Other good possibilities for meeting men are through clubs, co-ed classes, hobby groups, church organizations, employee social groups, drama or choral groups, volunteer work, or sports. Don't rule out a sport, such as tennis,

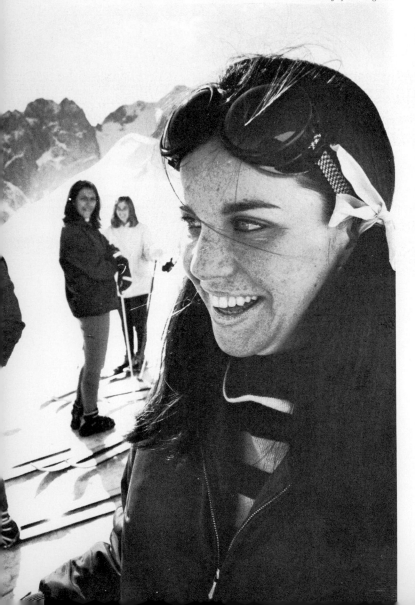

Courtesy of Ski Magazine

just because you've never tried it. Take some instruction or practice against a blank wall until your shots are sure enough for the public courts. If tennis or skiing or some other activity isn't to your liking, don't stick at it grimly in the hope of meeting new men. Your chances are much better when you're doing something you enjoy—enthusiasm acts as a magnet. But don't give up if you can't become an expert overnight. Being a novice is sometimes an asset. When you need help, a man has a natural opening to offer his experienced assistance.

In many of these ventures you'll feel more comfortable if your best girl friend comes along. But if you cling to each other, better forget about meeting men. A stranger who decides he wants to meet one of you won't know what to do with the other. Not many men think they can make friends with two girls at once.

Whether you're learning to ski or taking an evening course, don't pin your hopes on the instructor—or on any man who's already in the spotlight. The chances are that the competition is fierce; if anything, your indifference may make you stand out from the others. In the meantime, be charming to all.

❦ Dating Manners

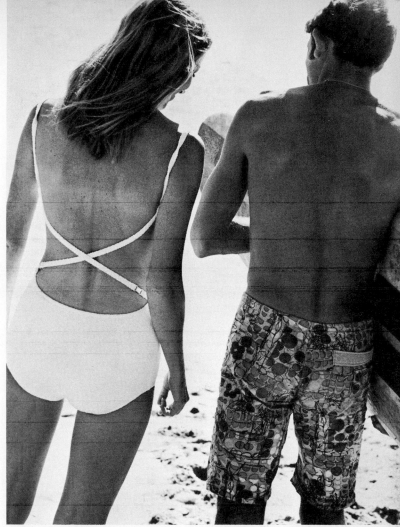

Courtesy of Bonne Bell Inc.

Many girls who are kind to old ladies and have impeccable behavior in most social matters sometimes treat the men in their lives in an off-hand, inconsiderate way. Remember that a man's feelings are every bit as sensitive as yours. He can be just as flattened by a rejection for a date as you can be by not being asked. In his role as the pursuer, he is in the vulnerable position of having to make the initial move. This sometimes requires a formidable amount of courage, and a tactless rejection can be pretty damaging to a delicate male ego. Even if he's the type who turns you off completely, answer him kindly. Treat all your dates with consideration. Word spreads quickly when a girl is unkind. Down goes her popularity rating

and down goes her rating as a human being.

To check yourself, see how you would rate in the following situations.

• If you are not particularly enthusiastic about a date, do you ever keep him dangling in hopes something better will come along? It's only fair to give him a definite answer the first time. If you play for time, you not only increase the hurt of your refusal, but the delay may spoil his chances with the girl who might be his second choice.

• Do you ever break a date to accept another? If you value your social life, don't. Not only is it unfair, but fellows talk to each other, too, and the word travels fast when a girl heartlessly juggles dates.

• If you don't want to accept a date, can you do it kindly and without getting yourself involved? The best strategy is to say simply that you'll be busy or have other plans. Don't trip yourself up by offering any concrete explanation that may keep you from accepting another date should another man call.

• If you already have a date when a second offer is made, can you refuse it without appearing smug? When you're already booked, don't rub it in, especially if you want to encourage the second fellow. Tell him you're very sorry you can't go (try to avoid mentioning the date you already have), and if you like him, suggest that perhaps you can make it some other time.

• If another girl wants you to go on a blind date, should you accept? Judge by the person who wants to introduce you and the caliber of the company she keeps. If you don't know the person very well or have any doubts about her, you can always reply "I can't make it this time, but perhaps I can later on." This will give you time to know her better.

• Are you ready when your date arrives? Every man appreciates promptness. He came to see you, not to sit around reading your magazines—or, worse yet, to make idle conversation with your roommates, parents, or kid sister.

• How considerate are you of your date's financial situation? Perhaps most of your dates seem fairly affluent, but before you write off a man as a miser or pressure him to spend more on you, consider his financial situation. Maybe he had to work his way through school and is still a long way from financial security. Perhaps in his field, salaries just aren't high. Follow his cue

If you live in a studio apartment, you have to be ready by the time he gets there.

B. D. Unsworth

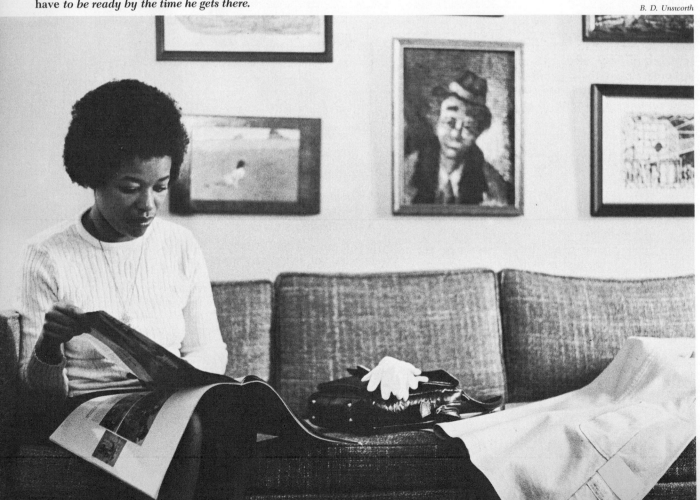

and you can't go wrong. If he suggests a bus instead of a cab, go along cheerfully. If he gets low-priced tickets for a show, don't point out that you could see more from better seats. If you know he'd like to take you out more often but can't afford it, offer some ideas for free fun. If the friendship stays casual, it won't hurt you to exercise such consideration. On the other hand, if you both become serious, he'll know that you don't equate pleasure with dollars spent, and he'll also feel that you won't be a hindrance to your family's financial security.

• At a party do you ever cling to your date? Or do you flirt with every man in sight in an effort to make your date jealous? While you should circulate at a party so that he has a little freedom, the girl who encourages the competition to too great a degree antagonizes not only her escort but also every other girl there. Since your date brought you to the affair, you owe him the courtesy of the major portion of your time and attention.

❦ Dating Dilemmas

Perhaps the least obvious dating pitfall is going steady. Always having a date is convenient. You know you won't have to sit home with a book on Saturday night—you can always count on being included in any plans the group makes. But when a relationship cools, yet drags on and on because neither partner has the courage to break it off, you are wasting valuable time. These are the years when you want to get to know as many men as possible and to acquire experience in getting along with many different types of dates so that you will be better able to judge the right man for marriage. Our personalities grow with each new close friendship. We can love several dates, each for a different reason. When you're ready for marriage, you will probably select someone who is a composite of all these; and you will have the experience to spot him and to appreciate him.

The prospect of getting back into circulation may not be encouraging, but spread the word among your girl friends and don't be afraid to be seen around alone. Go out and do things on your own. Go to different places, try new ac-

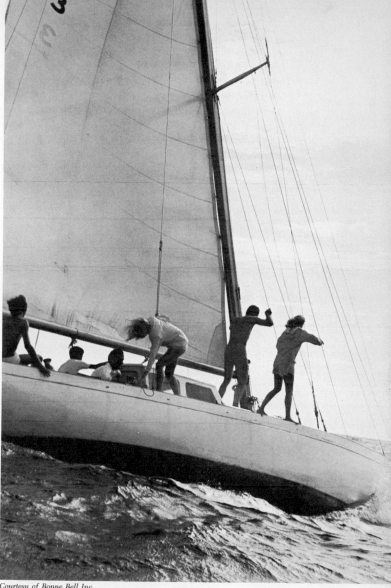

Courtesy of Bonne Bell Inc.

Don't be afraid to try new and different activities. You'll meet new people and make new friends.

tivities, meet new friends (girls as well as men)—anything that helps you forget the old routine and lets people know you're back in circulation. Stick at it and new prospects are sure to develop.

For the modern girl, the most serious dating dilemmas involve drinking, drugs, and sex.

389

How can you refuse without sounding like a prude? One good way to refuse a drink is to say that you have never liked the taste of liquor. Another approach is to develop the art of nursing a drink for a long period. Many people mistakenly think that eating a good deal while they drink will lessen the effect of alcohol; it may delay the impact of the liquor temporarily, but that is all. Another popular recommendation for allaying the effect of liquor is to substitute fruit juices for water or soda in mixing drinks. But be careful here! Whiskey sours and grasshoppers are fairly mild, but some fruit-juice

Dating is the best way to get to know lots of men, so that you can be a good judge when the right one comes along.

Courtesy of AT&T

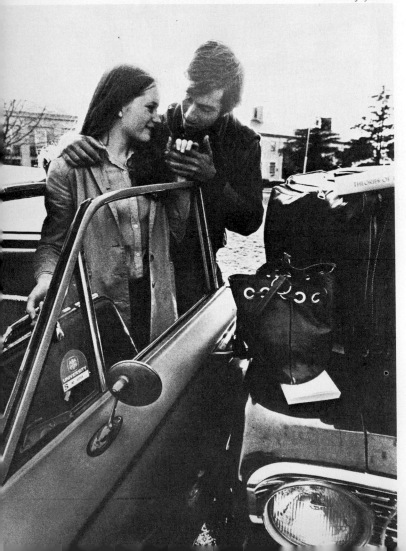

drinks are bolstered with extra quantities of liquor or with extra-strong liquor; they may taste mild but be very potent. The worst thing you can do is to order a martini or manhattan in an attempt to appear sophisticated. These drinks have a strong effect in a short time, so unless you are sure you can handle them, stay away.

As for drugs, the best advice is don't. Probably the best way to refuse is simply to say that you don't need them to feel good. Drugs are dangerous—sometimes lethal. Everyone's tolerance for them varies. The same dose that has a small effect on one person can be enough to kill another. Furthermore, many drugs have long-range psychological and physical effects that are just beginning to be discovered. In addition to the risk to your health and life, drugs are illegal. The person who takes them or associates with people who do runs the risk of getting into serous trouble.

The dating problem most often discussed is sex. You will probably meet your share of smooth operators, the boys who have all the arguments right at hand—and how convincing some of them can sound to the gullible girl when she is feeling more than a little bit in love or afraid that she will lose him. Just remember that men who try to seduce every girl they date are not capable of a deep and long-lasting love.

You have to be ready to recognize that behind those rationalizations is only one objective—and that is a selfish one. When a boy really cares for you, when he is thinking seriously about you and your feelings, he will not try to play on your emotions. If, on the other hand, he is just testing you (and his own powers of persuasion as well), your response will go a long way in determining what your mutual future will hold.

Everyone has to set up her own standards of conduct. The right boys will respect and admire you all the more if you maintain high standards and have the courage to stick to them. You don't need a long sermon to explain your stand; a tactful, polite—but firm—refusal will do. Never be afraid to be a little different from the crowd when you know you're right. If you've a pleasant personality, you'll always be popular.

❦ He Loves Me Not

If you're shy, perhaps you wish you had some dating problems to worry about. No matter how much some girls want to date, they fall apart when a desirable man talks to them. If this is your problem, take heart. Actually, many men prefer a girl who is a little shy, so all you need is a shot of self-confidence. If you haven't yet acted on what you've learned in this book, bolster your ego with a new hair style, some new clothes, perhaps more interesting eye makeup. Play up your individuality and concentrate on the assets you possess. Once you convince yourself of your own worth, it won't be hard to convince others.

Perhaps the most important secret of appeal that popular girls have is that they like boys. They show an interest in a man's ideas and in what he is doing. They let him know they appreciate his humor, his advice, his company. Any male dotes on a receptive audience, so forget yourself and your fears and try to concentrate on him. Practice on some of the men with whom you work. Soon your cordial attitude will seem natural, and you'll be ready to be your most charming self when the right man does appear.

---

1 *If you are going steady and can see no rosy future in the relationship, don't let it drag on any longer. This is the time to meet new men and to know as many as possible so that you can make the right permanent choice when the time comes.*

2 *If you would like to meet new men, see what activities you could join in your town or in nearby areas that would help you make new friends.*

3 *Experiment with ways to change your hairdo to make it a bit more festive for an important date.*

391

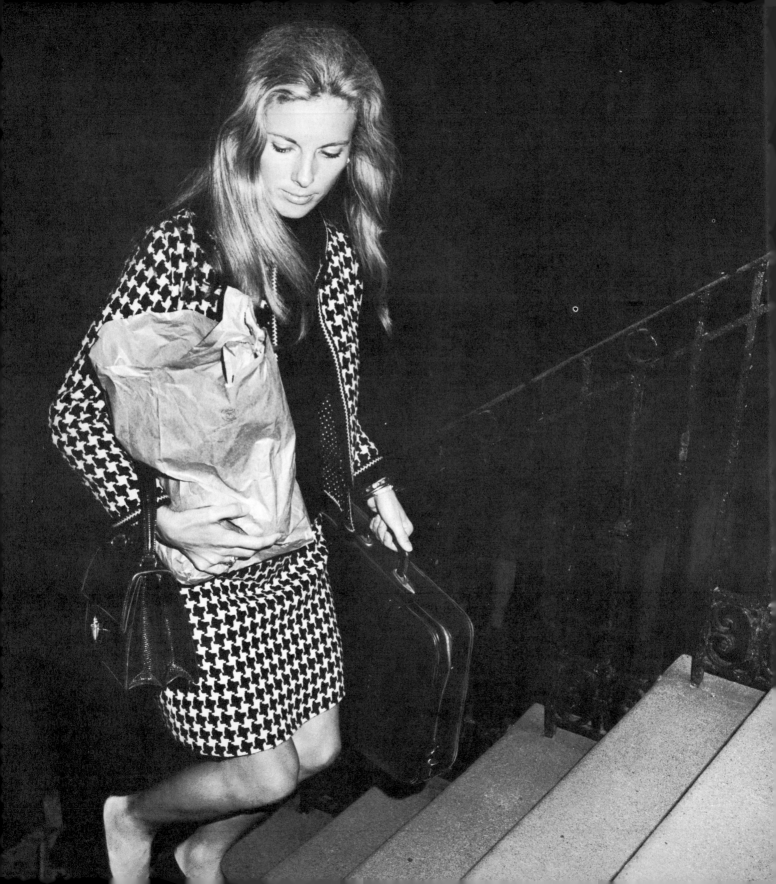

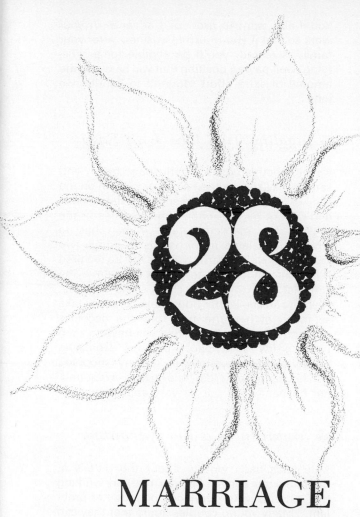

MARRIAGE
AND YOUR
CAREER

Once you've charmed the man of your choice into giving you his name, you may decide to take on the double job of marriage *and* a career. Then, more than ever, you'll need to apply all your techniques of charm and efficiency to keep life running smoothly. Your days will move at a swifter pace than ever before, but they can also be tremendously satisfying and purposeful.

Not too many years ago the married woman hesitated to work for fear that her action would be interpreted as a slur on her husband's earning power. But times have changed. Society has come to recognize that perhaps a woman might prefer to be active in the business world —she might like being good at something in addition to her housekeeping. Many women find that their jobs bolster their egos and give them a sense of importance and accomplishment that they never could achieve around the house. Work also has overcome the problem of loneliness and gives women the opportunity for companionship with people who have the same interests and who talk the same language.

Today almost one out of every three married women has a job. A girl no longer bids the boss good-bye just because she's taken a trip to the altar. She realizes that her education and skills can be put to good use to help finance the type of home and furnishings she wants and to accumulate savings for the advent of children. Even after the children arrive, she doesn't necessarily resign herself to becoming a permanent homebody. Many wives take part-time positions once the children reach school age, and an increasing number of women return to full-time employment when their children are grown.

❦ Careers Are for Keeping

With many work years added, it is possible for a woman, as well as a man, to have a worthwhile career. A job is no longer a brief stopgap between school and marriage. This makes it all the more important to secure a good education and to train yourself well to take part in work you will like. When you are planning a life career, selecting a job becomes more than a matter of taking whatever is most convenient. The long-term view should be considered if you want a job you might keep after marriage and perhaps return to in later years.

There are many jobs that a woman can do at home. Editing, writing, and a great deal of design work are done by wives who work on a free-lance basis.

B. D. Unsworth

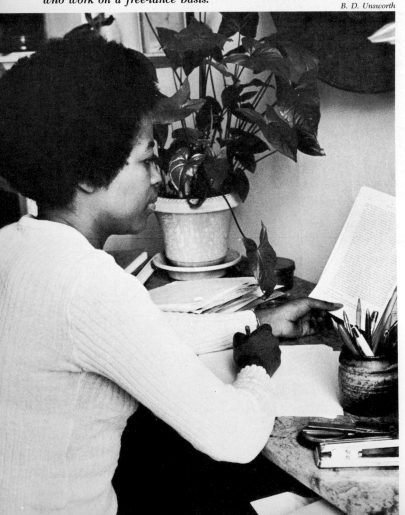

You'll also want to grow and advance in your work so that if you return to business after your family is reared, you'll be eligible for a satisfying, well-paying position that will be worth the amount of extra effort required to handle two jobs.

❦ Juggling Two Jobs Isn't Easy

Keeping both a boss and a husband happy and satisfied is likely to keep a career woman on the run. She owes definite responsibilities to each and cannot neglect one at the expense of the other. The married career woman has to stretch her talents if she wants to juggle two jobs with equal dexterity. She can't be too tired if her husband wants to go out at night. She can't let him run out of clean shirts or socks. Neither can she let her household concerns take so much of her attention that she becomes inattentive at the office. She will have to keep up a pretty swift pace, perhaps sacrificing lunch-hour gab sessions to grocery shopping and household errands. If overtime is required, her husband may not be very appreciative.

❦ Maturity Is a Big Advantage

Much has been written about the pitfalls of marrying too early. For the married working girl, extreme youth only compounds her problem. Many young couples figure that they can manage if the wife works for a while to help the marriage get on its feet, but some young girls find this much more difficult than they had expected. Here are factors every young girl would do well to consider before she decides to become a working wife.

• A youthful marriage has great financial pressures at the beginning. If *both* the husband and wife are young, they won't have the higher salaries that more job experience brings. Money will be scarce, and they won't be able to afford many of the timesaving appliances and other conveniences that make a wife's work easier. Life is much smoother for the couple who can save a little nest egg before marriage.

Then, too, if you have savings, the arrival of a baby will not be a financial problem.

• A working girl has a multitude of responsibilities. The married career girl no longer has Mother to handle household chores and to help care for her clothes. Even with a roommate, housekeeping is a 50-50 proposition. But after marriage she must keep her job running smoothly, she must take full charge of caring for herself and her wardrobe, and she must also take on the additional responsibilities of full care for her home and her husband. There will be *his* suits to press, *his* buttons to sew on, *his* laundry to do, as well as her own. The home must be kept attractive. Meals must be planned, shopped for, and prepared well. This alone can be a bit of a problem for the bride who hasn't had much experience in putting meals together.

• You may be forced to take on responsibility faster than you wish. Looking back, some girls who married young are a little resentful. They find themselves tired, suffering from nervous strain, and feeling a little sorry for themselves, especially if they weren't able to finish their education. An early marriage and the responsibility it entails deprives them of some of the fun they feel they ought to be having while they're young. They find themselves cleaning house and pinching pennies while their single friends are buying glamorous clothes and going on festive dates. Of course, marriage has many compensations, but the contrast may still hurt.

Some girls are ready for marriage earlier than others, but statistics prove that if a girl waits until she's 23 or 24, the odds for happiness are much greater. By this time she has had a chance for a little fling at life. When she settles down, she isn't afraid she may be missing her share of the fun. And neither will her husband.

• Much self-discipline is demanded. The wife who works has great need for well-controlled emotions and adult acceptance of responsibility. Rash behavior can multiply her difficulties.

Her husband also must be mature and understanding. She probably won't have time to cook and care for him as elaborately as his mother did. In fact, he will probably find that in order for them to have time for any fun together, he'll have to help with some of the household chores, too. Should he feel this to

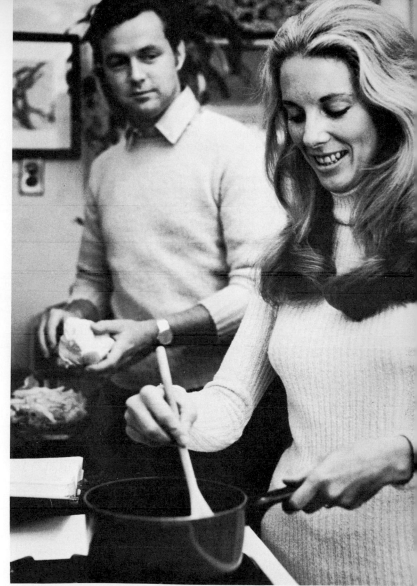

B. D. Unsworth

be beneath his masculine dignity, his bride will have a difficult time.

• If the husband's education has to be cut short, he may later be resentful when he realizes that he could have gone much further had he been able to finish. If he does try to continue his studies at night, there will be an even greater strain on the overworked household, because he will have little time to help his wife in any way and there will be less chance for relaxation and recreation together. The cost of tuition and books may also be a strain on the slim budget.

The couple who can hold off wedding bells until they have finished their education and have had time for both emotional and financial preparation are more likely to live happily ever after. Any new marriage takes a bit of doing, but when there is a little more time, money, and experience to give love a lift, the difficulties are easier to overcome.

❦ How to Swing It

The most important rule for success is to avoid trying to tackle too much—either too strenuous a job or too great a household load. If the job requires too much overtime or is so hectic that you come home exhausted, perhaps you had better try to find a less strenuous position. At home you'll have to accept the fact that there may sometimes be a little dust around, that meals won't be as elaborate as you'd wish, and that you won't have time for all the baking, curtain making, and other household fussing you might like. You may also have to get used to paying for some services you'd normally do yourself. Your time and energy are in great demand, and you will need to spend them where they provide the most benefit.

Many noted career women have found that one of the best ways to combine a successful career with a successful marriage is to form a definite separation between the two. Home problems shouldn't infringe on the job, and office problems shouldn't be brought home. Give your career its full due, but close the door promptly at quitting time and let your wifely concerns have full attention until you leave for work next morning. At home be careful not to monopolize the conversation with talk about *your* day. Your husband will want to tell you about *his* office adventures too.

Despite your busy schedule, your home must run as smoothly as possible. The working wife should try to provide appetizing meals, and they should be served on time. This may involve doing extra cooking on weekends or the night before and learning clever tricks with leftovers. A steady supply of TV dinners and delicatessen specialties is expensive as well as unappealing. Much as you're tempted to make excuses for yourself or to tell yourself you're too busy, don't. This won't pass with others. You'll have to budget each minute carefully if you want to find time to do the thoughtful little acts that make life more pleasant.

Maintaining your high grooming and beauty standards will also be more difficult. Many married women save time by resorting to simpler hairdos and by skipping nail polish for daily wear. Perhaps your beauty routine will need to be streamlined in a similar manner, but you must be careful that none of the important aspects of grooming are neglected. A good appearance is so vitally important both to success on the job and to pleasing a husband that no woman can ever afford to let down.

A good job is stimulating, it's true, but a well-rounded personality needs many interests. Your tight schedule may crowd out some of your former activities, but don't just bury your head in a hole of work, work, work. Take time for fun, spending your free moments carefully on worthwhile activities that give you a lift.

Although you will have to keep your social life within bounds, be ready for fun when your husband wants to go out or invites friends to drop in. Find some easy recipes for entertaining so that having company won't be too involved. Or, better yet, search out a store where you can buy something spectacular. You won't be at your social best that night if you get up at 5 a.m. to prepare some special delicacy before leaving for the office. Simplicity must be the rule in the working wife's household —simplicity of routine, simplicity of furnishings, simplicity of upkeep.

The person who can learn the trick of relaxing completely whenever she has an opportunity can do much to conserve her energy supply. If you commute to and from work, use this time to shut out all thoughts and to let your mind and body relax as completely as possible. When you get home, perhaps you can find fifteen minutes to lie down. Stretch out, close out the world, let yourself go limp, and imagine that your body feels very, very heavy. Some people use the trick of relaxing their bodies section by section: start with your left foot and concentrate on relaxing it completely; then do your calf, your knee, your thigh, then the other leg, and so on up your body until you are completely relaxed. Usually this will put you to sleep, so you had better set the alarm if your time is limited. Even a fifteen-minute catnap of this sort can be very refreshing and can make the evening a time you will enjoy.

When you are tired, give in to yourself and rest. With so much responsibility, you can't afford to let your health suffer. If you become ill, medical expenses can eat up a large chunk of the profits from your labors.

Above all, avoid developing a hurried, harried look. The truly charming woman maintains an air of calm serenity. She is never so rushed that she is brusque or thoughtless, that she skips the niceties of grooming or good manners, or that she cannot take a moment to be kind. You may be as busy or busier than anyone else, but try to conceal the pressure. Your accomplishments will be heightened by your untroubled look of peace and well-being—and you will seem all the more lovely.

ꙮ Handling the Finances

Two paychecks are quite pleasant. With a double income, the young couple will soon be able to buy many of the things they might otherwise have to wait years to afford. If the wife is planning to work for only a limited time after marriage, however, it's a good idea to set aside her earnings for some special purpose—furnishings, appliances, a car, a house, children—and to live on the husband's salary alone. Otherwise, it's all too easy to develop extravagant habits that may be more than his salary can stand. Unless this is done, there will be the unpleasant shock of having to trim their standards to manage on one paycheck when the wife retires. It's always easy to move up the financial scale, but hard to come down. ''Expenditure rises to meet income'' is a rule of thumb.

If you become very successful and earn more than your husband, you must be careful not to let this make him feel inferior. One girl whose student husband worked only part-time explained that they overcame this unequal income problem by lumping their earnings together and setting up a budget that allotted them each enough for their particular needs. She was careful that the term *our* money was always used, never *my* money.

Difficult though the career-marriage combination may be, thousands of women have mastered the techniques. It is a tribute to the modern woman that she has been able to do so much so well. A good part of her success can undoubtedly be ascribed to her charm. This all-important element plays a key role in her success both at home and in the office. Without it, neither job can bring the rewards it should.

Talk to some married couples who work full time. Find out what both the husbands and wives think of the arrangement. What problems and advantages result from the wife's job? How do they manage to have time for the details of home life and for fun together?

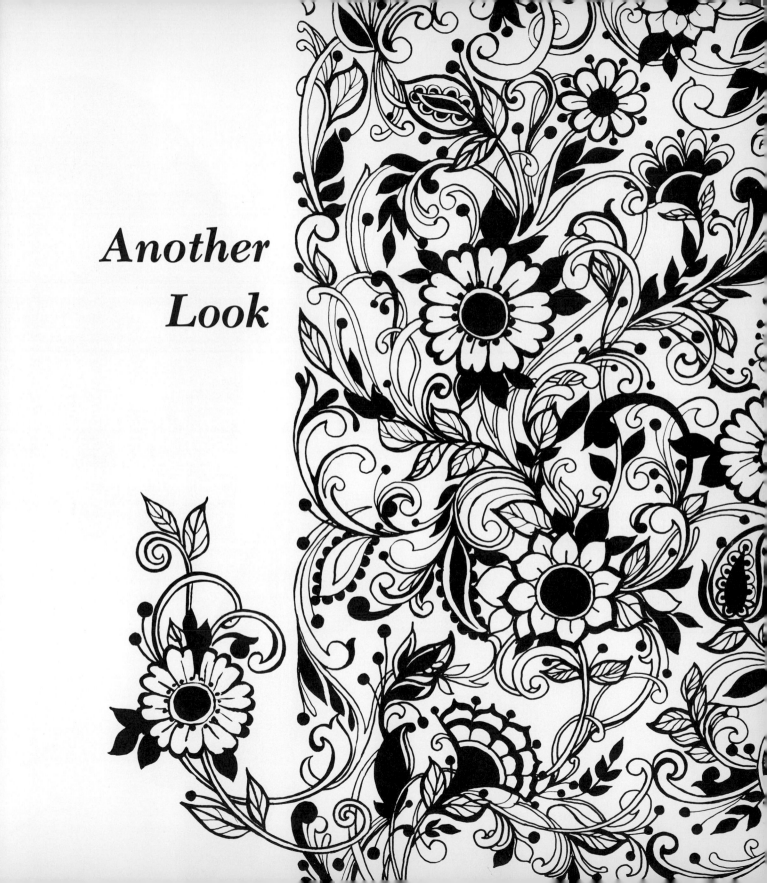

Another Look

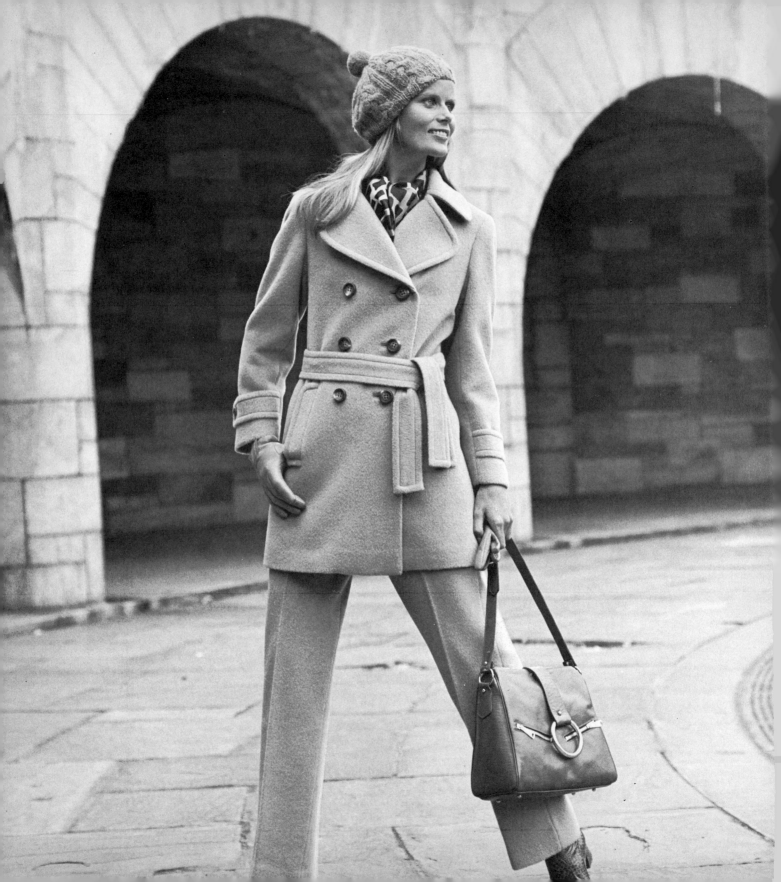

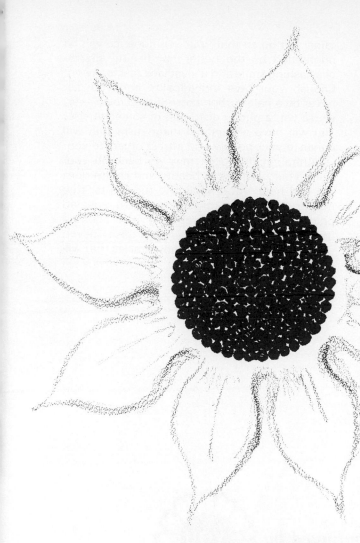

HAPPY ENDINGS

As you come to the end of these pages, pause for a moment to analyze the progress you've made so far. During this short time you have learned many ways to make yourself more beautiful, more appealing. If you have applied what you've learned, you are already enjoying a lovely improvement. Deep down inside, there is the blissful assurance that you are more confident, more poised, more happy with yourself. You are well on your way to a charmed life.

Beauty and charm are not easy goals to grasp. You must keep striving day after day until good habits are so deeply ingrained that they become a natural part of you. Now that you have made such a good start, keep up your progress. Constantly check your posture, your speech, your grooming, your attitudes. When necessary, turn back and reread pages that may help you.

Don't be discouraged, either, if your progress hasn't been all you wished. Some girls move ahead faster than others because they have more natural advantages to start with. Perhaps, for instance, you figure isn't yet a model's dream. Unfortunately, different molds were used to make some of us. Although you may never be the perfectly proportioned sylph you'd like to be, don't give up until you are convinced that you've done the very best you can with what Nature gave you. Then concentrate all the more on superb posture and the selection of the most flattering clothes you can find. Many beauties have merely learned well the tricks of diminishing less than perfect features and focusing attention where it does the most good.

Keep in mind that your aim is to create the best possible YOU—to develop your own individual capacities, talents, and assets . . . to perfect your own personal flair. Let this be expressed in your clothes, your grooming, your whole personality. Be the woman who is noted for exquisite taste: dramatic color combinations, clothing with an individual difference that is unfalteringly correct for her personality. Carry this personal flair through to your movements, your speech, your thoughts. Constantly strive to improve in every way possible, whether it be in exposing yourself to stimulating, vital thoughts, in moving ahead on the job, or in cultivating your capacity to give and receive love. Try to enjoy to the fullest everything you do so that your countenance will be brightened by the better-than-beauty sparkle of a flashing smile and a vivacious zest for living. Cherish your own individuality and you can never be a pale carbon copy of the crowd—or, worse yet, a phony distortion of someone else. You will have a personal magnetism that will enhance your beauty and attract others to you.

Although this book may go back on your shelf, your progress in beauty and charm does not end here. You know the rudiments; true mastery comes only through your own repeated practice. The most gratifying part about a quest for charm and beauty is that the more you work at it, the greater are the miracles that will be worked for you.

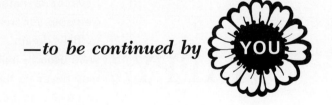

—to be continued by YOU

Index

406